3182273

ENDOCRINOLOGY
OF AGING

CONTEMPORARY ENDOCRINOLOGY

P. Michael Conn, SERIES EDITOR

ENDOCRINOLOGY OF AGING

Edited by

JOHN E. MORLEY, MB, BCH

*Saint Louis University Health
Sciences Center, St. Louis, MO*

and

LUCRETIA VAN DEN BERG, MB, BCH

*Saint Louis University Health
Sciences Center, St. Louis, MO*

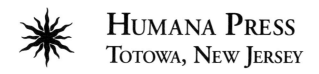

HUMANA PRESS
TOTOWA, NEW JERSEY

© 2000 Humana Press Inc.
999 Riverview Drive, Suite 208
Totowa, New Jersey 07512

For additional copies, pricing for bulk purchases, and/or information about other Humana titles,
contact Humana at the above address or at any of the following numbers: Tel: 973-256-1699;
Fax: 973-256-8341; E-mail: humana@humanapr.com; Website: http://humanapress.com

Cover design by Patricia F. Cleary

This publication is printed on acid-free paper. ∞
ANSI Z39.48-1984 (American National Standards Institute)
Permanence of Paper for Printed Library Materials.

Printed in the United States of America.   10 9 8 7 6 5 4 3 2 1

Endocrinology of Aging/edited by John E. Morley and Lucretia van den Berg.
      p.   cm.—(Contemporary endocrinology; 20)
    Includes index.
    ISBN 0-89603-756-8 (alk. paper)
    1. Aging—Endocrine aspects. 2. Endocrine glands—Aging. 3. Aged—Diseases—Endocrine Aspects
  4. Endocrine glands—Diseases—Age factors. I. Morley, John E. II. Van den Berg, Lucretia.
    III. Series: Contemporary endocrinology (Totowa, NJ) ; 20
    [DNLM: 1. Aging. 2. Endocrine Diseases—Aged. 3. Endocrine Glands—Physiology. WT 104 E5752 2000]
QP187.3 A34E532 2000
612.6'7—dc21
DNLM/DLC   97-18996
for Library of Congress   CIP

PREFACE

"To me, fair friend, you never can be old,
For as you were when first your eye I eyed,
Such seems your beauty still."
—**William Shakespeare**, *Sonnets* 104:1-3

The population of the world is aging. At the beginning of this century in the United States, people over the age of 65 accounted for only 4% of the population, whereas at the end of this millennium, they will comprise 14% of the population. This represents a growth of the older population in the United States from 30 million at present to approximately 55 million by the year 2030. Life expectancy in the United States has increased from a mere 49.2 years in 1900 to 75.7 years in 1991. However, it is not only the industrialized countries who are demonstrating this boom in their aging populations. Both China and India will have gained an additional 270 million persons over the age of 60 years by the year 2000, and in the year 2020, Mexico will have the ninth largest elderly population in the world. This graying of the world's populations makes it essential that physicians recognize the unique aspects of physiology and disease that are associated with the aging process.

Multiple physiological changes in hormones and the tissue responsiveness to hormones occur with aging. This has led to increasing attempts to explore the use of hormonal replacement as a modality to retard the aging process—the so-called "hormonal fountain of youth," although at present, only the use of estrogen in postmenopausal women has been proven to increase longevity. The era of hormonal replacement in older persons has opened up a veritable Pandora's box of exciting findings for the inquisitive endocrinologist.

Changes in the autoimmune system lead to an increased propensity for the aging person to develop endocrine failure syndromes. Further synergism toward the failure of hormonal production that accompanies aging comes from lifelong environmental insults and physiological changes.

The altered tissue responsiveness to hormones with aging results in altered manifestations of endocrine disease with aging. The classical presentation of any unusual manifestation of disease in older age is apathetic hypothyroidism. In addition, the physiological changes of aging often mimic the signs and symptoms of endocrine failure, making the diagnosis of endocrine disorders in older persons a biochemical rather than a clinical one. Polypharmacy is rampant in older persons and leads to alterations in hormonal levels and hormonal responsiveness, stretching the diagnostic imagination of even the most aware endocrinologist.

For all of these reasons, it is timely to include in the *Contemporary Endocrinology* series a volume concerning the *Endocrinology of Aging*. The first two chapters of this volume explore the basic mechanistic changes that result in the aging process and their physiological consequences. In addition, the putative role of hormonal replacement therapy to retard the aging process is examined. The next series of chapters examine the physiological changes in the hypothalamic pituitary axis that occur with aging and their clinical consequences. Two chapters deal with bone disease in older persons.

Paget's disease is almost an exclusive disease of the older person, making it a highly appropriate topic for inclusion in this volume.

The next three chapters examine the endocrinology of the sex hormone changes that occur with aging. Androgen Deficiency in Aging Males (ADAM) has now established itself as a real syndrome that occurs as men age. The potential use of testosterone replacement therapy in these men, though still in its infancy, has opened up an exciting panoply of possibilities. Gynecomastia occurs commonly in older males and has a variety of causes that need to be recognized by the physician. Menopause represents one of the most obvious aging changes and is an area where appropriate hormonal replacement therapy has gained widespread acceptance.

Nearly half of all Type II diabetes occurs in persons over the age of 65 years. The interaction of diabetes and cognitive function represents an extremely important area as persons age. There is increasing evidence of positive benefits from maintaining good control of glycemia into old age. The addition of the newer therapeutic agents to our armamentarium has now made this feasible.

The interaction of nutrition and metabolism in older persons is addressed in two chapters. The increasing awareness of the role of hypercholesterolemia in coronary artery disease and the effects of obesity on functional status and disease pathogenesis are highlighted. The physiological changes in food intake and nutrient metabolism with aging are then discussed. The role of these changes in producing the anorexia of aging and the increased prevalence of protein energy malnutrition in older persons is delineated. Alterations in vitamin and trace minerals with aging are discussed. In particular, the modern trend of utilizing vitamins as therapeutic agents in phamacological doses is highlighted.

Finally, the last two chapters discuss the alterations in the sympathetic nervous system with aging. Hypertension is rampant in older persons and the Systolic Hypertension in Elderly Persons (SHEP) trial and the European Working Party for Hypertension in the Elderly (EWPHE) have each demonstrated the importance of adequate blood pressure control in the young old. Alterations in the endocrine system play an integral role in the understanding and the development of appropriate management strategies of hypertension in older persons. Endothelin-producing tumors resulting in hypertension are a disease of old age.

Endocrinology of Aging has brought together a distinguished cast of international authors to highlight the importance of understanding the unique aspects of endocrinology in the aging process. It is our hope that endocrinologists, geriatricians, and practicing physicians will all find information in this book that will enhance the function of older persons throughout the world.

John E. Morley, MB, BCh
Lucretia van den Berg, MB, BCh

CONTENTS

CONTRIBUTORS

HAROLD E. CARLSON, MD, *Endocrinology Division, SUNY-Stony Brook, Stony Brook, NY*

IAN M. CHAPMAN, MBBS, PHD, *Royal Adelaide Hospital, Adelaide, South Australia, Australia*

GAYATHRI DUNDOO, MD, *Department of Geriatric Medicine, Saint Louis University Medical Center, St. Louis, MO*

JEROME M. HERSHMAN, MD, *Division of Endocrinology and Metabolism, UCLA School of Medicine, West Los Angeles VA Medical Center, Los Angeles, CA*

MICHAEL HOROWITZ, PHD, *Department of Medicine, University of Adelaide, Adelaide, South Australia*

HOSAM K. KAMEL, MD, *Division of Geriatric Medicine, Nassau County Medical Center, East Meadow, NY and SUNY Stony Brook School of Medicine, Stony Brook, NY*

AMY LEE, MD, *Division of Geriatric Medicine, Saint Louis University Health Sciences Center, St. Louis, MO*

DONGJIE LIU, MD, *Geriatric Division, Center for the Study of Aging and Human Development, Department of Medicine, Duke University Medical Center, Durham, NC*

KENNETH W. LYLES, MD, *Sarah W. Stedman Nutrition Center, Duke University Medical Center, Durham, NC*

GRAYDON S. MENEILLY, MD, FRCPC, *Division of Geriatric Medicine, Department of Medicine, University of Brititsh Columbia, Vancouver, BC, Canada*

MYRON MILLER, MD, *Division of Geriatric Medicine, Department of Medicine, Sinai Hospital of Baltimore, Baltimore, MD*

TANVEER MIR, MD, *Division of Geriatric Medicine, Department of Medicine, Nassau County Medical Center, SUNY Stony Brook School of Medicine, Long Island, NY*

ARSHAG D. MOORADIAN, MD, *Division of Endocrinology, Department of Internal Medicine, Saint Louis University Health Sciences Center, St. Louis, MO*

JOHN E. MORLEY, MB, BCH, *Division of Geriatric Medicine, Saint Louis University Health Sciences Center, St. Louis, MO*

HOWARD A. MORRIS, PHD, *Division of Clinical Biochemistry, Departments of Medicine and Pathology, Institute of Medical and Veterinary Science, Adelaide, South Australia*

ALLAN G. NEED, MD, *Division of Clinical Biochemistry, Departments of Medicine and Pathology, Institute of Medical and Veterinary Science, Adelaide, South Australia*

CHARLES B. NEMEROFF, MD, PHD, *Department of Psychiatry and Behavioral Sciences, Emory University School of Medicine, Atlanta, GA*

B. E. CHRISTOPHER NORDIN, MD, DSC, *Division of Clinical Biochemistry, Departments of Medicine and Pathology, Institute of Medical and Veterinary Science, University of Adelaide, Adelaide, South Australia*

MORRIS NOTELOVITZ, MD, PHD, *Women's Medical and Diagnostic Center, Gainesville, FL*

A. EUGENE PEKARY, PHD, *Division of Endocrinology and Metabolism, UCLA School of Medicine, West Los Angeles VA Medical Center, Los Angeles, CA*

EMILE D. RISBY, MD, *Department of Psychiatry and Behavioral Sciences, Emory University School of Medicine, Atlanta, GA*

MARY H. SAMUELS, MD, *Division of Endocrinology, Diabetes and Clinical Nutrition, Oregon Health Sciences University, Portland, OR*

JAMES R. SOWERS, MD, *Division of Endocrinology, Metabolism, and Hypertension, Wayne State University School of Medicine, Detroit, MI*

MARK A. SUPIANO, MD, *University of Michigan and Ann Arbor VA Health System-GRECC, Ann Arbor, MI*

DANIEL TESSIER, MD, FRCPC, *Division of Geriatric Medicine, Department of Medicine, University of Sherbroke, Sherbroke, Quebec*

DAVID R. THOMAS, MD, FACP, *Division of Geriatric Medicine, Saint Louis University Health Sciences Center, St. Louis, MO*

LUCRETIA VAN DEN BERG, MB, BCH, *Division of Geriatric Medicine, Saint Louis University Health Sciences Center, St. Louis, MO*

SCOTT P. VAN SANT, MD, *Department of Psychiatry and Behavioral Sciences, Emory University School of Medicine, Atlanta, GA*

1   Biological Theories of Aging

Hosam K. Kamel, MD,
Arshag D. Mooradian, MD,
and Tanveer Mir, MD

Contents

INTRODUCTION

Aging can be seen as an irreversible, time-dependent, functional decline that converts healthy adults into frail ones, with reduced capacity to adjust to everyday stresses, and increasing vulnerability to most diseases, and to death *(1)*. As far as anyone knows, the longest anyone has ever lived is 121 yr. The record-holder is Jeanne Calment, a French lady who celebrated her landmark birthday in 1996 *(2)*. Long lives always make us wonder: What is the secret behind it? Is there a maximum life-span beyond which we cannot live? What happens as we age? Would insight into longevity help us fight the diseases and disabilities associated with the aging process?

Concomitant with recent developments in molecular biology techniques, research activity into the mechanisms of aging at the cellular and molecular level has increased substantially. As a result, a myriad of theories explaining the aging phenomenon have been proposed, which can be grouped into two major categories (Table 1). The first includes the programmed theories, which emphasize internal biological clocks or programs. The second includes the wear-and-tear theories, which emphasize the role of wear and tear caused by random events over time. This chapter reviews the different theories of aging. The effect of caloric restriction on the aging process will also be reviewed in the context of theories of aging.

THEORIES BASED ON PROGRAMMED AGING

These theories are based on the notion that the aging process is governed by certain pacemakers at the organ system level or at the cellular level. Two organ systems, namely,

From: *Contemporary Endocrinology: Endocrinology of Aging*
Edited by: J. E. Morley and L. van den Berg © Humana Press Inc., Totowa, NJ

Table 1
Theories of Aging

Programmed theories
   Neuroendocrine
   Immune
   Finite cell division
Wear and tear theories
   Free radicals
   Rate of living
   Error catastrophe
   DNA damage
   Glycosylation

the neuroendocrine system and the immune system, have been the focus of these theories. This is mostly because these two systems influence an array of body functions.

Neuroendocrine Theory of Aging

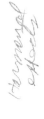

This theory proposes that biological clocks act through hormones to control the aging process *(3)*. In 1889, C. E. Brown-Sequard noted that a day would come when the degenerations of age could be mitigated by the use of testosterone, bringing fourth a rejuvenation that would approximate that of a younger individual *(4)*. Over the past century, understanding of hormonal changes with age and the effect of hormonal repletion in elderly individuals has increased dramatically. It is now established that a variety of hormonal changes occur with aging *(5;* Table 2). Among these, aging of the hypothalamic–pitutary–gonadal axis in women probably represents one of the best-studied models of programmed senescence. Although the precise mechanism of the menopause remains controversial, it is agreed that the neuroendocrine system orchestrates the loss of reproductive ability *(6)*. Estrogen replacement therapy alleviates the discomfort of menopause *(2)*. It also prevents the accelerated bone loss associated with the menopause *(7)*, and helps prevent cardiovascular disease in postmenopausal women *(8)*.

With aging, there is a decrease in the levels of plasma testosterone and bioavailable testosterone *(9)*. This is attributed not only to primary testicular changes, but also to changes, in the hypothalamic–pituitary axis *(10)*. Reproductive hormonal alterations in the aging male may have significant implications for the aging process *(9)*. Testosterone replacement therapy has been shown to reverse some of the phenotypic changes in older hypogonadal men *(11,12)*. It remains to be determined, however, whether the benefits of testosterone replacement therapy outweigh its long-term risks.

Dehydroepiandrosterone sulfate (DHEAS) is another reproductive hormone that decreases dramatically with aging *(13)*. Results from initial human studies suggest salutary effects of DHEAS on the aging process *(14–17)*. These effects, however, need to be confirmed by large-scale controlled studies.

Growth hormone (GH) is another hormone often implicated in the aging process. There are many similarities between the syndrome associated with the lack of GH in adults and the characteristics of normal older adults *(18,19)*. There is a progressive decline in GH and serum insulin-like growth factor (IGF)-I levels with aging *(20)*. Rudman et al. *(21)* demonstrated that administering recombinant human GH to a small group of elderly men with low GH levels reversed some signs of aging, resulting in increased lean

Table 2
Age-Related Changes in Serum Hormone Levels

Hormone	Change with aging[a]
Growth hormone	N in males; ↓ in females
Somatomedin C (insulin-like growth factor I)	↓
Adrenocorticotrophic hormone	N
Cortisol	N
Dehydroepinandrosterone	↓
Renin	N
Aldosterone	↓
Thyroid-stimulating hormone	N or ↑
Thyroxin	N
Triiodothyronine	↓
Parathyroid hormone	↑
Calcitonin	↓
1,25(OH)$_2$D	↓
Leuteinizing hormone	↑ or N male; ↑ in females
Follicle-stimulating hormone	↑ or N male; ↑ in females
Testosterone	↓ or N male; ↑ in females
Bioavailable testosterone	↓
Atrial natriuretic factor	↑
Insulin	↑
Glucagon	↓

[a]N, no change; ↑, increase; ↓, decreased.

body mass, decreased excess fat, and increased skin thickness. When the GH treatment was stopped, 3-mo later, these changes reversed, and the signs of aging returned. Researchers are continuing to explore whether or not GH therapy can also increase muscle strength (2). Prolonged administration of GH is complicated by the development of carpal tunnel syndrome, gynecomastia, and hyperglycemia (22).

Immune Theory of Aging

This theory proposes that the immune system is the pacemaker of the aging process (23). There are well-documented changes in the immune system with age (Table 3). The most remarkable of these is probably the universal involution of the thymic gland. Perhaps as a result, the T-cell-mediated responses are also impaired. Although the number of T-cells remains about the same, the proportion of the functioning T-cell population decreases (24). Most research on the aging immune system now centers on T-cells and their lymphokine products, notably the interleukins. Some, like interleukin (IL)-6, were found to rise with age; others, like IL-2, were found to fall with age (2). In addition, evidence now links IL-6 to the development of postmenopausal osteoporosis (25). Study of age-related immune changes may not only provide clues to the aging process, but may also shed light on the possible role of cytokines in the pathogenesis of age-related diseases.

Finite Cell Division Theory of Aging

In 1961, Hayflik and Morhead reported (26) that human fibroblasts in culture can only divide a limited number of times. These cells undergo approx 50 population doublings

Table 3
Age-Related Changes in Immune System

Thymic gland involution
Reduced T-helper and T-suppresser cells
Decreased cell-mediated cytotoxicity
Increased circulating autoantibodies
Increase in circulating immune complexes
Decreased levels of specific antibody response
Diminished delayed hypersensitivity
Diminished production of interleukin-2
Increased production of interleukin-6

before replicative ability ceases. In addition, fibroblasts "remember" how many divisions they have had, even after having been frozen at −20°C for prolonged periods (27). It was also observed that cell cultures derived from adult tissues consistently displayed a lower growth potential than those derived from fetal tissue (28,29). Furthermore, cells derived from individuals with certain genetic syndromes that display features of accelerated aging have diminished growth potential (30,31). The doubling potential of fibroblasts from diabetic subjects may also be reduced (32). In addition, it was observed that there was a positive correlation between the growth potential of a culture and the maximum life-span of the species from which it was derived (33). These observations collectively support the notion that cell doubling potential may be a biomarker of aging (32).

Researchers are discovering more clues to cellular senescence in the architecture of DNA. It became evident that each chromosome has tails at the end, named telomeres, which get shorter as cells divide (2). Tolemeres, composed of hundreds of repeated copies of a hexanucleotide (TTAGGG) (63), were found to shed 50–200 base pairs each replication cycle (64). As a result, these chromosome ends progressively shorten with each cell division, until the telomere region is gone and cell division ceases. This led researchers to believe that telomeres regulate cellular life-span in some way (2).

THEORIES BASED ON WEAR AND TEAR

Free Radicals Theory

A free radical is a molecule with an unpaired, highly reactive electron. A variety of free radicals are generated during normal cellular metabolism. These include superoxide, hydroxyl, lipid peroxy, purine, and pyrimidine radicals (32). Free radicals are implicated as an important cause of errors in cellular function (34). Free radicals may cause damage to cellular function through a scission reaction, such as DNA cleavage, mutations, addition reactions such as covalent bond formation, or aggregations of biomolecules through crosslinking reactions (32). In addition, a major stable product of free-radical-induced lipid peroxidation, malondiadehyde, can covalently bind to various proteins, resulting in changes in protein function or antigenicity (35).

The free radical theory of aging, first proposed by Denham Harman (36), holds that damage caused by oxygen radicals is responsible for many of the bodily changes that accompany aging. Researchers could demonstrate that an increase in the free radical level shortens the life-span of *Drosophila*, and leads to increase in the concentration of lipofuscin (37). Free radicals have been implicated not only in aging, but also in several conditions seen in aging, including atherosclerosis, Parkinson's disease, Alzheimer's disease, and immune deficiency of aging *(2)*.

Most of the support for the free radical theory comes from studies of antioxidants. One of these antioxidants, superoxide dismutase enzyme, converts oxygen radicals into hydrogen peroxide, which is then degraded by another enzyme, catalase, to oxygen and water *(38)*. Researchers have found that superoxide dismutase levels are directly related to life-span in several species, suggesting that the ability to fight free radicals has something to do with longer life-spans *(2)*. Higher levels of superoxide dismutase and catalase have been found in long-lived *Drosophila melanogaster (39)*. Furthermore, levels of superoxide dismutase in rat erythrocytes have been shown to decline with age *(40)*, but no correlation has been found between maximum life-span and levels of superoxide dismutase in primates *(41)*. Levels of other antioxidants, such as vitamin E and β-carotene, have also been correlated with life-span *(2)*.

The observation reported by Harman *(34)*, that mice treated with antioxidants had an extension of their life-span, raised hope that the aging process could be retarded by simply taking antioxidants. Subsequent studies, however, could not confirm the life-prolonging effect of antioxidants, even though age-related accumulation of cardiac lipofuscin was reduced *(42,43)*. More recently, it was found that treatment of rats with L-deprenyl, a monoamine oxidase-B (MAO-B) inhibitor, increased their life-span by 34%. The inhibition of MAO-B reduces the autoxidation of catecholamines, and subsequently reduces free-radical-induced tissue injury at critical sites in the nervous system *(32)*. Epidemiological studies provide evidence that increased dietary intake of antioxidants, such as vitamin A, vitamin E, and β-carotene, is associated with decreased risk of many cancers. Randomized clinical trials, however, have found that therapeutic levels of antioxidants do not reduce lung or skin cancer risk. Based on the currently available data, it is unlikely that dietary intake of antioxidants would fundamentally affect the aging process *(24,38,44)*.

Rate of Living Theory

The rate of living theory, proposed by Pearl in 1928 *(28)*, suggests that the life-span of an organism is inversely related to its metabolic rate. Support for this theory is mostly based upon observations that larger animals with lower metabolic rates generally live longer than smaller animals with higher metabolic rates, and that life-span is prolonged experimentally in lower species, such as invertebrates and fruit flies, when they are raised in cooler temperature *(24,45,46)*. These observations, however, are not universal. For example, bats have both high metabolic rates and long life-span, and marsupials have low metabolic rates and short lives *(1,47)*. Furthermore, recent studies have found poor correlation between metabolic rates and longevity *(24)*. It is now believed that the differences in longevity between species may not be associated with the metabolic rate, but rather with the balance of accumulation and detoxification of metabolic end products, such as free radicals *(24,48)*.

Error Catastrophe Theory

The error catastrophe theory, proposed by Orgel in 1963 *(49)*, is based on three general assumptions. The first assumption is that, as a function of age, nonfunctional proteins accumulate presumably because of errors in the transcription of genes and the translation of messenger RNA into proteins. The second assumption is that the error frequency increases with time, because, as errors in cellular function are made, the chances of making subsequent errors increase. The final assumption intrinsic to this theory is that, over time, the error frequency reaches a catastrophic threshold level that results in cell death. Orgel's theory has been studied in great detail experimentally *(50–53)*. Results from these experiments do not support a significant role for this theory in explaining the aging process *(32)*.

DNA Damage Theory

In the normal wear and tear of cellular life, DNA undergoes continued damage. This damage may be in the form of strand breaks, covalent modification, and/or chromosomal rearrangements *(2)*. Extrinsic factors, such as ionizing radiation and chemical mutagens, or intrinsic factors, such as the free radicals generated by oxidative metabolism, may be responsible for this damage *(38)*.This theory proposes that this DNA damage gradually accumulates and leads to malfunctioning genes, proteins, cells, and deteriorating tissues and organs *(54)*, and, thus, differences in longevity among species might be attributed to variations in the rate at which DNA damage occurs, or is repaired *(1)*.

In the cell, numerous enzyme systems operate to detect and repair damaged DNA. Hart and Setlow *(55)* demonstrated that rate of repair of DNA damage induced by ultraviolet light in cultured fibroblasts correlated with the life-span of the species from which the cell cultures were obtained. This has been demonstrated in both mammals *(55)* and primates *(56)*. Furthermore, patients with Warner's syndrome, a disease with several features of premature aging, have been found to have a defect in one of their enzyme repair systems, namely, the helicases *(2)*. Mitochondrial DNA, being in a highly oxidative environment, is more susceptible to damage than nuclear DNA *(2)*. This damage increases exponentially with age, and mutations in mitochondrial DNA have been associated with age-related disease, including ischemic heart disease and Parkinson's disease *(24)*.

Glycosylation Theory

The glycosylation theory proposes that, over time, proteins dehydrate and combine, nonenzymatically, with glucose, to form advanced glycosylated end products (AGEs) *(57)*. These AGEs have been linked to stiffening of collagen, hardening of arteries, cataracts, loss of nerve function, and less efficient kidney, all of which are age-related features *(2,32,58)*. These features also appear at younger ages in patients with diabetes who have high glucose levels. In fact, diabetes is now considered by some researchers as an accelerated model of aging. Not only do its complications mimic the physiological changes that can accompany old age, but its victims have shorter life expectancies *(2)*.

Glucose appears to react with cell constituents other than proteins. When DNA is incubated with glucose, nonenzymatic bonding occurs, altering its structure *(2)*. Studies in bacteria suggest that DNA altered in this manner may interfere with genetic functioning. Similar studies are currently underway to evaluate the effects of AGEs on human DNA *(32)*. Although glycosylation has been linked to the development of some age-related diseases, the precise role of glycation in the aging process itself is currently unknown.

Caloric Restriction and Modulation of Longevity

At the present time, dietary restriction appears to be the only intervention known to increase life-span in mammals *(59)*. Animals who live on restricted diet, being fed 30–40% fewer calories than normal (but inclusive of all necessary nutrients), survive months longer than those not on such dietary restriction *(2)*. Caloric restriction has increased the life-span of nearly every animal species studied, including protozoa, fruit flies, mice, rats, and other laboratory animals. Researchers are now investigating whether caloric restriction will affect aging in primates, humans' closest relatives in the animal kingdom *(2)*. Reducing caloric intake in rodents resulted in retarding the development of a broad range of age-associated physiologic changes, such as senescence of the reproductive system and deterioration of the immune system *(59)*. The timing of the institution of caloric restrictions affects the extent of its prolonging effect on life expectancy. Food restriction, started immediately in the postweaning period, prolongs life more effectively than dietary restrictions instituted later in life *(60)*.

The mechanisms by which calorie restriction prolongs the life-span are not exactly clear. Because caloric restrictions appear to affect the rate of aging, it is not surprising that the theories of aging discussed above are also implicated as possible mechanisms in the life-prolonging effect of caloric restriction *(32)*. Current evidence suggests that the effects of calorie restriction on the aging process may be mediated through a reduction in glycation *(61)*, oxidative damage, or alterations in specific gene expression *(62)*.

CONCLUSION

Although much is currently known about the aging process, much is yet to be explained. No single theory accounts for all the changes that take place as people age. Aging should be viewed as many processes, interactive and interdependent, that determine life-span and health. Currently, there are more questions than answers. However, with the current advances in molecular biological techniques, answers to most of these questions may be found in the near future.

REFERENCES

1. Miller RA. The biology of aging and longevity. In: Hazzard W, et al., eds. Principles of Geriatric Medicine and Gerontology, 3rd ed. McGraw-Hill, New York, 1994, pp. 3–18.
2. National Institute on Aging. In search of the secrets of aging. National Institutes of Health publication no. 93-2756, Washington, DC, 1996.
3. Lamberts SWJ, Van Den Beld AW, Van Der Lely AJ. The endocrinology of aging. Science 1997;278: 419–424.
4. Morley JE, Kaiser FE. Hypogonadism in the elderly man. Adv Endocrinol Metab 1993;4:241–261.
5. Mooradian AD, Morley JE, Korenman SG. Endocrinology in aging. Disease-a-Month 1988;34: 398–461.
6. Kamel H, Kaiser FE. The menopause: clinical aspects and current trends in therapy. In: Vellas B, Albarede L, Garry PJ, eds. Women, Aging and Health. Facts and Research and Intervention in Geriatrics Series. Serdi, Paris, 1998, pp. 105–143.
7. Cauly JA, Seeley DJ, Enrud K, Ettinger B, Black D, Cummings S., for the Study of Osteoporotic Fractures Research Group: Estrogen replacement therapy and fractures in older women. Ann Intern Med 1995;122:9–16.
8. Wild RA. Estrogen: effects on the cardiovascular tree. Obstet Gynecol 1996;87(Suppl 2):27S–35S.
9. Morley JE, Kaiser FE. Reproductive hormonal changes in the aging male. In: Timiras PS, Quay WD, Vernadakis A, eds. Hormones and Aging. Williams & Wiilkins, Baltimore, MA, 1995, pp. 153–166.
10. Morley JE, Kaiser FE, Perry HM 3rd, Patrick P, Morley PM, Stauber PM, Vellas B, Baumgartner RN, et al. Longitudinal changes in testosterone, luteinizing hormone, and follicle-stimulating hormone in healthy older men. Metabolism 1997;46:410–413.
11. Hajjar RR, Kaiser FE, Morley JE. Outcomes of long-term testosterone replacement in older hypogonadal males: a retrospective analysis. J Clin Endocrinol Metab 1997;82:3793–3796.

12. Sih R, Morley JE, Kaiser FE, et al. Testosterone replacement in older hypogonadal men: a 12-month randomized controlled trial. J Clin End Met 1997;82:1661–1667.
13. Morley JE, Kaiser F, Raum WJ, Perry HM 3rd, et al. Potentially predictive and manipulable blood serum correlates of aging in the healthy human male: progressive decrease in bioavailable testosterone, and dehydroepiandrosterone sulfate. Proc Natl Acad Sci USA 1997;94:7537–7542.
14. Horani MH, Morley JE. The viability of the use of DHEA. Clin Geriatr 1997;5:34–48.
15. Yen SSC, Morales AJ, Khorrram O. Replacement of DHEA in aging men and women: potential remedial effects. Ann NY Acad Sci 1995;774:128–142.
16. Wolkwitz OM, Reus VI, Robert E, et al. Antidepressant and cognitive-enhancing effects of DHEA in major depression. Ann NY Acad Sci 1995;774:337–339.
17. Szathmari M, Szucs J, Feher T, et al. Dehydroepiandrosterone sulphate and bone mineral density. Osteoporosis Int 1994;4:84–88.
18. Bouillanne O, Rainfray M, Tissandier O, et al. Growth hormone therapy in elderly people: an age-delaying drug? Fundam Clin Pharmacol 1996;10:416–430.
19. Martin FC, Yeo AL, Sonksen PH. Growth hormone secretion in the elderly: aging and the somatopause. Baillieres Clin Endocrinol Metab 1997;11:223–250.
20. Maheshwari H, Sharma L, Baumann G. Decline of plasma growth hormone binding protein in old age. J Clin Endocrinol Metab 1996;81:995–997.
21. Rudman D, Feller AG, Cohn L. Effects of human growth hormone on body composition in elderly men. Hormo Res 1991;36(Suppl 10):73–81.
22. Cohn L, Feller AG, Draper MW, Rudman IW, Rudman D. Carpal tunnel syndrome and gynecomastia during human growth hormone treatment of elderly men with low circulating IGF-1. Clin Endocrinol 1993;39:417–425.
23. Hayflik L. How and Why We Age, Ballantine, New York, 1994.
24. Shorr RI. Biology of aging. In: Reuben DB, Yoshikawa TT, Besdine RW, eds. Geriatric Review Syllabus, 3rd ed. Kendall/ Hunt, Dubuque, IA, 1996, pp. 6–11.
25. Passeeri G, Girasole G, Jilka RL, Manolagas SC. Increased interleukin-6 production by murine bone marrow and bone cells after estrogen withdrawal. Endocrinology 1993;133:822–828.
26. Hayflik L, Moorhead PS. The serial cultivation of human diploid cell strains. Exp Cell Res 1961;25: 585–621.
27. Hayflick L. The cell biology of aging. Clin Geriatr Med 1985;1:15–27.
28. Hayflick L. The limited in vitro lifetime of human diploid cell strains. Exp Cell Res 1965;37:614–636.
29. Hayflick L. The cellular basis of biological aging. In: Finch CE, Hayflick L, eds. Handbook of the Biology of Aging. Van Nostrand, New York, 1976, pp. 159–188.
30. Norwood TH. Cellular Aging. In: Cassel CK, et al., eds. Geriatric Medicine, 2nd ed. Springer-Verlag, New York, 1990, pp. 1–15.
31. Goldstein S. Human genetic disorders that feature premature onset and accelerated progression of biological aging. In: Schneider EL, ed. Genetics of Aging. Plenum, New York, 1978, pp. 171–224.
32. Mooradian AD. Molecular theories of aging. In: Morley JE, Glizk Z, Rubenstein LZ, eds. Geriatric Nutrition. A Comprehensive Review. Raven, New York, 1990, pp. 11–18.
33. Rohme D. Evidence for a relationship between longevity of mammalian species and life-spans of normal fibroblasts in vitro and erythrocytes in vitro. Proc Natl Acad Sci USA 1980;78:5009–5013.
34. Harman D. The aging process. Proc Natl Acad Sci USA 1981;78:7124–7128.
35. Lung CC, Pinnas JL, Yahya D, Meinke GC, Mooradian AD. Malondialdehyde modified proteins and their antibodies in the plasma of control and streptozotein induced diabetic rats. Life Sci 1993;52: 329–337.
36. Harman D. Aging: A theory based on free radical and radiation chemistry. J Gerontol 1956;11:298–300.
37. Miquel J, Lundgren PR, Bensch KG. Effects of oxygen-nitrogne (1:1) at 760 Torr on the life span and fine structure of Drosophila melanogaster. Mech Age Devel 1975;4:41–59.
38. Davies I. Theories and general principles of aging. In: Brocklehurst JC, Tallis RC, Fillit HM, eds. Textbook of Geriatric Medicine and Gerontology, 4th ed. New York, 1992, pp. 26–60.
39. Glass GA, Gershon D. Enzymatic changes in rat erythrocytes with increasing cell and donor age: loss of superoxide-dismutase activity associated with increases in catalytic defective forms. Biochem Biophys Res Commun 1981;103:1245–1253.
40. Tolmasoff JM, Ono T, Cutler RG. Superoxide dismutase correlation with life-span and specific metabolic rate in primate species. Proc Nat Acad Sci USA 1980;77:2777–2781.

41. Blackett AD, Hall DA. The effects of vitamin E on mouse fitness and survival. Gerontology 1981;27: 133–139.
42. Hall DA, Blackett AD, Zojac AR, Switala S, Airey CM. Changes in skinfold with increasing age. Age Aging 1981;10:191–195.
43. Pryor WA. The free-radical theory of aging revisited: A critique and a suggested disease-specific theory. In: Warner HR, et al., eds. Modern Biological Theories of Aging. Raven, New York, Aging 1987;31: 89–112.
44. Pearl R. The Rate of Living. University of London Press, London, 1928.
45. Clarke JM, Maynard-Smith J. Two phases of ageing in Drosophila subobscura. J Exp Biol 1961;38: 679–684.
46. Sohal RS, ed. Age Pigments. Elsevier/North Holland, Amsterdam, 1981, pp. 394.
47. Austad SN, Fischer KE. Mammalian aging, metabolism, and ecology: evidence from the bats and marsupials. J Gerontol Biol Sci 1991;46:B47.
48. Lints FA. The rate of living theory revisited. J Gerontol 1989;35:36–57.
49. Orgel LE The maintenance of the accuracy of protein synthesis and its relevance to ageing. Proc Natl Acad Sci USA 1963;49:517–521.
50. Heydari AR, Butler JA, Waggoner SM, Richardson A. Age-related changes in protein phophorylation by rat hepatocytes. Mech Aging Dev 1989;50:227–248.
51. Dingley F, Maynard-Smith J. Absence of life-shortening effect of amino acid analogues in adult *Drosophila*. Exp Gerontol 1969;4:145–149.
52. Bozcuk AN. Testing the protein error hypothesis of ageing in *Drosophila*. Exp Gerontol 1976;11: 103–112.
53. Ogrodnik JP, Wulf JH, Cutler RG. Altered protein hypothesis of mammalian ageing process. II. Discrimination ratio of methionine vs. ethionine in the synthesis of ribosomal protein and RNA of C57BL/6J mouse liver. Exp Gerontol 1975;10:119–137.
54. Tice RR, Setlow RB. DNA repair and replication in aging organisms and cells. In: Finch CE, Schneider EL, eds. Handbook of the Biology of Aging. Van Nostrand Reinhold, New York, 1985, pp. 173.
55. Hart RW, Setlow RB. Correlation between deoxyribonucleic acid excision repair and lifespan in a number of mammalian species. Proc Natl Acad Sci USA 1974;71:2169.
56. Hart RW, Daniel FB. Genetic stability in vitro and in vivo. Adv Pathobiol 1980;7:123.
57. Brownlee M. Advanced protein glycosylation in diabetes and aging. Ann Rev Med 1995;48:223–234.
58. Schnider SL, Kohn RR. Glycosylation of human collagen in aging and diabetes mellitus. J Clin Invest 1980;66:1179–1181.
59. Masoro EJ. Biology of aging. Current state of knowledge. Arch Intern Med 1987;147:166–169.
60. Ross MH. Length of life and caloric intake. Am J Clin Nutr 1972;25:834–838.
61. Masoro EJ, Katz MS, McMahan CA. Evidence for the glycation hypothesis of aging from the food-restricted rodent model. J Gerontol 1989;44:B20–B22.
62. Morley JE, Mooradian AD, Silver AJ, et al. Nutrition in the elderly. Ann Intern Med 1988;109:890–904.
63. Harley CB, Futcher AB, Greider CW. Telomeres shorten during aging of human fibroblasts. Nature 1990;345–358,460.
64. Baker TB III, Martin GR. Molecular and biologic factors in aging: the origins, causes, and prevention of senescence. In: Cassel CK, et al., eds. Geriatric Medicine, 3rd ed. Springer, New York, 1997, pp. 3–28.

2 Tithonusism

Is It Reversible?

John E. Morley, MB, BCH

CONTENTS

INTRODUCTION

Aurora, goddess of dawn, became particularly enthused about the qualities of her morning lover, Tithonus. She felt that losing him would be unbearable, and so she went to her father, Zeus, and asked him to bestow immortality on Tithonus. Unfortunately, she forgot to ask for eternal youth for him as well. Over the years, Tithonus lost his strength, had a decrease in his libido and potency, and eventually began to babble incessantly. Although she still loved him for what he had been to her, Aurora now found Tithonus' existence annoying and banished him to a far room in her castle, where she had him turned into a grasshopper.

The concept that chronological aging is associated with an inexorable physiological deterioration, which eventually leads to the development of frailty and a failure to thrive, is well encapsulated by the term "Tithonusism." Peak performance is reached by the third to fourth decade *(1)*, with biochemical (e.g., calmodulin *[2]*, testosterone *[3]*, and physiological changes, e.g., body fat *[4]*, VO_{2max}, and athletic performance *[5]*) being statistically present in the fifth to sixth decade (Fig. 1). It is clear that all aging individuals do not deteriorate at the same rate, and that the slippery downhill slope of aging, as originally postulated by Nathan Shock *(6)*, may, in fact, be punctuated by periods of no change or even periods of improvement, as shown by the longitudinal studies of creatinine clearance in the Baltimore Longitudinal Study on Aging *(7)*. The rate at which Tithonusism develops can be accelerated by the occurrence of disease and slowed by the success of the rehabilitation process following the disease (Fig. 2).

From: *Contemporary Endocrinology: Endocrinology of Aging*
Edited by: J. E. Morley and L. van den Berg © Humana Press Inc., Totowa, NJ

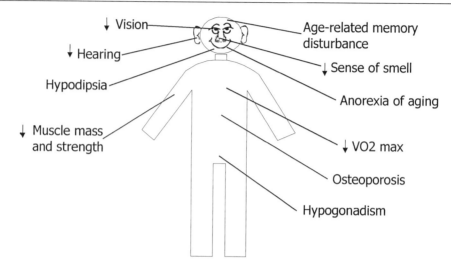

Fig. 1. Examples of the physiological changes of aging (Tithonusism).

Fries *(8)* has argued that the life-span is relatively fixed, and that, with appropriate health promotion and prevention, the quality of life can be improved, so that the illness and disability curve is rectangularized, with each person spending only a small portion of the end of their life in a state of frailty. Animal studies in both *Drosophila (9)* and *C. elegans (10)* have suggested that population life extension is feasible with genetic manipulation, and that, in these species, those animals with genetically increased life-spans have greater vitality and decreased sexual activity, but the populations continue to display a bell-shaped curve for survival, with no hint of rectangularization. This would suggest that, even in a genetically homogeneous population, the rate at which Tithonusism develops and progresses shows a wide variability.

The purpose of this review is to examine the evidence that the rate at which Tithonusism develops can be retarded. Rowe and Kahn *(11)* have argued for a focus on successful aging, i.e., examining the unique characteristics of highly functional aged individuals, but the approach that is suggested in this article leans toward examining how persons may age successfully, i.e., overcome their disabilities to allow continued enjoyment of the aging process, in the belief that this approach is more likely to result in a rectangularization of the curve of functional deterioration associated with aging. This concept of aging successfully was originally put forward by Eric Pfeifer *(12)* at a conference at Duke University in 1973, and is epitomized by Grandma Moses, who took up painting in late life, when she developed arthritis.

REVERSIBLE AND PREVENTABLE DISEASE PROCESSES

A number of studies *(13–15)* have suggested that health promotion and prevention programs for free-living older persons can improve their functional status. In addition, the controlled studies of geriatric evaluation and management units have demonstrated relatively dramatic improvements when intensive rehabilitation is targeted to specific groups of frail elderly (*see* ref. 16 for meta-analysis). Certain easily treatable endocrine disorders, such as hypothyroidism and vitamin B_{12} deficiency, occur at rates as high as 5% in persons over 80 yr of age *(17)*, and their diagnosis and treatment clearly improves functional status, including cognitive function *(18)*.

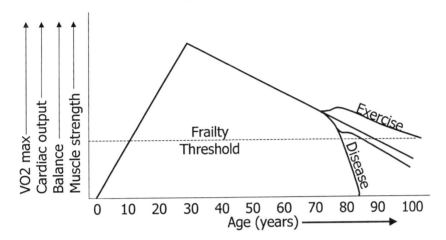

Fig. 2. Development of Tithonusism. Most performance parameters have peaked by 30 yr of age, after which they gradually decline. The onset of disease can increase the rate of decline, though adequate management may return the rate of decline to the previous slope. An exercise program may slow the rate of decline and may even temporarily enhance performance over previous levels. Eventually, the interaction of Tithonusism and disease leads to the individual slipping below the frailty threshold, with a marked deterioration in the individual's functional status.

Of all the treatable conditions whose diagnosis and treatment can produce the most dramatic improvements in function in older persons, depression is the most prominent. Depression is less common in older persons than younger persons *(19)*, but is less commonly diagnosed in older persons *(20)*. Depression is associated with increased mortality, even in nursing home residents, and has been demonstrated to be a major factor in predicting a poor response to rehabilitation therapy *(21)*. Screening for depression in older persons, utilizing the Beck Depression Inventory or the Yesavage Geriatric Depression Scale, represents a highly cost-effective approach to improving functional status in older persons.

EXERCISE

A number of articles have reviewed the benefits of exercise and the potential problems of disease and immobility in older persons *(22,23*; Fig. 3). Moderate exercise in epidemiological studies has been associated with enhanced longevity *(24)*, possibly because acute exercise bouts increase natural killer cell activity, and thus may enhance immune surveillance against cancer *(25)*. Endurance exercise can improve VO_{2max} and increase high density lipoprotein (HDL) cholesterol *(26)*. Strength exercises have been demonstrated to increase muscle mass and to enhance function, even in 90-yr-olds *(27)*. Balance deteriorates with aging, and has been implicated as a major cause of falls *(28)*. Deterioration of balance with aging is, in part, caused by alterations in adrenergic input to the cerebellum from the locus ceruleus, and by decreased β-adrenergic activity *(29)*. Animal studies have demonstrated that a physically stimulating environment can improve balance and induce new synaptic sprouting in old rodents *(30)*. Poor posture with aging can lead to a change in the locus of balance, and thus increase the potential of falling *(31)*. Posture exercises can prevent this from occurring, and may also prevent back strain. Flexibility also decreases with aging, and this deterioration can be prevented with appropriate flexibility exercises *(32)*.

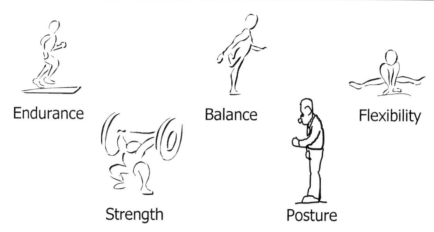

Endurance   Balance   Flexibility

Strength   Posture

Fig. 3. Cartoon representing the five forms of exercise necessary to slow the rate at which Tithonusism develops.

Clearly, prevention of disease and the avoidance of iatrogenic disuse, such as that produced by the use of physical restraints *(33)*, represents an important modality in delaying the onset of Tithonusism. Moderate, regular exercise, embracing all five of the aforementioned modalities (Fig. 2), is clearly the gold standard by which the success of all other interventions to slow the development of Tithonusism should be measured. The ancient Chinese martial arts exercise form, Tai Chi, is an exercise approach that embodies all the components of exercise necessary to slow Tithonusism *(34)*.

NUTRITION

It is now well recognized that in old age there is a J-shaped curve linking body mass index (BMI) with mortality *(35,36)* and the presence of disability *(37)*. Overall low BMI appears to be a better predictor of poor outcomes than high BMI, though it has been suggested that the most important predictor is weight loss from middle age *(38)*. Part of the risks associated with low BMI appear to result from the profound deleterious effects of protein energy undernutrition (PEU) in older persons. PEU produces a variety of negative effects on immune function, including a decrease in the $CD_4^+:CD_8^+$ ratio *(39)*. Much of the PEU that occurs in old age is the result of treatable disorders *(40)*. Increasing evidence suggests that depression is the commonest treatable cause of PEU *(41,42)*.

Based on the evidence from the National Health and Nutrition Examination Survey (NHANES) studies that there is a decrease in caloric consumption with advancing age *(43)*, it was postulated that there is a physiological anorexia of aging *(44)*. Rodent studies have demonstrated that decreased food intake with advancing age is associated with a decrease in endogenous opioid (dynorphin) feeding drive *(45)* and an increase in the satiation effect of the gastrointestinal hormone, cholecystokinin *(46)*. In healthy humans, it has recently been established that older persons develop satiation more rapidly following a meal, and have a greater decrease in hunger than younger persons *(47)*. These changes appear to be related to the delay in gastric emptying that occurs with aging. Changes in taste and olfaction, which occur in many but not all older persons, decrease the hedonic qualities of food *(44)*. These physiological changes make older persons particularly vulnerable to developing weight loss and PEU in response to physical or psychological illness or social deprivation.

Older persons have also been demonstrated to develop a hypodipsia that makes them relatively insensitive to cues that normally induce drinking *(48)*. Based on animal *(49)* and human *(50)* studies, this hypodipsia appears to result from a lack of the endogenous μ opioid receptor drinking drive. This decrease in thirst drive with aging places older persons at high risk for developing dehydration when exposed to infection, with increased insensible water loss, or when they develop diabetes mellitus, with its associated osmotic diuresis, or secondary to diuretic therapy.

Overall, the physiological changes leading to the anorexia and hypodipsia of aging place older persons particularly at risk for developing PEU and dehydration.

TROPHIC FACTORS: THE HORMONAL FOUNTAIN OF YOUTH

The most dramatic of the hormonal changes associated with aging occurs in the female at the menopause, when exhaustion of the ovarian follicles leads to estrogen deficiency. Estrogen replacement following the menopause has been demonstrated to increase life expectancy, despite the fact that it increases endometrial cancer risk 2–15-fold *(51)*, and possibly breast cancer relative risk by 1.3 times *(52)*. Estrogen replacement at the menopause clearly maintains bone density and decreases future fracture risk *(53)*, enhances HDL cholesterol levels *(54)*, decreases angiographically defined coronary artery disease *(55–57)*, reduces stroke *(57)*, and possibly reduces coronary artery disease *(58)*. The benefit of estrogen replacement beyond 10 yr following menopause, and its utility in ethnic groups with less predisposition to bone disease, remains to be proven. The Women's Health Initiative Study may provide the answers to some of these questions.

It has long been recognized that estrogen, although demonstrating the most dramatic decline, is not the only hormone to decrease with aging. Many of the changes classically associated with aging are similar to the changes observed with endocrine deficiency. This has led to the concept that aging results from a hormonal menopause, and to the hypothesis that hormonal replacement may prevent the onset of Tithonusism. A cautionary note is raised by the studies of dietary restriction in rodents. Dietary restriction prolongs life in rodents. However, one of the early changes observed with dietary restriction are hormonal changes that parallel the hormonal changes seen in old rodents *(59*; Table 1). This raises the possibility that the hormonal deficiencies seen with aging are protective rather than detrimental.

Both growth hormone (GH) and insulin-like growth factor-I (IGF-I) levels are reduced with aging *(60)*. The decrease in the hypothalamic–GH–IGF axis is predominantly caused by an increase in hypothalamic somatostatin activity *(61)*. To explore the effectiveness of GH at reversing age-associated deficits, Rudman et al. *(62,63)* treated 45 healthy older males between 61 and 80 yr of age with 0.03 mg/kg recombinant growth hormone 3× a week. This study found an increase in lean body mass, skin thickness, liver volume, and spleen volume with a decrease in adipose mass. Nine of 28 of the GH-treated individuals developed bilateral carpal tunnel syndrome, and four developed gynecomastia, necessitating withdrawal from the study. Other approaches to restoring the integrity of the GH axis include the administration of GH releasing hormone, which restores the IGF-I axis and improves muscle strength in older men *(64)*. A preliminary *(65)* study has shown that short-term administration of IGF-I to healthy older women results in nitrogen retention and an increase in lean body mass. However, long-term IGF-I administration may result in the development of hypoglycemia *(66)*. At present, restoration of the GH axis in

Table 1
Effects of Aging and Dietary Restriction in Rodents

Hormone	Aging	Dietary restriction
Insulin	Decrease	Decrease
Insulin receptor mRNA	Increase	Increase
Insulin growth factor I	Decrease	Decrease
Growth hormone	Decrease	Decrease
Thyroxine	Decrease	Decrease
Triiodothyronine	Decrease	Decrease
Luteinizing hormone	Decrease	Decrease
Testosterone (males)	Decrease	Increase
Estradiol (females)	Decrease	Decrease
25-Hydroxy vitamin D	Decrease	No change
Parathormone	Increase	Decrease

Adapted with permission from ref. 59.

healthy elderly persons does not appear to be a feasible approach to the reversal of Tithonusism. A number of studies have suggested that short-term administration of GH to malnourished, critically ill patients will improve their nutritional status (67–69). Studies are still necessary to determine if this approach will improve functional outcomes in older persons.

In males, testosterone levels decrease with aging, albeit in a much less dramatic way than is seen with the female menopause (70). Fifty percent of healthy males over 50 yr of age have bioavailable testosterone levels less than those seen in healthy younger males (3). The decline in testosterone is caused by a decrease in testicular production of testosterone, coupled with a failure of the hypothalamic–pituitary axis to appropriately detect and respond to this fall by increasing luteinizing hormone secretion (71). Besides potential effects of testosterone replacement on muscle strength, libido energy, and potency (72), Flood et al. (73) have reported animal data suggesting that testosterone may improve age-related impairment of visuospatial-associated memory. Testosterone deficiency is associated with minimal trauma hip fracture in nursing home residents (74).

Three placebo-controlled testosterone treatment studies in older persons have been reported. In two 3-mo studies, testosterone increased hematocrit, and lowered low-density lipoprotein cholesterol (75,76). One of these studies also found an increase in lean body mass (75), and the other, an increase in right-hand grip strength (76). Sih et al. (77) have reported their data on 1 yr treatment with testosterone cypionate (200 mg every 2 wk). Besides the expected increase in hematocrit, they found an increase in right and left grip strength, and an improvement in balance. These relatively short-term studies have not reported any side effects. Potential side effects include prostatic growth (hyperplasia and cancer) and stroke secondary to the increased hematocrit. Although interventional studies with testosterone look promising as an approach to the reversal of Tithonusism, their short-term nature forces the conservative conclusion that the role of testosterone is not yet proven.

A number of steroid hormones decrease with aging in healthy older persons. These include pregnenolone and dehydroepiandrosterone (DHEA) (78, and unpublished observations). Both of these steroids enhance memory in mice (73). DHEA has been demonstrated to have positive effects on the immune system (74), and correlative studies suggest potential benefits associated with bone mass and cardiovascular disease (51).

Studies by Yen et al. *(96–98)* have suggested that DHEA may improve mood, strength in men, and perhaps activate the immune system. More interventional studies with both pregnenolone and DHEA are needed before any conclusions can be made.

With aging, there are numerous reasons for a decrease in vitamin D and its efficacy *(80)*, including utilization of sunblock to prevent skin cancer, decreased skin syntheses of cholecalciferol, decreased conversion of 25(OH) vitamin D to $1,25(OH)_2$ vitamin D, and altered receptor function. Genetic studies have suggested a pivotal role for the vitamin D receptor in the development of osteoporosis *(81)*. Chapuy et al. *(82)* have demonstrated that vitamin D and calcium markedly decrease hip fracture risk in nursing home residents. Other studies have suggested that vitamin D may play an important role in macrophage function and immunosurveillance for diseases such as tuberculosis *(83)*. Adequate vitamin D status is clearly an important player in delaying the onset of Tithonusism.

Available information allows no clear cut conclusions concerning the ability of hormone replacement to reverse Tithonusism. Testosterone in males may, like estrogen in females, have a limited role in retarding the aging process. GH's role may be limited to short-term use in those persons with PEU. Evidence is accumulating for a central role for vitamin D in maintaining bone mass.

PERSONAL NEUROCHEMISTRY ADJUSTMENT

Although there are many tasks that older persons can perform, it is clear that age-related memory impairment is a real phenomenon *(84)*. Early animal and human studies concentrated on the role of acetylcholine in memory function *(85)*, which led to attempts to stimulate cholinergic function by utilizing acetylcholine precursors, such as lecithin or choline *(86)*. These attempts have been fundamentally disappointing. Tacrine, a drug that inhibits acetylcholine breakdown, has a miniscale improvement in memory function in patients with mild Alzheimer's disease *(87,88)*. This degree of improvement may be no better than that seen in some studies involving nootropics, such as piracetam and hydergine *(89,90)*.

Numerous other neurotransmitters have been demonstrated to modulate memory, including neuropeptides such as neuropeptide Y *(91)* and β-endorphin *(92)*, the *N*-Methyl-D-aspartic acid receptor *(93)*, γ-amino butyric acid *(94)*, and neurosteroids *(73)*. This suggests that it may be possible to individualize neurotransmitter adjustments to improve age-related memory deficits.

Another area of potential intervention in memory dysfunction is the modulation of amyloid-β protein production and effects. β-Amyloid (1-28) has been demonstrated to produce amnesia in mice *(94)*. Antagonists thata prevent the amnesia produced by β-amyloid (1-28) have been synthesized *(95)*. Eventually, genetic manipulation of β-amyloid protein should be feasible.

At present, the concept of a personalized neurochemistry adjustment to rectify age-related memory disturbances is science fiction, but it would seem fairly certain that, early in the next century, this will become a relatively simple task.

GERIATRIC VISION 2020: MODULATION OF TITHONUSISM

This chapter has provided glimpses of the potential to modulate the rate at which the physiological aging process occurs. At present, the major focus of the wise clinician should be to identify and appropriately manage treatable disorders such as depression

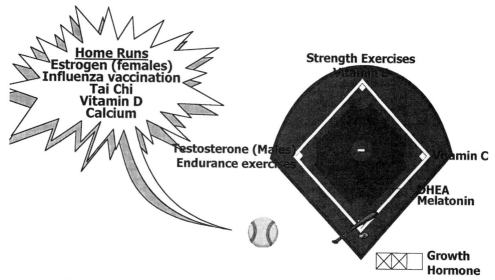

Fig. 4. Report card on the modalities available to prevent Tithonusism.

and PEU. Clearly, a prudent exercise program remains the best preventive technique to delay the onset of Tithonusism and frailty. Only the future will tell whether some of the more innovative approaches to the retardation of the aging process will become a reality in the next century. Finally, it is recognized that this article has not discussed the potential of immune enhancement with cytokine analogs, and the role of transplantation and artificial joint replacement in the modulation of Tithonusism. Figure 4 demonstrates current ability to modulate Tithonusism. Unlike Zeus, we cannot bestow immortality on the human race, but it is possible that the geriatrics of the future may better approximate the eternal youth (rectangularity of the morbidity curve) that was never bestowed on Tithonus.

REFERENCES

1. Kenney RA. Physiology of aging. Clin Geriatr Med 1985;1:37–59.
2. Morley JE, Levine AS, Beyer HS, Mooradian AD, Kaiser FE, Brown DM. The effect of aging and diabetes mellitus on human red and white cell calmodulin levels. Diabetes 1984;33:77–80.
3. Korenman SG, Morley JE, Mooradian AD, Davis SS, Kaiser FE, Silver AJ, Viosca SP, Garza D. Secondary hypogonadism in older men: its relationship to impotence. J Clin Endocrinol Metab 1990;71:963–969.
4. Silver AJ, Guillen CP, Kahl MJ, Morley JE. Effect of aging on body fat. J Am Geriatr Soc 1993;41: 211–213.
5. Morley JE, Reese SS. Clinical implications of the aging heart. Am J Med 1989;86:77–86.
6. Shock NW. Age changes in physiological changes in the total animal: the role of tissue loss. In: Strehler BL, ed. Biology of Aging. American Institute of Biological Sciences, Washington DC, 1960.
7. Rowe JW, Andres R, Tobin JD, et al. The effect of age on creatinine clearance in men: a cross-sectional and longitudinal study. J Gerontol 1976;31:155–163.
8. Fries JF. Aging, natural death and the compression of morbidity. New Engl J Med 1980;303:130–135.
9. Rose MR, Nusbaum TJ, Fleming JE. Drosophila with postponed aging as a model for aging research. Lab Anim Sci 1992;42:114–118.
10. Johnson TE, Lethgow GJ. The search for the genetic basis of aging: the identification of gerontogenes in the nematode, Caenorrhabditis elegans. J Am Geriatr Soc 1992;40:936–949.
11. Rowe JW, Kahn RL. Human aging: usual and successful. Science 1987;237:143–149.
12. Pfeifer E. Successful Aging. Duke University Center for Aging, Durham, NC, 1974.
13. Farbacher D, Josephson K, Pietruzska F, Linderbom K, Morley JE, Rubenstein LZ. An in-home preventive assessment program for independent older adults: a randomized controlled trial. J Am Geriatr Soc 1994;42:630–638.

14. Fries JF, Bloch DA, Harrington H, et al. Two-year results of a randomized controlled trial of a health promotion program in a retiree population. The Bank of America Study. Am J Med 1993;94:455–462.

15. Hendricksen C, Lund E, Stomgard E. Consequences of assessment and intervention among elderly people: a three-year randomized controlled trial. Br Med J 1984;289:1522–1524.

16. Stuck AE, Siu AL, Wieland GD, et al. Comprehensive geriatric assessment: a meta-analysis of controlled trials. Lancet 1993;342:1032–1036.

17. Mooradian AD, Morley JE, Korenman SG. Endocrinology in aging. Disease-a-Month 1988;34:395–461.

18. Martin DC, Francis J, Protech J, Huff FJ. Time dependency of cognitive recovery with cobalamin replacement: report of a pilot study. J Am Geriatr Soc 1992;40:168–172.

19. Fitten LJ, Morley JE, Gross PL, et al. Depression. J Am Geriatr Soc 1989;37:459–472.

20. Miller DK, Morley JE, Rubenstein LZ, et al. Formal geriatric assessment instruments and the care of elderly general medical outpatients. J Am Geriatr Soc 1990;38:645–651.

21. Parikh RM, Robinson RG, Lipsey JR, et al. The impact of poststroke depression on recovery in activities of daily living over a 2-year follow-up. Arch Neurol 1990;47:785–789.

22. Shepard RJ. The scientific basis of exercise prescribing in the very old. J Am Geriatr Soc 1990;38: 62–70.

23. Edward K, Larson EB. Benefits of exercise for older adults. A review of existing evidence and current recommendations for the general population. Clin Geriatr Med 1992;8:35–50.

24. Paffenbarger RS, Hyder RT, Wing AL, Hsieh CC. Physical activity, all-cause mortality and longevity of college alumni. N Engl J Med 1986;314:605–613.

25. Fiatarone MA, Morley JE, Bloom ET, Benton D, Solomon GF, Makinodan T. The effect of exercise on natural killer cell activity in young and old subjects. J Gerontol Med Sci 1989;44:M37–M46.

26. Schwartz RS, Cain KC, Shuman WP, et al. Effect of intensive endurance training on lipoprotein profiles in young and older men. Metabolism 1992;41:649–654.

27. Fiatarone MF, Marks EC, Ryan ND, et al. High-intensity strength straining in nonagenerians: effects on skeletal muscle. JAMA 1990;263:3029–3034.

28. Robbins AS, Rubenstein LZ, Josephson KR, et al. Predictors of falls among elderly people: results of two population-based studies. Arch Intern Med 1989;149:1628–1632.

29. Rosenthal MJ, Morley JE, Flood JF, Scarpace PJ. Relationship between behavioral and motor responses of mature and old mice and cerebellar adrenergic receptor density. Mech Age Dev 1988;45:231–237.

30. Black JE, Isaacs KR, Anderson BJ, et al. Learning causes synaptogenesis, whereas motor activity causes angiogenesis in cerebellar cortex of adult rats. Proc Natl Acad Sci USA 1990;87:5568–5572.

31. Herning MM. Posture improvement in the frail elderly. In: Perry HM III, Morley JE, Coe RM, eds. Aging and Musculoskeletal Disorders. Springer, New York, 1993, pp. 334–353.

32. Adrian MJ. Flexibility in the aging adult. In: Smith EL, Serfass RC, eds. Exercise and Aging: the Scientific Basis. Enslow, Hillside, NJ, 1981, pp. 45–58.

33. Evans LK, Strumpf NE. Tying down the elderly: a review of the literature on physical restraints. J Am Geriatr Soc 1989;37:65–74.

34. Wolf SL, Coogles CE, Green RC, et al. Novel interventions to prevent falls in the elderly. In: Perry HM III, Morley JE, Coe RM, eds. Aging and Musculoskeletal Disorders. Springer, New York, 1993, pp. 178–195.

35. Harris T, Cook EF, Garrison R, et al. Body mass index and mortality among nonsmoking older persons. JAMA 1988;259:1520–1524.

36. Tayback M, Kumanijika S, Chee E. Body weight as a risk factor in the elderly. Arch Intern Med 1990; 150:1065–1072.

37. Galanos AN, Pieper CF, Cornoni-Huntley J, et al. Nutrition and function: is there a relationship between body mass index and functional capabilities of community-dwelling elderly? J Am Geriatr Soc 1994; 42:368–373.

38. Rumpel C, Harris TB, Madans J. Modification of the relationship between Quetelet index and mortality by weight loss history among older women. Ann Epidemiol 1993;3:448–450.

39. Kaiser FE, Morley JE. CD_4^+ lymphopenia in older persons. J Am Geriatr Soc 1994;42:1291–1294.

40. Morley JE. Why do physicians fail to recognize and treat malnutrition in older persons? J Am Geriatr Soc 1991;39:1139–1140.

41. Morley JE, Kraenzle DK. Causes of weight loss in a community nursing home. J Am Geriatr Soc 1994; 42:583–585.

42. Katz IR, Beaston-Wimmer P, Parmlee P, et al. Failure to thrive in the elderly: exploration of the concept and delineation of psychiatric components. J Geriatr Psychiatr Neurol 1994;6:161–169.

43. Subar AF, Harlan LC, Mattson M. Food and nutrient intake differences between smokers and non-smokers in the US. J Public Health 1990;80:1323–1329.
44. Morley JE, Silver AJ. Anorexia in the elderly. Neurobiol Aging 1988;9:9–16.
45. Gosnell BA, Levine AS and Morley JE. The effects of aging on opioid modulation of feeding in rats. Life Sci 1983;32:2793–2799.
46. Silver AJ, Flood JF, Morley JE. Effect of gastrointestinal peptides on ingestion in young and old mice. Peptides 1988;9:221–226.
47. Clarkston WK, Pantano MM, Morley JE, et al. Evidence for the anorexia of aging: correlations with gastric emptying in healthy elderly vs healthy young adults. Am J Physiol 1997;272:R243–R248.
48. Phillips PA, Rolls BJ, Ledingham JG, et al. Reduced thirst after water deprivation in healthy elderly men. N Engl J Med 1986;311:753–759.
49. Silver AJ, Flood JF, Morley JE. Effect of aging on fluid ingestion in mice. J Gerontology 1991;46: B117–B121.
50. Silver AJ, Morley JE. Role of the opioid system in hypodipsia associated with aging. J Am Geriatr Soc 1992;40:556–560.
51. Villareal DT, Morley JE. Trophic factors in aging. Should older people receive hormonal replacement therapy? Drugs Aging 1994;4:492–509.
52. Steinburg LL, Stephen TB, et al. A meta-analysis of the effect of estrogen replacement therapy on the risk of breast cancer. JAMA 1991;265:1985–1990.
53. Genant HK, Baylink DJ, Gallagher JC. Estrogens in the prevention of osteoporosis in postmenopausal women. Am J Obstet Gynecol 1989;161:1842–1846.
54. Gruchow HW, Anderson AJ, Barboriak JJ, Sobocinski KA. Postmenopausal use of estrogen and occlusion of coronary arteries. Am Heart J 1988;115:954–963.
55. McFarland KF, Boniface ME, Hornung CA, et al. Risk factors and noncontraceptive estrogen use in women with and without coronary disease. Am Heart J 1989;117:1209–1214.
56. Sullivan JM, van der Zwaag R, Lemp GF, et al. Postmenopausal estrogen use and coronary atherosclerosis. Arch Intern Med 1988;108:358–363.
57. Falkeborn M, Persson I, Terent A, et al. Hormone replacement therapy and the risk of stroke: follow-up of a population-based cohort in Sweden. Arch Intern Med 1993;153:1201–1209.
58. Barrett-Connor E, Bush TL. Estrogen and coronary heart disease in women. J Am Med Assoc 1991;265: 1861–1867.
59. Morley JE. Aging. In: Bagdale JW, ed. Yearbook of Endocrinology. Mosby, St. Louis, MO, 1993, pp. 61–93.
60. Kelijman M. Age-related alterations of the growth hormone/insulin-like growth factor I axis. J Am Geriatr Soc 1991;39:295–307.
61. Ghigo E, Goffi S, Nicolosi M, et al. Growth hormone (GH) responsiveness to combined administration of arginine and GH-releasing hormone does not vary with age in man. J Clin Endocrinol Metab 1990;71: 1481–1485.
62. Rudman D, Feller AG, Nagraj HS, et al. Effects of human growth hormone in men over 60 years old. New Engl J Med 1990;323:1–6.
63. Cohn L, Feller AG, Draper MW, et al. Carpal tunnel syndrome and synecomastia during growth hormone treatment of elderly men with low circulating IGF-I concentrations. Lin Endocrinol 1993;39: 417–425.
64. Vittone J, Harman SM, Rodgers M, et al. Effects of growth hormone releasing hormone (GHRH) in healthy elderly men. Clin Res 1994;42:216A.
65. Thompson J, Butterfield G, Marcus R, et al. Hormonal and metabolic changes in IGF-1 treatment of aging women. Clin Res 1994;42:12A.
66. Guler H-P, Zapf J, Froesen ER. Short term effects of recombinant human insulin-like growth factor I in healthy adults. N Engl J Med 1987;317:137–140.
67. Kaiser FE, Silver AJ, Morley JE. The effect of recombinant human growth hormone on malnourished older individuals. J Am Geriatr Soc 1991;39:235–240.
68. Douglas RG, Humberstone DA, Haystead A, Shaw JHF. Metabolic effects of recombinant human growth hormone: isotopic studies in the postabsorptive state and during total parenteral nutrition. Br J Surg 1990;77:785–790.
69. Binnerts A, Wilson JHP, Lamberts SW. The effects of human growth hormone administration in elderly adults with recent weight loss. J Clin Endocrinol Metab 1988;67:1312–1316.
70. Gray A, Berlin JA, McKinley JB, Longcope C. An examination of research design effects on the association of testosterone and male aging: results of a meta-analysis. J Clin Epidemiol 1991;44:1671–1684.

71. Morley JE, Kaiser FE. Hypogonadism in the elderly male. Adv Endocrinol Metab 1993;4:241–262.

72. Mooradian AD, Morley JE, Korenman SG. Biological actions of androgens. Endocr Rev 1987;8:1–28.

73. Flood JF, Morley JE, Roberts E. Memory enhancing effects in male mice of pregnenolone and steroids metabolically derived from it. Proc Natl Acad Sci USA 1992;89:1567–1571.

74. Stanley HL, Schmitt BP, Poses RM, Deiss WP. Does hypogonadism contribute to the occurrence of a minimal trauma hip fracture in elderly men? J Am Geriatr Soc 1991;39:766–771.

75. Tenover JS. Effects of testosterone supplementation in the aging male. J Clin Endocrinol Metab 1992; 75:1092–1098.

76. Morley JE, Perry HM III, Kaiser FE, Kraenzle D, Jensen JM, Houston KA, Mattammal M, Perry HM Jr. Effect of testosterone replacement therapy in old hypogonadal males. J Am Geriatr Soc 1993;41: 149–152.

77. Sih R, Morley JE, Kaiser FE, Perry HM III, Patrick P, Ross C. Testosterone replacement in older hypogonadal men: a 12-month randomized controlled trial. J Clin Endocrinol Metab 1997;82:1661–1677.

78. Orentreich N, Brind JL, Vogelman JH, et al. Long-term longitudinal measurements of plasma dehydro-epiandrosterone sulfate in normal men. J Clin Endocrinol Metab 1992;75:1002–1004.

79. Daynes RA, Araneo BA, Ershler WB, et al. Altered regulation of IL-6 production with normal aging. Possible linkage to the age-associated decline in dehydroepiandrosterone and its sulfated derivative. J Immunol 1993;150:5219–5230.

80. Morley JE. A place in the sun does not guarantee adequate vitamin D. J Am Geriatr Soc 1989;37: 663–664.

81. Morrison NA, Cheng QI, Toketa A, et al. Prediction of bone density from vitamin D receptor alleles. Nature 1994;367:284–287.

82. Chapuy MC, Arlot ME, Duboeuf F, et al. Vitamin D_3 and calcium to prevent hip fractures in elderly women. N Engl J Med 1992;327:1637–1642.

83. McMurray DN, Bartow RA, Mentzer CL, Hernandez-Fontera F. Micronutrient status and immune function in tuberculosis. Ann NY Acad Sci 1990;587:58–69.

84. Albert MS. Cognition and aging. In: Hazzard WR, et al., eds. Principles of Geriatric Medicine and Gerontology. McGraw-Hill, New York, 1990, pp. 913–919.

85. Bartus RT. Drugs to treat age-related neurodegenerative problems. The final frontier of medical science? J Am Geriatr Soc 1990;38:680–695.

86. Goodnick P, Gershon S. Chemotherapy of cognitive disorders in geriatric subjects. J Clin Psychiat 1984; 45:196–209.

87. Knapp MJ, Knapman DS, Solomon PR, et al. A 30-week randomized controlled trial of high dose tacrine in patients with Alzheimer's disease. The Tacrine study group. JAMA 1994;985–991.

88. Wilcock GK, Surmon DJ, Scott M, et al. An evaluation of the efficacy and safety of tetra hydroamino-cridine (THA) without lecithin in the treatment of Alzheimer's disease. Age Aging 1993;22:316–324.

89. Thompson TL 2nd, Filley CM, Mitchell WD, et al. Lack of efficacy of hydergine in patients with Alzheimer's disease. N Engl J Med 1991;324:197–198.

90. Whitehouse PJ. Treatment of Alzheimer disease. Alzheimer Dis Assoc Disord 1991;S:S1:S32–S36.

91. Flood JF, Baker ML, Hernandez EN, Morley JE. Modulation of memory processing by neuropeptide Y varies with brain injection site. Brain Res 1989;503:73–82.

92. Gallagher M. Behavioral significance of opioid peptides in relation to hippocampal function. National Institute of Drug Abuse (NIDA). Research Monograph Series 1988;82:118–132.

93. Flood JF, Morley JE, Lanthorn TH. Effect on memory processing by D-cycloserine, an agonist of the NMDA/glycine receptor. Eur J Pharmacol 1992;221:249–254.

94. Flood JF, Morley JE, Roberts E. Amnestic effects in mice of four synthetic peptide homologous to amyloid β-protein from Alzheimer disease. Proc Natl Acad Sci USA 1991;88:3363–3366.

95. Flood JF, Roberts E, Sherman MA, Kaplan BE, Morley JE. Topography of a binding site for small amnestic peptides deduced from structure-activity studies. Relation to amnestic effect of amyloid β-protein. Proc Natl Acad Sci USA 1994;91:380–384.

96. Khorram O, Vu L, Yen SSC. Activation of immune function by dehydroepiandrosterone (DHEA) in age-advanced men. J Gerontol Biol Sci Med Sci 1997;52:M1–M7.

97. Morales AJ, Nolan J, Nelson G, Yen SSC. Effects of replacement dose of dehydroepiandrosterone (DHEA) in men and women of advancing age. J Clin Endocrinol Metab 1995;80:2799.

98. Yen SS, Morales AJ, Khorram O. Replacement of DHEA in aging men and women. Potential remedial effects. Ann NY Acad Sci 1995;774:128–142.

3

Hypothalamic Growth Hormone–IGF-I Axis

Ian M. Chapman, MBBS, PHD

CONTENTS

INTRODUCTION
NORMAL PHYSIOLOGY OF GH–IGF-I AXIS
EFFECT OF AGING ON GH–IGF-I AXIS
STRATEGIES TO REJUVENATE GH–IGF-I AXIS IN OLDER PEOPLE
SUMMARY
REFERENCES

INTRODUCTION

Human aging is associated with a decline in circulating concentrations of both growth hormone (GH) and insulin like growth factor I (IGF-I). Substantial numbers of older people are GH-deficient, by young adult standards. Many of the symptoms and biochemical and body composition changes that accompany human aging are similar to those that accompany organic, adult, GH deficiency (for example, in people who have had surgical removal of the pituitary), including a decrease in lean tissue and muscle strength, and an increase in body fat. Severe organic adult GH deficiency is now an approved indication for GH replacement therapy in a number countries, including the United States. By extension, it has been suggested that normal human aging is a form of functional GH deficiency, and that the elderly population, or selected elderly people who are particularly deficient, may benefit from treatments that rejuvenate the GH–IGF-I axis. The results of several short- to medium-term (≤6 mo) studies of GH, IGF-I, or GH secretatogue administration to healthy older people have now been reported. This chapter will provide a brief overview of the physiology of the GH–IGF-I axis, and summarize the effects of aging on the GH–IGF-I axis, the cause(s) and effects of these changes, and results of the therapeutic studies reported to date.

NORMAL PHYSIOLOGY OF THE GH–IGF-I AXIS

GH is a peptide hormone synthesized and stored in somatotroph cells of the anterior pituitary gland, from which it is secreted into the peripheral circulation in pulses. This pulsatile release results from interacting stimulatory and inhibitory inputs from the

From: *Contemporary Endocrinology: Endocrinology of Aging*
Edited by: J. E. Morley and L. van den Berg © Humana Press Inc., Totowa, NJ

23

hypothalamus, which is in turn affected by negative feedback effects of GH *(1–3)* and IGF-I *(4–7)*. Somatostatin (SS) is the principal hypothalamic inhibitor of GH release; growth hormone releasing hormone (GHRH) is the major stimulator. Both hormones are secreted at the median eminence into the hypothalamic–pituitary portal circulation, for transport to the anterior pituitary, where they interact. SS–GHRH interactions also occur in the hypothalamus, where there are anatomical connections between SS and GHRH neurons *(8,9)*. GHRH binds to receptors on the somatotroph membrane, and increases both GH synthesis and secretion by stimulating adenylate cyclase and increasing intracellular cyclic adenosine monophosphate and calcium concentrations *(10–12)*. SS binding to specific receptors on the somatotrophs has the opposite effects on adenylate cyclase and intracellular calcium *(13)*, but blocks only GH release without affecting ongoing synthesis *(14)*. In humans, SS inhibits both basal GH release and GH release induced by a variety of stimuli, including GHRH, sleep, exercise, arginine, and insulin-induced hypoglycemia.

A potent hexapeptide that stimulates GH secretion, growth hormone releasing peptide (GHRP), has been developed *(15,16)*. It acts through a unique receptor *(15,17)*, located in both the hypothalamus and pituitary. The presence of this receptor suggests that an endogenous GHRP-like ligand for this receptor may exist, but such a ligand has not yet been identified.

Insulin-like Growth Factor I and IGF-Binding Proteins

GH mediates many of its metabolic effects by stimulating hepatic, as well as local, production of IGF-I, previously called somatomedin-C. The other IGF, IGF-II, is much less important. GH has direct actions independent of IGF-I *(18,19)*, and GH and IGF-I also act synergistically to stimulate growth, and to produce the other metabolic effects of GH *(20)*. Consistent with the predominant role that IGF-I plays in mediating the metabolic actions of GH, circulating IGF-I and GH concentrations are significantly correlated across the range from GH deficiency to acromegaly. The IGF-I receptor (IGF-IR) mediates most of the biological actions of IGF-I, and has a high degree of homology with the insulin receptor. It is found in a wide variety of tissues, including the pituitary and hypothalamus. In both the circulation and the tissues, IGF-I is associated with specific binding proteins (IGFBPs), which bind most of the circulating IGFs. In the basal state, only about 1% of IGF-I is free. Approximately 75% of IGF -I circulates as part of a 150-kDa ternary complex, which consists of IGF-I or -II, plus IGFBP-3 and an 85-kDa acid-labile subunit. This ternary complex is unable to leave the vascular compartment, and binding of the IGFs in this complex leads to a dramatic prolongation of circulating IGF half-life, from about 10 min to 12-15 hr for IGF-I *(21)*. Serum IGFBP-3 levels are increased in acromegaly and decreased in hypopituitarism *(22)*; measurement of IGFBP-3 has been recommended as a diagnostic test for GH deficiency in both children *(23)* and adults *(24)*.

Growth Hormone Actions

GH exerts its actions by binding to transmembrane receptors on the plasma membranes of hepatocytes and other cells, and also to cytosolic receptors, which may represent internalized or newly formed receptors *(25)*. The binding of GH to its receptor leads to receptor dimerization, followed by hormone-receptor internalization and degradation *(26)*. The subsequent signal transduction mechanisms have not been fully defined, but involve the tyrosine phosphorylation of multiple intracellular proteins, including Jak 2 *(27,28)* and the signal transducers and activators of transcription (STATs) 1, 3, and 5 *(29)*. As its name implies, GH plays an important role in stimulating linear growth during childhood. In addition, it has a number of metabolic effects that persist throughout life. High-dose GH administration results in hyperinsulinemia, accompanied by varying degrees of glucose intolerance *(30,31)*; diabetes mellitus develops in about 20% of people with acromegaly. GH is also anabolic. Administration of GH to GH-deficient children *(32)*, normal and obese adults *(33)*, and adults with a variety of catabolic states, including burns *(34)*, high-dose glucocorticoid treatment *(35)*, and chronic obstructive lung disease *(36)*, results in positive nitrogen balance. Muscle mass is increased in GH-deficient children given GH *(37)*, and GH treatment increases lean body mass in GH-deficient adults *(38)*. GH administration has been found to increase muscle size in highly trained non-GH-deficient adult athletes *(39)*, but the effects on muscle strength in such GH-sufficient subjects have not been reported, nor have beneficial effects on performance in GH-replete individuals. Despite a lack of evidence that GH is beneficial, a number of athletes, including some competing at the highest levels, are apparently using it in an attempt to improve strength and performance.

The net effect of GH on fat metabolism is lipolytic, with a decrease in fat deposition and an increase in fat mobilization. GH deficiency is associated with an increase in percentage body fat, and redistribution of that fat to central sites. GH replacement therapy reduces body fat in GH-deficient subjects. In addition, GH deficiency is associated with abnormalities in circulating lipid profiles, including decreases in high-density lipoprotein and increases in low-density lipotrotein and total cholesterol levels, which favor the development of atherosclerosis *(38,40,41)*. These effects are reversible with GH therapy *(38,42,43)*. It has been suggested that GH deficiency increases overall mortality by increasing deaths caused by cardiovascular disease (CVD) *(44)*. Bone mineral density is increased by GH treatment in GH-deficient subjects, although these effects are rather small *(45,46)*, and most GH-deficient subjects are not osteoporotic. GH also exerts a number of effects on the immune system, apparently via production of IGFs, including stimulatory effects on thymic development, mitogen-induced lymphocyte proliferation, and natural killer cell activity. However, no clinical symptoms or syndromes associated with immune dysfunction have been described in GH-deficient humans *(47,48)*.

EFFECT OF AGING ON GH–IGF-I AXIS

GH is secreted throughout life in healthy humans. Circulating GH concentrations are relatively stable during childhood, then peak during the pubertal growth spurt. After puberty, increasing age is associated, on average, with declining GH secretion and parallel reductions in circulating GH and IGF-I concentrations *(45,49–51)*. Much of this decrease occurs between the ages of 20 and 40 yr (Fig. 1), and mean GH concentrations of adults 60–80 yr of age are reported to be, on average, one-fourth to two-thirds those of adults in their twenties *(49–52)*. It has been estimated, using deconvolution analysis, that the GH production rate decreases by 14% with each advancing decade during adulthood *(50)*. Increased GH clearance may be another cause of reduced circulating GH concentrations in the elderly *(50)*. GH secretion is reduced proportionally across the day in the elderly; nocturnal release, although lower than in young subjects, is still more than

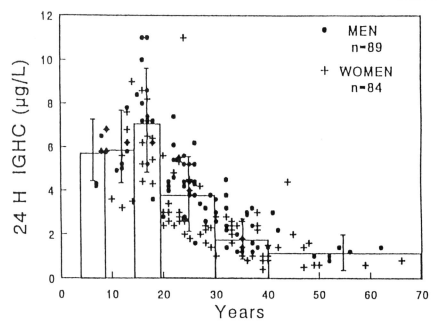

Fig. 1. Relationship between 24-h integrated growth hormone concentration (IGHC) and age in 89 normal men (●) and 84 normal women (+). Reprinted with permission from ref. *52.*

twice the daytime GH release, as in younger adults *(51,53)*. Until recently, GH assays were too insensitive to permit meaningful investigation of the effects of aging on GH secretion. Even in young adults, serum GH concentrations were undetectable for a substantial amount of the time, corresponding to the troughs between GH pulses: This was even more common in older people. Ultrasensitive GH assays have now been developed, with detection limits as low as 1 pg/L *(54–56)*, which effectively allow measurement of GH concentrations at all times, and have greatly aided study of the hyposomatotropism of aging.

Responses to stimuli of GH release are variably affected by aging. The acute GH response to exercise is reduced *(57,58)*. Most, but not all *(59)*, studies report a reduced GH response to GHRH, and the response to insulin-induced hypoglycemia is either reduced or unchanged *(60,61)*. The acute GH response to arginine, an amino acid postulated to stimulate GH secretion by inhibiting SS action *(62)*, is unaltered *(63,64)*.

Etiology of Age-Related Decline in GH Secretion

The mechanisms responsible for the decline in GH secretion with aging have not been determined, and may be multiple. Possible causes include one or more of the following: reduced pituitary function, increased SS activity, reduced GHRH activity, reduced activity of the endogenous ligand of GHRP, and increased feedback effects of GH, IGF-I, or other inhibitory factors. Reduced pituitary function is probably a cause, although apparently not a major one. Although people 40–55 yr of age were found to have significantly fewer and smaller somatotrophs than people 16–37 yr of age, in one autopsy study *(65)*, somatotroph function appears to be relatively intact in the elderly. This is indicated by the ability of arginine, which is thought to act at the hypothalamic and not at the pituitary level, to restore the GH response to GHRH in elderly adults to that of young adults *(64)*. The effects of aging are probably exerted mostly at the hypothalamic level. There is evidence from both animal and human studies (including the aforementioned arginine study), to suggest that SS tone increases with age. GHRH input to the pituitary may also be reduced. This is indicated by the partial reversal of the reduced GH response to GHRH in elderly subjects by repetitive administration of GHRH (66,67), the increased serum GH and IGF-I concentrations observed in older men after 14 d of sc GHRH treatment (51), and the larger rise in plasma GH in young than older subjects after withdrawal of a SS infusion (68). Because of the evidence that GHRH can induce slow-wave sleep, the phase most strongly associated with GH release, it is possible that the decreased GH secretion and sleep fragmentation that accompany aging are both related to decreased GHRH activity. Little is known about the effect of age on the sensitivity to negative feedback effects of inhibitory factors, such as circulating free fatty acids, insulin, and GH itself, but there is evidence that the sensitivity to the negative feedback effects of endogenous IGF-I does not increase with age (69).

Numerous factors, such as gender, body composition, nutrition, exercise, and physical fitness, affect GH secretion, presumably by modulating neurotransmitter and other inputs to the hypothalamus and pituitary. Premenopausal women have mean GH concentrations and GH secretion rates approx 20–50% higher than those of age-matched men (49,70). Stimulatory effects of endogenous estrogen appear to be the major cause of gender differences in GH secretion. Testosterone also stimulates GH release, and serum testosterone levels correlate with measures of GH secretion in adult men (71). However, it appears that testosterone stimulates GH release only after aromatization to estrogens (72,73). Serum levels of endogenous estradiol correlate with the increased GH secretion in girls during puberty (74), and serum-free and total estradiol (but not testosterone) concentrations chiefly account for the higher, 24-h integrated GH concentrations in adult women, compared to men (49). Oral estrogen increases basal and stimulated GH serum concentrations in postmenopausal women (75). Declining sex hormone effects are unlikely, however, to contribute much to the often dramatic decline in GH secretion that occurs between puberty and about age 40. Nevertheless, the abrupt decline in circulating estrogen concentrations in women at the menopause, and the more gradual age-related decline in testosterone in men throughout adult life, probably do contribute substantially to the decrease in GH secretion present in most elderly people.

Increased adiposity, particularly central, visceral adiposity (50,70,76,77), and decreased activity levels are independently associated with decreased GH secretion rates. Both changes tend to accompany normal aging in Western societies. Acute GH responses to aerobic and resistance exercise correlate positively with the physical fitness level, both in young and older adults (57) and older adults have a lower GH response to exercise than young adults (57,78), possibly because of reduced fitness levels. There is also evidence that physical fitness influences GH secretion at times not associated with exercise. After controlling for the effects of age and body fat, physical fitness significantly correlates with basal GH secretion in young men, and the correlation in young women approaches significance (79). One year of exercise training at an intensity above the lactate threshold has been shown to double 24-h mean GH concentrations on nonexercise days in young women, despite little change in body composition (80). It is not known whether obesity and reduced activity levels precede and cause the decline in GH secretion that accompanies aging, whether the aging-associated decline in GH secretion is itself a major cause of the body composition changes and reduced activity levels observed in older people, or whether a combination of both applies.

Effects of Age-Related Decline in GH–IGF-I Axis

Aging is associated with significant changes in body composition. Between the ages of 30 and 75 yr, the mean percentage body fat increases by up to 100%, muscle mass decreases by 20–50%, and bone mass by 20% *(81)*. The decrease in muscle mass is associated with a reduction in muscle strength. In addition, fat is redistributed from peripheral to central sites and total body water decreases. The same qualitative body composition changes are present in younger adults who are GH-deficient as a result of pituitary or hypothalamic disease, and these changes can be at least partially reversed by GH treatment *(38,82)*. Similarly, GH treatment of young adults with organic GH deficiency increases bone density *(83)*, and bone density is proportional to circulating IGF-I concentrations in elderly women *(84)*, suggesting that GH–IGF-I deficiency may contribute to the decline in bone density and increased incidence of osteoporosis that accompanies normal aging. It has been proposed that GH-deficient adults have a greater overall mortality rate than non-GH-deficient adults, because of death from CVD *(44)*. By analogy from these younger adults with true GH-deficiency, it has been suggested that functional GH deficiency may be a cause of the changes in body composition and increased risk of CVD that accompany normal aging *(81)*. The inescapable implication of this is that stimulation of the GH–IGF-I axis in older people may reverse some of the effects of aging and possibly prolong life by reducing the incidence and/or severity of CVD. This prospect has raised many expectations and aroused much excitement. A number of pharmaceutical companies are expending considerable time, money, and effort to develop oral GH secretagogues.

Another component of the GH/IGF-I axis that has recently been implicated in the aging process is the IGF-IR *(85)*. Activation of this receptor by IGF-I stimulates cell proliferation and protects the cell from programmed cell death (apoptosis). Postreceptor signaling is mediated through the phosphatidyl inositol 3' kinase and Ras/Raf/mitogen-activated protein kinase pathways *(86)*. In addition, there is evidence that IGF-I induces the expression of an antiapoptotic protein, bcl-xL *(87)*. These findings provide evidence for antiaging effects of IGF-I at the cellular level, and a further rationale for attempts to stimulate the GH–IGF-I axis in older people. The prize of rejuvenation may be won at a high price, however. The stimulation of cell proliferation and inhibition of apoptosis by IGF-I-induced activation of the IGF-IR also promotes malignant change and tumor growth *(88)*. Disruption of the IGF-IR inhibits tumor growth and prevents metastases in experimental animals *(89)*. This would be consistent with the increased incidence of tumors, particularly malignant tumors of the colon, observed in people with acromegaly *(90)*, and a recent report that men with plasma IGF-I concentrations in the top quartile of the normal range are 2–4× more likely to develop prostate cancer than those with concentrations in the lowest quartile *(91)*. Given that tumors of many types develop more frequently with increasing age, the possibility that stimulation of the GH–IGF-I axis promotes tumor growth will need to be carefully considered if long-term therapeutic stimulation of this axis is to be undertaken in older people.

STRATEGIES TO REJUVENATE GH–IGF-I AXIS IN OLDER PEOPLE

Nonpharmacological Methods

Theoretically, the circulating GH concentrations of older people can be increased by a number of nonpharmacological means. Because body fat stores are negatively related to GH secretion, loss of adipose tissue induced by diet and/or increased exercise could have this effect. Exercise has the added potential benefit that it stimulates GH secretion independent of its effects on body weight, acutely and probably also chronically (*see* above). Old, physically untrained men are reported to have significantly lower mean plasma IGF-I concentrations than old, physically trained men matched for weight, height, and body mass index *(92)*. The acute GH secretory response to exercise is less in elderly than young adults *(57,78)*, and increases less after an exercise training program *(93)*. It might be expected, therefore, that spontaneous GH secretion, at times unassociated with exercise, would not be increased as much by improvements in physical fitness in the elderly as in young adults. Consistent with this, one group of elderly men and women, who completed a resistance exercise training program in which they performed weight-lifting exercises 3× per week for 1 yr, showed no increase in basal or stimulated GH release during this time *(94)*; there was no significant increase in circulating IGF-I concentrations in a group of healthy older men and women who underwent a 6-mo endurance training program that significantly increased maximal aerobic power and decreased body fat mass *(95)*. Further studies are underway to evaluate the effects of chronic exercise programs on the GH–IGF-I axis and body composition in older people, and to compare the functional effects of exercise alone with those of GH therapy alone, and the two combined (M. Hartman, personal communication).

Another way the elderly could potentially increase their GH secretion is by changing how and what they eat. Fasting from food for 2–5 d increases mean 24-h serum GH concentrations 3–5-fold in normal-weight, obese, and older individuals *(96–98)*, because of a reduction in IGF-I negative feedback *(99)*, suppression of secretion of insulin (which inhibits GH secretion) *(79)*, and, possibly, also a combination of reduced SS and increased GHRH secretion *(100)*. However, an increase in GH secretion may not be desirable, if it comes at the cost of decreased IGF-I secretion. Moreover, the effects of less dramatic and more chronic reductions of energy intake on GH secretion in older people are not known, and such reductions in energy intake are not necessarily desirable *(101)*. Although little is known about the effects of long-term variations in the macronutrient composition, rather than the amount, of food eaten, changes in dietary composition could be a more feasible way of stimulating GH secretion in older people. Acute administration of carbohydrates suppresses both GH secretion *(56)* and the GH response to GHRH *(102)*, free fatty acids acutely suppress the GH secretory response to GHRH *(103)*, and prior ingestion of meals high in fat (but not glucose) reduces the acute GH response to exercise. On the other hand, administration of amino acids, such as arginine and lysine, acutely stimulates GH release *(103)*. Amino acid supplements, particularly arginine, are promoted as chronic stimulators of the GH–IGF-I axis, and are apparently used by some older people for this purpose. The area has been little investigated, and may warrant further study. However, the few available data do not support this use: Combined twice daily oral administration of arginine and lysine (6 g/d of each) for 14 d to older men (mean age 69 yr) was found to be without effect on spontaneous or GHRH-stimulated GH release, or on serum IGF-I *(104)*.

Pharmacological Methods

GROWTH HORMONE

The administration of recombinant human GH to elderly adults increases circulating GH and IGF-I concentrations (the latter often into the young adult normal range), increases lean tissue mass, decreases adipose tissue mass, and increases parameters of bone turn-over *(105,106)*. Rudman et al. *(45)* were among the first to demonstrate an effect of GH treatment on body composition in older people. They administered GH by sc injection 3 d/wk for 6 mo to healthy men 61–81 yr old, selected on the basis of having a plasma IGF-I concentration less than 350 U/L. This treatment increased plasma IGF-I levels into the youthful range of 500–1500 U/L, and was associated with a significant 14.4% decrease in adipose tissue mass, 8.8% increase in lean body mass, and 1.6% increase in bone density in the lumbar vertebrae; bone density in the radius and femur was not affected. Skin thickness increased 7.1% ($P = 0.07$). These favorable effects of GH treatment on body composition in elderly men have been confirmed in other studies *(107,108)* and also occur in older women *(105,109,110)*. Subsequent studies have not, however, confirmed a stimulatory effect of GH therapy on BMD in older people. In a study by Erdtsieck et al. *(110)*, BMD in a group of postmenopausal women with osteoporosis was not increased by 6-mo treatment with GH. A further 6-mo GH treatment actually inhibited the increase in bone density produced by pamidronate treatment. Similarly, in another study, the addition of GH treatment to a 16-wk resistance exercise program did not further increase BMD in a group of older men with normal bone density, despite GH-induced increases in serum osteocalcin and IGF-I *(111)*. Cuttica et al. *(112)* administered low-dose GH to a small group of healthy, elderly subjects for 6 mo, and found a trend toward decreased bone density, despite increases in lean tissue mass and decreased fat tissue. Systemic administration of GH does not therefore appear to be useful in either the prevention or treatment of osteoporosis in the elderly. This is in contrast to the proven ability of GH treatment to increase bone density in young adults with organic GH deficiency, and suggests that the two conditions may be qualitatively, as well as quantitatively, different.

It has not been established that the improvements in body composition in the elderly produced by GH therapy are accompanied by functional benefits. Six-mo GH treatment increased muscle strength in one small study involving five elderly subjects *(112)*, but other studies have not confirmed this. Papadakis et al. *(107)* administered GH for 6 mo to healthy, elderly men with low baseline IGF-I levels, in a dose that produced significant favorable effects on body composition, but was without effect on knee or hand-grip strength, or on systemic endurance. Two studies have examined the combined effects of GH treatment and exercise training on musculoskeletal function in the elderly. In one *(113)*, an exercise program was combined with GH treatment for 16 wk. In the other *(108)*, the exercise program started 16 wk before, and continued throughout, 10 wk of GH administration. In neither study did GH treatment augment the effects of exercise alone on muscle strength. The seeming inability, or very limited ability, of GH treatment to improve musculoskeletal function in the elderly, despite restoration of circulating IGF-I concentrations to young adult levels, is perhaps consistent with the poor baseline correlation between either body composition *(114)* or musculoskeletal function *(115)* and IGF-I levels in this age group.

There has been limited investigation of the effects of GH therapy on cognitive and immune function in the elderly. In the study of Papadakis et al. *(107)*, GH therapy significantly improved the mean Trials B score, but was without effect on Digit Symbol Substitution Test, and produced a deterioration in performance on the Mini-Mental Status Examination, nonsignificantly worse than the improvement in the placebo-treated group. Aging is associated with a decline in immune function *(116)*. Administrations of GH and IGF-I, alone and combined, for 7 wk to aged female rhesus monkeys, activated the immune system, with increases in T-cell numbers, the ratio of CD4:CD8 T-cells, and an enhanced in vivo response to tetanus toxoid *(117)*. Natural killer T-cell activity increased in postmenopausal women after 14-d GH treatment *(105)*. The functional effects, if any, of these changes, are not known. The effect of GH treatment on cardiovascular risk factors and the incidence and outcome of CVD in the elderly have not been reported.

Elderly subjects seem particularly prone to suffer side effects from GH therapy, and, in some studies *(45)*, the majority of subjects have experienced some side effects, including carpal tunnel syndrome, gynecomastia, fluid retention, lethargy, joint pains and swelling, and headaches *(109,118)*. However, these side effects are mostly dose-related, and accumulating experience with GH therapy in the elderly has demonstrated that the dose, and hence rate of side effects, can be reduced substantially without loss of the beneficial effects on body composition *(112)*.

INSULIN-LIKE GROWTH FACTOR I

It remains unclear how important direct effects of GH, as opposed to those of IGF-I, are in exerting the metabolic effects of GH: In most situations, circulating concentrations of the two hormones are positively related, and any treatment that increases circulating GH concentrations almost always has the same effect on IGF-I. Administration of IGF-I alone exerts a negative feedback effect to suppress circulating GH concentrations *(6,69)*. Recombinant human IGF-I (rhIGF-I) is now available. It increases growth in GH-deficient rodents, but not as much as GH treatment. In humans, rhIGF-I stimulates growth in children with Laron dwarfism, and produces short-term increases in nitrogen retention in a variety of catabolic conditions, including HIV/AIDS. However, rhIGF-I is very expensive, and there is little convincing evidence that treatment with IGF-I alone produces significant, sustained anabolic effects in GH–IGF-I-replete young adults. Little is known of the effects of rhIGF-I treatment in elderly humans. In one uncontrolled study, healthy, elderly women (mean age 71.9 yr) were treated for 4 wk with sc rhIGF-I, 0.015 or 0.06 mg/kg twice daily *(109)*. Body fat stores decreased significantly (5.7–6.6%) with both doses, and lean body mass increased significantly (8.8%) with the higher, but not lower, dose. However, side effects, including headache, lethargy, bloating, and Bell's palsy, occurred in a third of subjects on the low dose, and in all of the subjects on the higher dose of rhIGF-I. The effects of longer-term IGF-I administration on body composition, or other measures, have not been reported. As with GH, short-term systemic administration of IGF-I increases bone remodeling and turnover *(119,120)*, and GH and IGF-I appear to act on bones via separate mechanisms at the cellular level; IGF-I enhanced short term formation of collagen type I more than did GH in one study *(121)*. The effects of IGF-I treatment on bone density in older people have not been reported. Combined short-term administration of IGF-I and GH to young adults has been shown to be more anabolic than either alone *(122)*. Studies to investigate the effect of combined GH and IGF-I administration in older people may therefore be indicated.

GROWTH HORMONE RELEASING HORMONE

Elderly people probably have an attenuated GH secretory response to GHRH *(64, 123,124)*. Nevertheless, continuous sc infusions of GHRH for 14 d have been shown to increase circulating GH and IGF-I levels in old men *(125)*, and twice daily sc injections of GHRH increase serum IGF-I and GH concentrations in old men to approximate those of young men *(126)*. In a recent study, sc injection of GHRH nightly for 6 wk, in a dose that had increased GH when infused continuously, increased nocturnal GH secretion, but was without effect on serum IGF-I in healthy, nonobese elderly men *(127)*. Two of six measures of muscle strength, and a test of muscle endurance, improved. Dual-energy X-ray absorptiometry measures of fat and muscle were unchanged, although the study period was probably too short to exclude a long-term effect of this treatment on body composition. Administration of GHRH to elderly people has also been shown to stimulate the immune system. Khorran et al. *(121)* reported that 16-wk treatment, with nightly sc injections of GHRH, activated the immune system, as well as increased GH secretion and serum IGF-I concentrations in 19 healthy elderly men and women. There was a significant (30%) increase in the number of B-cells and cells expressing T-cell receptors in the peripheral blood, enhanced sensitivity to B-cell mitogens, and functional activation of T-cells. As with GH treatment, it is not yet known whether this stimulation of the immune system has beneficial effects on the health of older people. Nevertheless, these results provide some hope that GHRH, if administered in an optimum fashion, may reverse some of the effects of aging on musculoskeletal and immune function in the elderly.

GROWTH HORMONE RELEASING PEPTIDE AND ITS ANALOGS

All of the above agents (GH, IGF-I, and GHRH) are expensive, and must be administered by injection. This limits their potential widespread use in the healthy elderly population, even if they are shown to provide significant functional benefits. The GHRPs were developed by Bowers et al. *(17,128)* in the early 1980s, specifically as GH secretagogues. They are small, synthetic peptide molecules, created by modifying the structure of metenkephalin, and include GHRP-6 (His-D-Tryp-Ala-Trp-D-Phe-Lys-NH$_2$), -1, -2, and hexarelin. In contrast to the effects of GH, IGF-I, and, to a lesser extent, GHRH, these agents and their recently developed analogs, which have greater oral bioavailability, offer the potential advantages of amplifying normal pulsatile GH secretion. They are potent stimulators of GH secretion. The acute GH secretory response of older people to an iv injection of the GHRP, hexarelin, although less than that of young adults, is greater than that to a maximum dose of GHRH in both young and old subjects *(129)*. In elderly women, an oral dose of GHRP-6 produces a higher GH rise than that induced by a maximal dose of iv GHRH *(130)*. Moreover, 15-d treatment with oral hexarelin, 3/d, produced a small (10%), but statistically significant, increase in IGF-I levels *(131)*. Nonpeptide GHRP analogs have been developed that stimulate pulsatile GH secretion in older people, when infused continuously *(132)* or administered intermittently. One of these, MK-677, has a long duration of action and can be administered daily. Daily oral administration of MK-677 for 28 d to 32 healthy subjects, 64–81-yr-old, produced dose-responsive stimulation of pulsatile GH secretion (Fig. 2), and increases in mean 24-h serum GH, IGF-I, and IGFB-3 concentrations *(133)*. The highest dose, 25 mg, produced a 97% increase in GH levels at 2 wk, and a 88% increase in IGF-I levels at 4 wk; eight of the 10 subjects given this dose had serum IGF-I concentrations below the normal young adult range at baseline; the IGF-I levels of eight of the 10 were within the normal young range at 4 wk (Fig. 3). The drug was well tolerated, with three reports of mild abdominal pain and five of mild appetite stimulation, although body wt did not change significantly. There were no effects on thyroid function tests or cortisol levels, but the highest dose increased serum prolactin concentrations within the normal range, and increased fasting glucose and insulin concentrations, suggesting a possible enhancement of insulin resistance. Studies are now under way to determine whether longer-term admin-

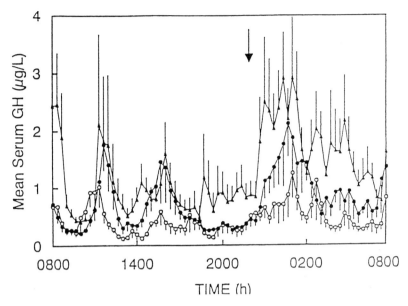

Fig. 2. Mean (±SE) serum GH concentrations (μg/L) in older subjects after 2 wk of treatment with placebo (O; $n = 10$), 10 mg/d MK-677 (●; $n = 12$), and 25 mg/d MK-677 (▲; $n = 10$). Evening treatment time (between 2200 and 2300 h) is indicated by an arrow. Reproduced with permission from ref. *133.*

istration of this drug can attenuate the body composition, musculoskeletal function, and cardiovascular changes accompanying aging. GHRP and GHRH have synergistic effects on GH secretion *(16)*, and arginine has been shown to enhance the GH secretory response to GHRPs in elderly, but not young, adults *(129)*. Therefore, combinations of GHRP analogs, GHRH, and arginine may provide even greater stimulation of GH secretion.

Estrogen

Treatment of postmenopausal women with oral estrogens increases spontaneous GH secretion and circulating GH concentrations, probably by reducing the negative feedback effects of IGF-I; serum IGF-I concentrations are suppressed by oral estrogen treatment *(134,135)*. At conventionally prescribed doses, transdermal estrogen has minimal effects of the GH–IGF-I axis *(135)*, but very high doses probably have the same effects as oral estrogen *(134)*. Neither form of estrogen therapy is capable of completely reversing the aging-related decline in GH secretion. Because the increase in GH secretion is associated with a decrease in IGF-I secretion, it is unclear whether the net effect of estrogen therapy is to stimulate or inhibit the metabolic actions of the GH–IGF-I axis. The effects of testosterone therapy on the GH–IGF-I axis in older men have not, to the author's knowledge, been reported.

SUMMARY

Aging represents a form of functional GH deficiency, although the reduction in GH and IGF-I levels is heterogeneous, and not as severe as in most younger adults with organic GH deficiency. By analogy with organic GH deficiency and its favorable response to GH therapy, elderly people may benefit from therapies that rejuvenate the GH–IGF-I axis.

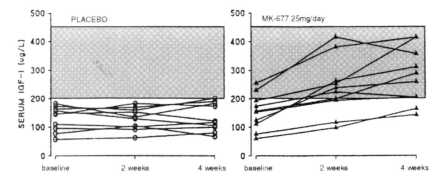

Fig. 3. Serum IGF-I concentrations (μg/L) of individual subjects at baseline and after 2 and 4 wk of treatment with daily evening oral placebo (O; $n = 10$; left panel) or 25 mg MK-677 (▲; $n = 10$; right panel). The shaded zone represents the assay normal range for adults 21–25 yr old (202–453 μg/L). Reproduced with permission from ref. *133.*

In recent years, a number of treatments, including GH, GHRH, and GHRP and its analogs, have been shown to be capable of restoring GH and IGF-I levels of the elderly to those of young adults, and producing favorable body composition changes. It is not yet clear, however, that these changes are accompanied by functional benefits, or whether the long-term use of such treatments will be associated with reductions in morbidity or mortality. It is possible that stimulation of the GH–IGF-I axis in the elderly may induce new tumors or potentiate the growth of existing ones. Although the possibility of reversing some of the effects of aging by stimulation of the GH–IGF-I axis is exciting, and is attracting much interest, further studies are clearly needed to determine just how realistic this prospect is, and whether it can be realized safely. A conservative interpretation of available data is that there is insufficient evidence to recommend any pharmaceutical method of GH–IGF-I axis rejuvenation to older people at the present time.

REFERENCES

1. Ab H, Molitch ME, Van W, Underwood LE. Human growth hormone and somatomedin C suppress the spontaneous release of growth hormone in unanesthetized rats. Endocrinology 1983;113:1319–1324.
2. Abrams RL, Grumbach MM, Kaplan SL. The effect of administration of human growth hormone on the plasma growth hormone, cortisol, glucose and free fatty acid response to insulin: evidence for growth hormone autoregulation in man. J Clin Invest 1971;50:940–950.
3. Rosenthal J, Hulse JA, Kaplan SL. Exogenous growth hormone inhibits growth hormone releasing factor-induced growth hormone secretion in normal men. J Clin Invest 1986;77:176–180.
4. Guler HP, Zapf J, Froesch ER. Short-term metabolic effects of recombinant human insulin-like growth factor in healthy adults. N Engl J Med 1987;317:137–140.
5. Zenobi PD, Graf S, Ursprung H, Froesch ER. Effects of insulin-like growth factor I on insulin secretion and renal function in normal human subjects. Proc Natl Acad Sci USA 1992;86:2868–2872.
6. Hartman ML, Clayton PE, Johnson ML, Celniker A, Perlman AJ, Alberti KGMM, Thorner MO. A low dose euglycemic infusion of recombinant human insulin-like growth factor I rapidly suppresses fasting-enhanced pulsatile growth hormone secretion in humans. J Clin Invest 1993;91:2453–2462.
7. Bermann M, Jaffe CA, Tsai W, DeMott-Friburg R, Barkan AL. Negative feedback regulation of pulsatile growth hormone secretion by insulin-like growth factor I. Involvement of hypothalamic somatostatin. J Clin Invest 1994;94:138–145.
8. Horvath S, Palkovits M, Gorcs T, Arimura A. Electron microscopic immunoctochemical evidence for the existence of bidirectional synaptic connections between growth hormone releasing hormone and somatostatin neurons in the hypothalamus of the rat. Brain Res 1989;481:8–15.

9. McCarthy GF, Beaudet A, Tannenbaum GS. Colocalization of somatostatin receptors and growth hormone-releasing factor immunoreactivity in neurons of the rat arcuate nucleus. Neuroendocrinology 1992;56:18–24.

10. Cronin MJ, Rogol AD, Dabney LG, Thorner MO. Selective growth hormone and cyclic AMP stimulating activity is present in human pancreatic islet cell tumor. J Clin Endocrinol Metab 1982;55:381–383.

11. Cronin MJ, Hewlett EL, Evans WS, Thorner MO, Rogol AD. Human pancreatic tumor growth hormone (GH)-releasing factor and cyclic adenosine 3',5'-monophosphate evoke GH release from anterior pituitary cells: the effects of pertussis toxin, cholera toxin, forskolin, and cycloheximide. Endocrinology 1984;114:904–913.

12. Holl RW, Thorner MO, Leong DA. Intracellular calcium concentration and growth hormone secretion in individual somatotropes: effects of growth hormone-releasing factor and somatostatin. Endocrinology 1988;122:2927–2932.

13. Holl RW, Thorner MO, Mandell GL, Sullivan JA, Sinha YN, Leong DA. Spontaneous oscillations of intracellular calcium and growth hormone secretion. J Biol Chem 1988;263:9682–9685.

14. Herman V, Weiss M, Becker D, Melmed S. Hypothalamic hormonal regulation of human growth hormone gene expression in somatotroph adenoma cell cultures. Endocr Pathol 1990;1:236–244.

15. Bowers CY, Momany FA, Reynolds GA, Hong A. On the in vitro and in vivo activity of a new synthetic hexapeptide that acts on the pituitary to specifically release growth hormone. Endocrinology 1984; 114:1537–1545.

16. Bowers CY, Reynolds GA, Durham D, Barrera CM, Pezzoli SS, Thorner MO. Growth hormone (GH)-releasing peptide stimulates GH release in normal men and acts synergistically with GH-releasing hormone. J Clin Endocrinol Metab 1990;70:975–982.

17. Bowers CY, Sartor AO, Reynolds GA, Badger TM. On the actions of the growth hormone-releasing hexapeptide, GHRP. Endocrinology 1991;128:2027–2035.

18. Skottner A, Clark RG, Robinson IC, Fryklund L. Recombinant human insulin-like growth factor: testing the somatomedin hypothesis in hypophysectomized rats. J Endocrinol 1987;112:123–132.

19. Guler HP, Zapf J, Scheiwiller E, Froesch ER. Recombinant human insulin-like growth factor I stimulates growth and has distinct effects on organ size in hypophysectomized rats. Proc Natl Acad Sci USA 1988;85:4889–4893.

20. Green H, Morikawa M, Nixon T. A dual effector theory of growth-hormone action. Differentiation 1985;29:195–198.

21. Guler HP, Zapf J, Schmid C, Froesch ER. Insulin-like growth factors I and II in healthy man. Estimations of half-lives and production rates. Acta Endocrinol 1989;121:753–758.

22. Baxter RC, Martin JL. Radioimmunoassay of growth hormone-dependent insulin-like growth factor binding protein in human plasma. J Clin Invest 1986;78:1504–1512.

23. Blum WF, Ranke MB. Use of insulin-like growth factor-binding protein 3 for evaluation of growth disorders. Horm Res 1990;33(Suppl):31–37.

24. de Boer H, Blok G-J, Van Der Veen EA. Clinical aspects of growth hormone deficiency in adults. Endocr Rev 1995;16:63–86.

25. Roupas P, Herington AC. Cellular mechanisms in the processing of growth hormone and its receptor. Mol Cell Endocrinol 1989;61:1–12.

26. Leung DW, Spencer SA, Cachianes G, Hammonds RG, Collins C, Henzel WJ, et al. Growth hormone receptor and serum binding protein: purification, cloning and expression. Nature 1987;330:537–543.

27. Argetsinger LS, Campbell GS, Yang X, Witthuhn BA, Silvennoinen O, Ihle JN, Carter-Su C. Identification of JAK2 as a growth hormone receptor-associated kinase. Cell 1993;74:237–244.

28. Silva CM, Lu H, Weber MJ, Thorner MO. Differential tyrosine phosphorylation of JAK1, JAK2, and STAT1 by growth hormone and interferon-gamma in IM-9 cells. J Biol Chem 1994;269:27,532–27,539.

29. Waxman DJ, Ram PA, Park S-H, Choi HK. Intermittent plasma growth hormone triggers tyrosine phosphorylation and nuclear transcription of a liver-expressed, stat 5-related DNA binding protein. J Biol Chem 1995;22:13,262–13,270.

30. Sherwin RS, Schulman GA, Hendler R, Walesky M, Belous A, Tamborlane W. Effect of growth hormone on oral glucose tolerance and circulating metabolic fuels in man. Diabetologia 1983;24: 155–161.

31. Rosenfeld RG, Wilson DM, Dollar LA, Bennett A, Hintz RL. Both human pituitary growth hormone and recombinant DNA-derived human growth hormone cause insulin resistance at a postreceptor site. J Clin Endocrinol Metab 1982;54:1033–1038.

32. Dahms WT, Owens RP, Kalhan SC, Kerr DS, Danish RK. Urea synthesis, nitrogen balance and glucose turnover in growth deficient children before and after GH administration. Metabolism 1989;38: 197–203.

33. Manson JM, Wilmore DW. Positive nitrogen balance with human growth hormone and hypocaloric intravenous feeding. Surgery 1986;100:188–197.

34. Soroff HS, Pearson E, Green NL, Artz CP. The effect of growth hormone on nitrogen balance at various levels of intake in burned patients. Surg Gynecol Obstet 1960;111:259–273.

35. Horber FF, Haymond MV. Human growth hormone prevents the protein catabolic side effects of prednisone in humans. J Clin Invest 1990;86:265–272.

36. Pape GS, Friedman M, Underwood LE, Clemmons DR. The effect of growth hormone on weight gain and pulmonary function in patients with chronic obstructive lung disease. Chest 1991;99:1495–1500.

37. Cheek DB, Hill DE. Muscle and liver cell growth: role of hormone and nutritional factors. Fed Proc 1970;29:1503–1509.

38. Salomon F, Cuneo RC, Hesp R, Sonksen PH. The effects of treatment with recombinant human growth hormone on body composition and metabolism in adults with growth hormone deficiency. N Engl J Med 1989;321:1797–1803.

39. Crist DM, Peake GT, Egan PA, Waters DL. Body composition response to exogenous GH during training in highly conditioned adults. J Appl Physiol 1988;65:579–584.

40. Rosen T, Eden S, Larson G, Wilhelmsen L, Bengtsson BA. Cardiovascular risk factors in adult patients with growth hormone deficiency. Acta Endocrinol 1993;129:195–200.

41. de Boer H, Blok GJ, Voerman HJ, Phillips M, Schouten JA. Serum lipid levels in growth hormone-deficient men. Metabolism 1994;43:199–203.

42. Blackett PR, Weech PK, McConathy WJ, Fesmire JD. Growth hormone in the regulation of hyperlipidemia. Metabolism 1982;31:117–120.

43. Asayama K, Amemiya S, Kusano S, Kato K. Growth hormone-induced changes in postheparin plasma lipoprotein lipase and hepatic triglyceride lipase activties. Metabolism 1984;33:129–131.

44. Rosen T, Bengtsson BA. Premature mortality due to cardiovascular disease in hypopituitarism. Lancet 1990;336:285–288.

45. Rudman D, Feller AG, Nagraj HS, Gergans GA, Lalitha PY, Goldberg AS, et al. Effects of human growth hormone in men over 60 years old. N Engl J Med 1990;323:1–6.

46. Baum HBA, Biller BMK, Oppenheim DS, Baker KE, Lord J, Klibanski A. Long-term physiologic growth hormone (GH) replacement improves bone density and body composition in men with adult-onset GH deficiency. Proceedings of the 77th Meeting of the Endocrine Society 1995;P2–261:356 (Abstract).

47. Gala RR. Prolactin and growth hormone in the regulation of the immune system. Proc Soc Exp Biol Med 1991;198:513–527.

48. Wit JM, Kooiijman R, Riskers GT, Zegers BJ. Immunological findings in growth hormone-treated patients. Horm Res 1993;39:107–110.

49. Ho KY, Evans WS, Blizzard RM, Veldhuis JD, Merriam GR, Samojlik E, et al. Effects of sex and age on the 24-hour profile of growth hormone secretion in man: importance of endogenous estradiol concentrations. J Clin Endocrinol Metab 1987;64:51–58.

50. Iranmanesh A, Lizzarralde G, Veldhuis JD. Age and relative adiposity are specific determinants of the frequency and amplitude of GH secretory bursts and the half-life of endogenous GH in healthy men. J Clin Endocrinol Metab 1991;73:1081–1088.

51. Corpas E, Harman SM, Pineyro MA, Roberson R, Blackman MR. GHRH 1-29 twice daily reverses the decreased GH and IGF-I levels in old men. J Clin Endocrinol Metab 1992;75:530–535.

52. Zadik Z, Chalew SA, McCarter RJ Jr, Meistas M, Kowarski AA. The influence of age on the 24-hour integrated concentration of growth hormone in normal individuals. J Clin Endocrinol Metab 1985;60: 513–516.

53. Vermeulen A. Nyctohemeral growth hormone profiles in young and aged men: correlation with somatomedin-C levels. J Clin Endocrinol Metab 1987;64:884–888.

54. Hattori N, Shimatsu A, Kato Y. Growth hormone responses to oral glucose loading measured by highly sensitive enzyme immunoassay in normal subjects and patients with glucose intolerance and acromegaly. J Clin Endocrinol Metab 1990;70:771–776.

55. Goji K. Pulsatile characteristics of spontaneous growth hormone (GH) concentration profiles in boys evaluated by an ultrasensitive immunoradiometric assay: evidence for ultradian periodicity of GH secretion. J Clin Endocrinol Metab 1993;76:667–670.

56. Chapman IM, Hartman ML, Straume M, Johnson ML, Veldhuis JD, Thorner MO. Enhanced sensitivity growth hormone (GH) chemiluminescence assay reveals lower postglucose nadir GH concentrations in men than women. J Clin Endocrinol Metab 1994;78:1312–1319.
57. Hagberg JM, Seals DR, Yerg JE, Gavin J, Gingerich R, Bhartur P, Holloszy J. Metabolic responses to exercise in young and old athletes and sedentary men. J Appl Physiol 1988;65:900–908.
58. Craig BW, Brown R, Everhart J. Effects of progressive resistance training on growth hormome and testosterone levels in young and elderly subjects. Mech Aging Dev 1989;49:159–169.
59. Corpas E, Harman SM, Blackman MR. Human growth hormone and human aging. Endocr Rev 1993; 14:20–39.
60. Kalk WJ, Vinik AI, Pimstone BL, Jackson PU. Growth hormone response to insulin hypoglycemia in the elderly. J Gerontol 1973;28:431–433.
61. Muggeo M, Fedele D, Tiengo A, Molinari M, Crepaldi G. Human growth hormone and cortisol response to insulin stimulation in aging. J Gerontol 1975;30:546–551.
62. Ghigo E, Bellone J, Mazza E, Imperiale E, Procopio M, Valente F, et al. Arginine potentiates the GHRH- but not the pyridostigmine-induced GH secretion in normal short children. Further evidence for a somatostatin suppressing effect of arginine. Clin Endocrinol (Oxford) 1990;32:763–767.
63. Blichert-Toft M. Stimulation of the release of corticotrophin and somatotrophin by metyrapone and arginine. Acta Endocrinol 1975;195(Suppl):65–85.
64. Ghigo E, Goffi E, Nicolosi M, Arvat E, Valente F, Mazza E, Ghigo C, Camanni F. Growth hormone (GH) responsiveness to combined administration of arginine and GH-releasing hormone does not vary with age in man. J Clin Endocrinol Metab 1990;71:1481–1485.
65. Sun YK, Xi YP, Fenoglio CM, Pushparaj N, O'Toole KM, Kledizik GS, Nette EG, King DW. The effect of age on the number of pituitary cells immunoreactive to growth hormone and prolactin. Hum Pathol 1984;15:169–180.
66. Iovino M, Monteleone P, Steardo L. Repetitive growth hormone-releasing hormone administration restores the attenuated growth hormone (GH) response to GH-releasing hormone testing in normal aging. J Clin Endocrinol Metab 1989;69:910–913.
67. Franchimont P, Urbain-Choffray D, Lambelin P, Fontaine MA, Frangin G, Reginster JY. Effects of repetitive administration of growth hormone-releasing. Acta Endocrinol 1989;120:121–128.
68. degli Uberti EC, Ambrosio MR, Cella SG, Margutti AR, Trasforini G, Rigamonti AE, Petrone E, Muller EE. Defective hypothalamic growth hormone (GH)-releasing hormone activity may contribute to declining GH secretion with age in man. J Clin Endocrinol Metab 1997;82:2885–2888.
69. Chapman IM, Hartman ML, Pezzoli SS, Thorner MO. Evidence against increased sensitivity to IGF-I negative feedback as a cause of the aging-associated decline in GH secretion. Proceedings of the 77th Meeting of the Endocrine Society 1995;OR20–5:73 (Abstract).
70. Weltman A, Weltman JY, Hartman ML, Abbott RD, Rogol AD, Evans WS, Veldhuis JD. Relationship between age, percentage body fat, fitness, and 24-hour growth hormone release in healthy young adults: effects of gender. J Clin Endocrinol Metab 1994;78:543–548.
71. Iranmanesh A, Lizarralde G, Veldhuis JD. Age and relative adiposity are specific negative determinants of the freqency and amplitude of growth hormone (GH) secretory bursts and the half-life of endogenous GH in healthy men. J Clin Endocrinol Metab 1991;73:1081–1088 (Abstract).
72. Weissbeger AJ, Ho KK. Activation of the somatotropic axis by testosterone in adult males: evidence for the role of aromatization. J Clin Endocrinol Metab 1993;76:1407–1412.
73. Metzger DL, Kerrigan JR. Estrogen receptor blockade with tamoxifen diminishes growth hormone secretion in boys: evidence for a stimulatory role of endogenous estrogens during male adolescence. J Clin Endocrinol Metab 1994;79:513–518.
74. Plotnick LP, Thompson RG, Beitins I, Blizzard RM. Integrated concentrations of growth hormone correlated with stage of puberty and estrogen levels in girls. J Clin Endocrinol Metab 1974;38:436–439.
75. Dawson Hughes B, Stern D, Goldman J, Reichlin S. Regulation of growth hormone and somatomedin-C secretion in postmenopausal women: effect of physiological estrogen replacement. J Clin Endocrinol Metab 1986;63:424–432.
76. Veldhuis JD, Iranmanesh A, Ho KK, Waters MJ, Johnson ML, Lizarralde G. Dual defects in pulsatile growth hormone secretion and clearance subserve the hyposomatotropism of obesity in man. J Clin Endocrinol Metab 1991;72:51–59.
77. Williams T, Berelowitz M, Joffe SN, Thorner MO, Rivier J, Vale W, Frohman LA. Impaired growth hormone responses to growth hormone-releasing factor in obesity. A pituitary defect reversed with weight reduction. N Engl J Med 1984;311:1403–1407.

78. Pyka G, Wiswell RA, Marcus R. Age-dependent effect of resistance exercise on growth hormone secretion in people. J Clin Endocrinol Metab 1992;75:404–407.

79. Yamashita S, Melmed S. Effects of insulin on rat anterior pituitary cells: inhibition of growth hormone secretion and mRNA levels. Diabetes 1986;35:440–447.

80. Weltman A, Weltman JY, Schurrer R, Evans WS, Veldhuis JD, Rogol AR. Endurance training amplifies the pulsatile release of growth hormone: effects of training intensity. J Appl Physiol 1992;72:2188–2196.

81. Rudman D. Growth hormone, body composition, and aging. J Am Geriatr Soc 1985;33:800–807.

82. Johannsson G, Rosen T, Bosaeus L, Bengtsson BA. The effects of 2 years treatment with recombinant human growth hormone on body composition and metabolism in adults with growth hormone deficiency. Proceedings of the 76th Meeting of the Endocrine Society 1994;A18 (Abstract).

83. Baum HB, Biller BM, Finkelstein JS, Cannistraro KB, Oppenhein DS, Schoenfeld DA, et al. Effects of physiologic growth hormone therapy on bone density and body composition in patients with adult-onset growth hormone deficiency. A randomized, placebo-controlled trial. Ann Intern Med 1996; 125:883–890.

84. Boonen S, Lesaffre E, Dequeker J, Aerssens J, Nijs J, Pelemans W, Bouillon R. Relationship between baseline insulin-like growth factor-I (IGF- I) and femoral bone density in women aged over 70 years: potential implications for the prevention of age-related bone loss. J Am Geriatr Soc 1996;44:1301–1306.

85. Rosen CJ, Conover C. Growth hormone/insulin-like growth factor-1 axis in aging: a summary of a National Institutes of Aging-sponsored symposium. J Clin Endocrinol Metab 1997;82:3919–3922.

86. Parrizas M, Saltiel AR, LeRoith D. Insulin-like growth factor 1 inhibits apoptosis using the phosphatidylinositol 3'-kinase and mitogen-activated protein kinase pathways. J Biol Chem 1997;272:154–161.

87. Parrizas M, LeRoith D. Insulin-like growth factor-1 inhibition of apoptosis is associated with increased expression of the bcl-xL gene product. Endocrinology 1997;138:1355–1358.

88. Lahm H, Suardet L, Laurent PL, Fischer JR, Ceyhan A, Givel JC, Odartchenko N. Growth regulation and co-stimulation of human colorectal cancer cell lines by insulin-like growth factor I, II and transforming growth factor alpha. Br J Cancer 1992;65:341–346.

89. D'Ambrosio C, Ferber A, Resnicoff M, Baserga R. A soluble insulin-like growth factor I receptor that induces apoptosis of tumor cells in vivo and inhibits tumorigenesis. Cancer Res 1996;56:4013–4020.

90. Jenkins PJ, Fairclough PD, Richards T, Lowe DG, Monson J, Grossman A, Wass JA, Besser M. Acromegaly, colonic polyps and carcinoma. Clin Endocrinol (Oxford) 1997;47:17–22.

91. Chan JM, Stampfer MJ, Giovannucci E, Gann PH, Ma J, Wilkinson P, Hennekens CH, Pollack M. Plasma insulin-like growth factor-I and prostate cancer risk: a prospective study. Science 1998;279: 563–566.

92. Horber FF, Kohler SA, Lippuner K, Jaeger P. Effect of regular physical training on age-associated alteration of body composition in men. Eur J Clin Invest 1996;26:279–285.

93. Craig BW, Brown R, Everhart J. Effects of progressive resistance training on growth hormone and testosterone levels in young and elderly subjects. Mech Aging Dev 1989;49:159–169.

94. Pyka G, Taaffe DR, Marcus R. Effect of a sustained program of resistance training on the acute growth hormone response to resistance exercise in older adults. Horm Metab Res 1994;26:330–333.

95. Vitiello MV, Wilkinson CW, Merriam GR, Moe KE, Prinz PN, Ralph DD, Colasurdo EA, Schwartz RS. Successful 6-month endurance training does not alter insulin-like growth factor-I in healthy older men and women. J Gerontol A Biol Sci Med Sci 1997;52:M149–M154.

96. Ho KY, Veldhuis JD, Johnson ML, Furlanetto R, Evans WS, Alberti KG, Thorner MO. Fasting enhances growth hormone secretion and amplifies the complex rhythms of growth hormone secretion in man. J Clin Invest 1988;81:968–975.

97. Hartman ML, Veldhuis JD, Johnson ML, Lee MM, Alberti KGMM, Samojlik E, Thorner MO. Augmented growth hormone (GH) secretory burst frequency and amplitude mediate enhanced GH secretion during a two day fast in normal men. J Clin Endocrinol Metab 1992;74:757–765.

98. Clasey JL, Hartman ML, Pezzoli SS, Weltman A, Veldhuis JD, Thorner MO. The hyposomatotropism associated with obesity is reversed by five days of fasting. Proceedings of the 77th Meeting of the Endocrine Society 1995;P1–172:155 (Abstract).

99. Clemmons DR, Klibanski A, Underwood LE, McArthur JW, Ridgway EC, Beitins IZ, Van Wyk JJ. Reduction of plasma immunoreactive somatomedin-C during fasting in humans. J Clin Endocrinol Metab 1981;53:1247–1250.

100. Hartman ML, Kanaley JA, Weltman A. Growth hormone economy in menopausal women: effects of age. In: Adashi EY, Thorner MO, eds. The Somatotrophic Axis and the Reproductive Process in Health and Disease. Springer-Verlag, New York, 1995, pp. 142–159.

101. Morley JE, Silver AJ. Anorexia in the elderly. Neurobiol Aging 1988;9:9–16.
102. Masuda A, Shibasaki T, Nakahara M, Imaki T, Kiyosawa Y, Jibiki K, et al. The effect of glucose on growth hormone (GH)-releasing hormone-mediated GH secretion in man. J Clin Endocrinol Metab 1985;60:523–526.
103. Reichlin S. Regulation of somatotropic hormone secretion. In: Handbook of Physiology. American Physiological Society, Washington, DC, 1974, pp. 405–407.
104. Corpas E, Blackman MR, Roberson R, Scholfield D, Harman SM. Oral arginine-lysine does not increase growth hormone or insulin-like growth factor-I in old men. J Gerontol 1993;48:M128–M133.
105. Crist DM, Peake GT, Mackinnon LT, Sibbitt WLJ, Kraner JC. Exogenous growth hormone treatment alters body composition and increases natural killer cell activity in women with impaired endogenous growth hormone secretion. Metabolism 1987;36:1115–1117.
106. Marcus R, Butterfield G, Holloway L, Gilliland L, Baylink DJ, Hintz RL, Sherman BM. Effects of short term administration of recombinant human growth hormone to elderly people. J Clin Endocrinol Metab 1990;70:519–527.
107. Papadakis MA, Grady D, Black D, Tierney MJ, Gooding GA, Schambelan M, Grunfeld C. Growth hormone replacement in healthy older men improves body composition but not functional ability. Ann Intern Med 1996;124:708–716.
108. Taaffe DR, Pruitt L, Reim J, Hintz RL, Butterfield G, Hoffman AR, Marcus R. Effect of recombinant human growth hormone on the muscle strength response to resistance exercise in elderly men. J Clin Endocrinol Metab 1994;79:1361–1366.
109. Thompson JL, Butterfield GE, Marcus R, Hintz RL, Van Loan M, Ghiron L, Hoffman AR. The effects of recombinant human insulin-like growth factor-I and growth hormone on body composition in elderly women. J Clin Endocrinol Metab 1995;80:1845–1852.
110. Erdtsieck RJ, Pols HA, Valk NK, van Ouwerkerk BM, Lamberts SW, Mulder P, Birkenhager JC. Treatment of post-menopausal osteoporosis with a combination of growth hormone and pamidronate: a placebo controlled trial. Clin Endocrinol (Oxford) 1995;43:557–565.
111. Yarasheski KE, Campbell JA, Kohrt WM. Effect of resistance exercise and growth hormone on bone density in older men. Clin Endocrinol (Oxford) 1997;47:223–229.
112. Cuttica CM, Castoldi L, Gorrini GP, Peluffo F, Delitala G, Filippa P, Fanciulli G, Giusti M. Effects of six-month administration of recombinant human growth hormone to healthy elderly subjects. Aging Milano 1997;9:193–197.
113. Yarasheski KE, Zachwieja JJ, Campbell JA, Bier DM. Effect of growth hormone and resistance exercise on muscle growth and strength in older men. Am J Physiol 1995;268:E268–E276.
114. Harris TB, Kiel D, Roubenoff R, Langlois J, Hannan M, Havlik R, Wilson P. Association of insulin-like growth factor-I with body composition, weight history, and past health behaviors in the very old: the Framingham Heart Study. J Am Geriatr Soc 1997;45:133–139.
115. Papadakis MA, Grady D, Tierney MJ, Black D, Wells L, Grunfeld C. Insulin-like growth factor 1 and functional status in healthy older men. J Am Geriatr Soc 1995;43:1350–1355.
116. Miller RA. Aging and immune function. Int Rev Cytol 1991;124:187–215.
117. LeRoith D, Yanowski J, Kaldjian EP, Jaffe ES, LeRoith T, Purdue K, et al. The effects of growth hormone and insulin-like growth factor I on the immune system of aged female monkeys. Endocrinology 1996;137:1071–1079.
118. Cohn L, Feller AG, Draper MW, Rudman IW, Rudman D. Carpal tunnel syndrome and gynaecomastia during growth hormone treatment of elderly men with low circulating IGF-I concentrations. Clin Endocrinol (Oxford) 1993;39:417–425.
119. Ebeling PR, Jones JD, O'Fallon WM, Janes CH, Riggs BL. Short-term effects of recombinant human insulin-like growth factor I on bone turnover in normal women. J Clin Endocrinol Metab 1993;77: 1384–1387.
120. Ghiron LJ, Thompson JL, Holloway L, Hintz RL, Butterfield GE, Hoffman AR, Marcus R. Effects of recombinant insulin-like growth factor-I and growth hormone on bone turnover in elderly women. J Bone Miner Res 1995;10:1844–1852.
121. Johansson AG, Lindh E, Blum WF, Kollerup G, Sorensen OH, Ljunghall S. Effects of growth hormone and insulin-like growth factor I in men with idiopathic osteoporosis. J Clin Endocrinol Metab 1996;81: 44–48.
122. Kupfer SR, Underwood LE, Baxter RC, Clemmons DR. Enhancement of the anabolic effects of growth hormone and insulin-like growth factor I by use of both agents simultaneously. J Clin Invest 1993;91: 391–396.

123. Ghigo E, Goffi S, Nicolosi M, Arvat E, Valente F, Mazza E, Ghigo MC, Camanni F. Growth hormone (GH) responsiveness to combined administration of arginine and GH-releasing hormone does not vary with age in man. J Clin Endocrinol Metab 1990;71:1481–1485.
124. Arvat E, Gianotti L, Ragusa L, Valetto MR, Cappa M, Aimaretti G, et al. The enhancing effect of pyridostigmine on the GH response to GHRH undergoes an accelerated age-related reduction in Down syndrome. Dementia 1996;7:288–292.
125. Corpas E, Harman SM, Pineyro MA, Roberson R, Blackman MR. Continuous subcutaneous infusions of growth hormone (GH) releasing hormone 1-44 for 14 days increase GH and insulin-like growth factor-I levels in old men. J Clin Endocrinol Metab 1993;76:134–138.
126. Corpas E, Harman SM, Pineyro MA, Roberson R, Blackman MR. Growth hormone (GH)-releasing hormone-(1-29) twice daily reverses the decreased GH and insulin-like growth factor-I levels in old men. J Clin Endocrinol Metab 1992;75:530–535.
127. Vittone J, Blackman MR, Busby Whitehead J, Tsiao C, Stewart KJ, et al. Effects of single nightly injections of growth hormone-releasing hormone (GHRH 1-29) in healthy elderly men. Metabolism 1997;46:89–96.
128. Bowers CY, Momany F, Reynolds GA, Chang D, Hong A, Chang K. Structure–activity relationships of a synthetic pentapeptide that specifically releases growth hormone in vitro. Endocrinology 1980;106:663–667.
129. Arvat E, Gianotti L, Grottoli S, Imbimbo BP, Lenaerts V, Deghenghi R, Camanni F, Ghigo E. Arginine and growth hormone-releasing hormone restore the blunted growth hormone-releasing activity of hexarelin in elderly subjects. J Clin Endocrinol Metab 1994;79:1440–1443.
130. Ghigo E, Arvat E, Rizzi G, Goffi S, Grottoli S, Mucci M, Boghen MF, Camanni F. Growth hormone-releasing activity of growth hormone-releasing peptide-6 is maintained after short-term oral pretreatment with the hexapeptide in normal aging. Eur J Endocrinol 1994;131:499–503.
131. Ghigo E, Arvat E, Gianotti L, Grottoli S, Rizzi G, Ceda GP, et al. Short-term administration of intranasal or oral Hexarelin, a synthetic hexapeptide, does not desensitize the growth hormone responsiveness in human aging. Eur J Endocrinol 1996;135:407–412.
132. Chapman IM, Hartman ML, Pezzoli SS, Thorner MO. Enhancement of pulsatile growth hormone secretion by continuous infusion of a growth hormone-releasing peptide mimetic, L-692,429, in older adults—a clinical research center study. J Clin Endocrinol Metab 1996;81:2874–2880.
133. Chapman IM, Bach MA, Van Cauter E, Farmer M, Krupa D, Taylor AM, et al. Stimulation of the growth hormone (GH)-insulin-like growth factor I axis by daily oral administration of a GH secretogogue (MK-677) in healthy elderly subjects. J Clin Endocrinol Metab 1996;81:4249–4257.
134. Friend KE, Hartman ML, Pezzoli SS, Clasey JL, Thorner MO. Both oral and transdermal estrogen increase growth hormone release in postmenopausal women—a clinical research center study. J Clin Endocrinol Metab 1996;81:2250–2256.
135. Bellantoni MF, Vittone J, Campfield AT, Bass KM, Harman SM, Blackman MR. Effects of oral versus transdermal estrogen on the growth hormone/insulin-like growth factor I axis in younger and older postmenopausal women: a clinical research center study. J Clin Endocrinol Metab 1996;81:2848–2853.

4

Hypothalamic–Pituitary–Thyroid Axis in Aging

Mary H. Samuels, MD, A. Eugene Pekary, PHD, and Jerome M. Hershman, MD

CONTENTS

THYROID PHYSIOLOGY

Dietary iodine (I) is essential for synthesis of thyroid hormone (TH). The usual dietary I intake is 150–250 µg/d. Iodine is absorbed in the upper gastrointestinal tract, enters the blood stream, and is actively transported into thyroid cells by the sodium (Na^+)/iodide (I^-) symporter (NIS), a membrane transport protein. The I^- that is not concentrated by the thyroid, is rapidly cleared by the kidneys. The trapped I^- is oxidized by thyroid peroxidase and hydrogen peroxide to an unstable intermediate, which is rapidly incorporated into tyrosine, to form monoiodotyrosine (MIT) and diiodotyrosine (DIT) in peptide linkage within the thyroglobulin molecule. The iodotyrosines couple to form thyroxine (3,5,3′,5′-tetraiodothyronine, T_4) or triiodothyronine (3,5,3′-triiodothyronine, T_3), a reaction that is also catalyzed by thyroid peroxidase. Once iodinated, thyroglobulin containing newly formed iodothyronines is stored in the follicular lumen. The T_4:T_3 ratio within the thyroid is about 10.

The pituitary thyrotroph cells secrete thyrotropin (thyroid-stimulating hormone [TSH]), which binds to the TSH receptor on the thyroid cell membrane, and exerts its stimulatory action by activation of adenylate cyclase and increase of cyclic adenosine monophosphate (cAMP). TSH causes the release of T_4 and T_3 by proteolytic digestion of thyroglobulin, and stimulates all of the metabolic processes within the thyroid, including growth and hormone (GH) TH synthesis.

The daily production of T_4 is about 80 µg, and that of T_3 is 32 µg. Only 8 µg of T_3 is secreted directly by the thyroid gland. The other 24 µg arises from outer ring deiodination of T_4 in other tissues, such as the liver and kidney. There are two 5′-deiodinases in

From: *Contemporary Endocrinology: Endocrinology of Aging*
Edited by: J. E. Morley and L. van den Berg © Humana Press Inc., Totowa, NJ

peripheral tissues. Outer ring deiodination of T_4 is a pathway of activation that produces the more active hormone, T_3; inner ring deiodination is a pathway of inactivation yielding $3,3',5'-T_3$, called reverse T_3, which is metabolically inactive. These processes are carefully regulated.

Regulation of TH secretion is through a negative feedback loop involving the hypothalamus, the anterior pituitary, and the thyroid gland. Thyrotropin-releasing hormone (TRH), synthesized and stored within the hypothalamus, stimulates the release of TSH from the anterior pituitary gland. In turn, T_4 and T_3 from the serum feed back on the pituitary and the hypothalamus, to inhibit TSH and TRH secretion. The inhibition of TSH secretion and production by T_3 and T_4 is the most important step in regulation of the system.

STUDIES IN EXPERIMENTAL ANIMALS
Hypothalamic Effects of Aging
HISTOLOGY

In mice, closely juxtaposed tanycytes, specialized ependymal cells that line the floor of the third ventricle, gradually separate with aging, leaving only fine cytoplasmic processes to interconnect them (1). This loss of tight gap junctions between tanycytes may cause gradual impairment of the integrity of the blood–brain–cerebrospinal fluid barrier with aging, although evidence for such impairment was lacking in 26-mo-old rats, as judged by trypan blue staining and antibody-binding criteria (2). In rats, dopamine and cAMP-regulated phosphoprotein mr 32 (DARPP-32) and glial fibrillary acidic protein (GFAP) immunoreactivities (IR) were investigated in tanycytes of the arcuate nucleus by means of semiquantitative immunocytochemistry (3). These two markers showed opposite changes during aging: DARPP-32 IR decreased by 70%; GFAP IR increased by 300% in 24-mo-old vs 3-mo-old rats. These changes were accompanied by a progressive loss in the number of tanycytes, measured by counting of their long processes in the arcuate nucleus. These observations indicate that the tanycytic population of the arcuate nucleus undergoes important modifications during aging, which include cell loss, impairment in the intracellular signaling cascade linked to DARPP-32, and hypertrophy. These changes may be related to the alterations in the neuroendocrine systems known to occur during aging (3). The nuclear volume of neurons in most regions of the rat hypothalamus decline with aging (4). The sexual difference in nuclear volume of neurons from different hypothalamic nuclei tends to diminish with age (4). The first signs of ultrastructural change in hypothalamic neurons with aging was observed in mitochondria (5). Morphologic changes were most prominent in dendrites of medium size (5). A significant decrease in the number of neurons per unit area was noted in the ventral medial and arcuate nuclei. However, no significant changes in the number and type of cells in the paraventricular nucleus of the rat hypothalamus were detected in aging rats (6).

BIOCHEMISTRY

Prepro-TRH messenger RNA (mRNA) levels in whole rat hypothalamus do not change significantly during aging. Because these levels represent an average over many different hypothalamic nuclei, significant regional changes may be obscured by extracting the entire hypothalamus. The content and secretion rate of hypothalamic TRH decline with aging in rats, and the pituitary TRH receptor level approximately doubles (7,8). Passive immunization with TRH antisera leads to a rapid and nearly quantitative suppression of TSH secretion in the euthyroid adult *(9)* and 24-mo-old (M Simard, AE Pekary, unpublished results) male rat. These results indicate that the inhibitory influences on TSH secretion in the euthyroid state, which are predominantly caused by T_4 and T_3 negative feedback at the pituitary thyrotroph, are dominant, and that hypothalamic TRH secretion and serum TH levels determine the set point of TSH release.

Cold exposure stimulates TSH release in rats, which can be blocked by passive immunization with TRH antiserum *(10)*. The TSH response to cold stress decreases with aging, as a result of declining norepinephrine production in the hypothalamus *(11)*. The responsiveness of body temperature to intraventricular administration of TRH and other neurotransmitters decreases with aging *(12)*. Circadian changes in brain serotonin decrease with aging *(13)*.

Pituitary Effects of Aging

HISTOLOGY

Ultrastructural changes in the normal rat anterior pituitary appear to be most prominent in the thyrotrophs, somatotrophs, and gonadotrophs *(14)*. These consist of atrophy of the Golgi apparatus, appearance of cytoplasmic vacuoles, lipid and lipofuscin granules, secondary lysosomes, and damage to the inner mitochondrial membrane. Aging in male rats results in a marked reduction in TSH cell number, and the volume density and surface density of TSH immunoreactive secretory vesicles. On the other hand, cell surface area increased significantly *(15)*.

BIOCHEMISTRY

In man, a pronounced increase in serum TSH levels occurs in the late evening, and is inhibited by the onset of sleep *(16)*. This nocturnal rise in TSH gradually declines with aging *(17,18)*. The specific biological activity of TSH extracted from aged humans and other mammals is reduced, and has an altered pattern of glycosylation *(19–22)*. Because of technical and ethical constraints, it is not possible to sample portal blood in humans, to determine whether the nocturnal rise in TSH levels is caused by an actual increase in hypothalamic TRH release to the pituitary, or an increased pituitary sensitivity to TRH-induced TSH release, perhaps caused by a reduction in hypothalamic release of somatostatin or dopamine, which are known to inhibit TSH release. In rats, a diurnal variation in serum TSH levels has also been observed, but, because they are nocturnal animals, this rise is observed during the middle of the day *(23,24)*.

The essential role that TRH plays in regulating the biosynthesis, as well as the release, of TSH has recently been shown in mice that have had their prepro-TRH gene disrupted by a targeted mutation *(25)*. These mice were mildly hypothyroid, as expected, but they also had an elevated TSH level, which was not expected, because TRH is the only known positive stimulus for TSH secretion. It was shown that the TSH response to TRH administration was normal, but the thyroidal response to endogenous TSH in these TRH knockout mice was impaired. On the other hand, their response to exogenous rat TSH was normal. This clearly indicates that the biological potency of the endogenously released TSH was reduced.

Advanced age in rats is associated with a progressive age-dependent loss in in vivo responsivity of the thyrotroph to synthetic TRH, and paradoxically augmented response of GH to this peptide in the oldest rats *(26)*. The number of thyrotrophs in the TRH knock-out mice was reduced, demonstrating that TRH is an important mitogen for thyrotroph growth *(25)*. Thus, the decline in the pituitary thyrotroph responsiveness with aging may result, at least in part, from a reduction in the number of thyrotrophs, despite an increase in the number of TRH receptors *(8)*.

The pituitary of rats becomes progressively more sensitve to TH suppression of TSH secretion with aging *(22)*. This effect is attributable in part to an increase in the rate of conversion of T_4 to T_3 within the anterior pituitary *(27)*. Sex differences in the number of nuclear T_3 receptors and concentration of T_3 in the anterior pituitary have been noted, which change differentially with aging *(8)*. Adult female rats have a greater density of pituitary T_3 receptors and concentration of T_3 in the pituitary and plasma, and a lesser concentration of pituitary and plasma TSH than do male rats. In male rats, the number of T_3 nuclear receptors increases, but the pituitary T_3 and plasma TSH remained unchanged with aging. In old females, on the other hand, there was no significant increase in T_3 receptors, but pituitary T_3 was reduced, and plasma TSH was greater than in young females *(28)*. Pituitary 5'-deiodinase declined with aging in female rats *(29)*.

Thyroidal Effects of Aging

HISTOLOGY

Detailed histomorphometric studies of changes in thyroid glands with aging have been carried out in a number of mammalian species, with consistent findings *(30)*. In the rat, which has been studied most extensively, the total number of cells remains constant throughout life. Colloid volume increases, follicular cells lining the colloid become progressively flattened, and signs of colloid resorption decrease, including the size and morphology of pseudopods and the number of cytoplasmic colloid droplets. In young thyroid cells, microtubules run longitudinally from the apical region to the basal region, intersecting with each other. Microtubules and microfilaments appear in the pseudopods after TSH injection. In hypophysectomized or aged rats, thyroid follicular epithelial cells decreased in height, and immunofluorescent labeling against tubulin and microfilaments were markedly decreased *(31)*. The rough endoplasmic reticulum was less developed, and mitochondria were swollen and abnormally shaped. Lysosomal dense bodies accumulate, many cells become overloaded with pigment-lipid granules, and polyploid nuclei increase with aging. Radioactive I^- uptake appears to be normal in the aged thyroid, but the rate of resorption of radiolabeled thyroglobulin from the colloid declines to a small fraction of that for young adults. The extent of sympathetic innervation of the thyroidal blood supply and follicles, although quite variable among species, decreases with age *(32)*. Somatostatin immunoreactive cells, which are widely distributed in the thyroid of young rats, increase in number with aging, and occur in small clusters *(33)*.

BIOCHEMISTRY

Direct sampling of thyroid venous blood and systemic arterial blood in young (6–8 mo), middle-aged (25–26 mo), and aged (28–30 mo) male Wistar rats demonstrated that thyroidal T_4 secretion rate remains constant throughout life, but the T_3 secretion rate in middle-aged and aged rats rises to 1.6–1.7× the rate in adult rats *(34)*. Serum T_4 levels have been almost universally reported to decline significantly in male and female rats with aging *(7,28,35)*. In male rats, at least part of this fall is caused by a decline in TH-binding proteins *(22)*. Binding proteins do not appear to be affected by aging in female rats, which show a progressive fall in free T_4 levels (36). Serum T_3 concentrations have been reported to remain unchanged in rats (7,28), although evidence for a decline in both total and free T_3 levels has also been presented (33). In female rats, free T_3, but not total T_3, declines with aging (36). Thyroid 5'-deiodinase did not fall with aging in female rats, and this may be responsible for maintaining serum T_3 levels (29).

The number of TSH binding sites of high affinity in old rats is about one-half that in young rats; the number of low-affinity binding sites is not affected by aging (37). TSH induced a significant increase in cAMP formation by thyroid membranes from young rats, but not in old rats. In contrast, the stimulation of cAMP formation by guanosine triphosphate (GTP) or forskolin, two direct stimulators of adenylate cyclase, was similar in both groups of rats (37).

IN VITRO STUDIES

Fisher Rat Thyroid Line 5 Cells

Development of the Fisher Rat Thyroid Line (FRTL) cells, which can be maintained in 5% calf serum (FRTL-5) with a mixture of six hormones, including bovine TSH, insulin, somatostatin, hydrocortisone, transferrin, and glycyl-histidyl-lysine, has revolutionized the study of thyroid cell function and regulation (38). In vivo experiments, along with studies of primary cell cultures, however, remain indispensible. The long-sought development of the stable FRTL-5 cell line, which retains almost all of the differentiated functions of normal thyroid cells, including a dependence on TSH for viability and growth, TSH-induced I^- uptake, and inhibition of growth by I^-, have permitted the independent variation of growth factor and second-messenger systems, which is not possible in an in vivo model. FRTL-5 cells appear to lack only one essential thyroid cell function: the ability to produce significant amounts of THs. This may be attributable to the inability of these cells to organize into follicles in response to TSH stimulation, as do most mammalian thyroid cells in culture (39,40), and to a mutation in the thyroid peroxidase (TPO) gene (41).

In the lumen of normal follicles, thyroglobulin and I^- accumulate. TPO, anchored in the extracellular surface of the apical membrane of thyrocytes lining the colloid, oxidizes I^-, resulting in the iodination of thyroglobulin and condensation of MIT and DIT residues, to form T_4 and T_3. Iodinated thyroglobulin is then phagocytized by the thyrocytes, and digested by lysozomal enzymes, which release THs, as well as MIT and DIT. An abnormal splice donor site in one allele of the TPO gene in FRTL-5 cells introduces a premature stop codon, resulting in a truncated form of TPO lacking enzymatic activity (41). Thus, FRTL-5 cells could not organify I^-, even if they were able to form follicles. This block in TH formation does not necessarily diminish the relevance of studies showing that the TSH-induced growth and I^- transport by FRTL-5 cells is mediated, at least in part, by profound changes in the production and release of important autocrine-derived growth factors, including insulin-like growth factor I (IGF-I), epidermal growth factor (EGF), and transforming growth factor β_1 (TGF-β_1).

Role of IGF-I, EGF, and TGF-β_1
in Normal and Abnormal Thyroid Cell Growth and Function

IGF-I, EGF, and TGF-β_1 are produced by subconfluent porcine thyroid follicular cells in vitro (42). IGF-I and EGF facilitate TSH-induced thyroid cell growth and I^- uptake, but TGF-β_1 inhibits these responses *(43–46)*. TSH stimulates the production and secretion of IGF-I *(42)*. I^- inhibits follicular cell growth through stimulation of TGF-β_1 synthesis and secretion *(42,47)*. Heterogenetity in the sensitivity to the growth-inhibitory effect of TGF-β_1 develops in FRTL-5 cells with increasing passage number, as well as in normal thyroid cells in vivo. This gradual loss of growth inhibition by TGF-β_1, which is probably the predominant inhibitor of thyroid cell growth in vivo, has been hypothesized to be responsible for the development of nodular goiter in susceptible individuals *(42,48)*.

Effect of Aging on Thyroid Cell Function

Rat thyroid cells in vivo and in tissue culture gradually lose their ability to take up radioactive I^- with increasing numbers of cell divisions *(49)*. This effect correlates with an increased level of TGF-β mRNA, and increased synthesis and secretion of all three isoforms of TGF-β (types 1, 2, and 3) during in vivo and in vitro aging of rat thyroid (FRTL-5) cells *(50)*. TGF-β_1 reduces the expression and activity of Na^+/K^+-adenosine triphosphatase, which is needed for the maintenance of the inward-directed Na^+ electrochemical gradient that is essential for I uptake, as well as for other essential transport processes *(51)*. TGF-β_1 also reduces the NIS mRNA levels in FRTL-5 cells *(49)*. The NIS mRNA levels of aged FRTL-5 cells (defined as more that 40 passages in vitro) was 2% that of young cells with less than 20 passages *(49)*.

Effect of Aging on Thyroid Cell Growth

The growth rate of thyroid follicular cells, which line the thyroid follicular colloid, slows with aging in vivo. Thyroid follicles develop a progressively thinner, squamous-appearing, layer of thyrocytes. The multifunctional proteins of the TGF-β family have a potent antiproliferative effect on thyroid follicular cell growth *(52)*. Increased expression of TGF-β in proliferating thyroid cells and in thyroid tumors has been described. These remain sensitive to the inhibitory effect of TGF-β on I^- uptake, but the growth rate of a subset of cells is no longer suppressed by this cytokine. The doubling time for aged (>40 passages) FRTL-5 cells is actually less than that for young (<20 passages) cells *(50)*. This selective escape by FRTL-5 cells from the growth inhibitory effect of TGF-β is not the result of a change in cell karyotype *(44)*, TGF-β_1 receptor number, or subtype, because the only functional TGF-β receptor consists of a heteroduplex of TGF-β_1 receptors type I and type II *(53)*. Apparently some change in the responsiveness to the second-messenger signaling pathway regulating growth is involved.

CLINICAL THYROID DISEASES

TSH and Thyroid Hormone Levels in the Elderly

The hypothalamic–pituitary–thyroid (HPT) axis has been extensively studied in aging human subjects *(54–57)*. Many early studies of the elderly reported significant alterations in circulating TH and TSH levels, as well as blunted TSH responses to TRH. However, further studies revealed that most of these alterations are caused by the effects of illness and medications on the HPT axis *(58)*. Acute or chronic nonthyroidal illness leads to decreases in serum T_3 levels, with more severe illness also causing decreases in serum T_4 levels. Serum TSH levels are usually normal in illness, but can be low, and TSH responses to TRH are blunted. In addition, medications, including I-containing compounds, nonsteroidal anti-inflammatory agents, glucocorticoids, dopamine, amiodarone, and radiocontrast agents, can affect TH or TSH levels *(59,60)*. Therefore, care must be taken when reviewing studies of thyroid function in the elderly, to exclude those studies that do not adequately screen elderly subjects for nonthyroidal illness or medication use.

Studies that include only healthy elderly subjects have in general shown the following changes in the HPT axis *(54–57)*: T_4 production decreases by approx 25% in the elderly, but serum T_4 levels are unchanged, because of concomitant reductions in T_4 clearance. T_3 production and degradation decrease by approx 30%; and serum T_3 levels may be slightly lower, compared to young subjects, but remain in the normal range. Basal TSH levels are normal in the elderly *(61)*, excluding subjects with subclinical thyroid disease, which is common in elderly populations. However, several studies showed decreased 24-h mean serum TSH levels, and a decreased nocturnal TSH rise in a small group of healthy elderly men, suggesting that 24-h TSH secretion may be decreased in the elderly *(17,18,62)*. The clinical significance of this finding is uncertain. TSH responses to TRH are normal or decreased in elderly subjects.

Clinical Presentation of Thyroid Disease in the Elderly

HYPOTHYROIDISM

It is a common impression that the typical clinical features of hypothyroidism are less pronounced in the elderly. One study systematically addressed this question, and found that most symptoms and signs of hypothyroidism were present to similar degrees in young and old patients with biochemically proven hypothyroidism *(63)*. Specifically, fatigue, weakness, mental status changes, depression, hoarseness, dry skin, decreased heart rate, and slowed deep tendon reflexes were equally common in both groups. However, elderly patients did have fewer complaints of weight gain, cold intolerance, parasthesias, and muscle cramps. From these data, it appears that the major difficulty in diagnosing hypothyroidism in the elderly is not the lack of symptoms, but rather their nonspecific nature. Clinical findings of hypothyroidism in the elderly are often attributed to medical illnesses, medication use, depression, or the aging process itself.

HYPERTHYROIDISM

A number of reports have shown that elderly hyperthyroid subjects do not manifest the same degree of adrenergic symptoms and signs as younger hyperthyroid subjects *(64–68)*. Older patients with hyperthyroidism have decreased rates of fatigue, weakness, nervousness, sweating, heat intolerance, hyperphagia, diarrhea, tremor, tachycardia, and hyperactive reflexes, compared to young patients with hyperthyroidism. Instead, they have high rates of confusion, anorexia, and atrial fibrillation as presenting symptoms of hyperthyroidism. This phenomenon has been termed "apathetic hyperthyroidism" in the elderly *(69)*. Such patients can be mistakenly diagnosed with cancer, heart disease, dementia, or gastrointestinal illness, rather than hyperthyroidism.

Diagnosis of Thyroid Disease in the Elderly

Based on the above discussion, it is evident that a high index of suspicion must be maintained for the possibility of thyroid disease in elderly patients. When thyroid disease is suspected in a healthy ambulatory elderly subject, it is usually sufficient to obtain a serum TSH level, utilizing a sensitive TSH assay able to distinguish low from normal values. In this setting, a normal TSH level will essentially rule out primary thyroid dysfunction. An abnormal serum TSH level should lead to repeat measurement of TSH, along with measurement of serum free T_4. In some cases, the TSH will have returned to normal, and no further action is necessary. If the TSH is still abnormal on repeat measurement, the free T_4 level will assist in determining the severity of the thyroid disorder. All patients with persistent abnormalities in serum TSH levels, especially if accompanied by abnormal free T_4 levels, require further evaluation, and possible treatment.

Many elderly subjects are not healthy, but have concurrent illnesses and medication use that confound the interpretation of a single serum TSH level *(58–60)*. If possible, TSH levels should not be measured during acute illness (when TSH may be low), or during recovery from acute illness (when TSH may be transiently elevated). In chronically ill elderly patients, it is often helpful to obtain a serum free T_4 level initially, in addition to the serum TSH level. Serum T_3 levels should rarely be obtained, because they are often low because of illness or decreased caloric intake. TRH stimulation tests are not recommended for the diagnosis of thyroid disease in the elderly population, because they do not provide any additional information over the basal serum TSH level. Abnormal free T_4 or TSH levels in chronically ill patients may require consultation with a specialist, to assess the presence and severity of thyroid disease.

Prevalence of Thyroid Dysfunction in the Elderly

When discussing the prevalence of thyroid disease in the elderly population, it is helpful to distinguish between overt and subclinical thyroid disease *(70,71)*. Overt thyroid disease is present when both serum TSH and free T_4 levels are outside the normal range (with the rare exception of pituitary disease causing thyroid dysfunction, in which case, serum TSH levels may be normal, despite overt hypothyroidism or hyperthyroidism). In subclinical thyroid disease, only the serum TSH is abnormal; serum free T_4 levels are within the normal range. Changes in TH levels in overt and subclinical thyroid disease are as follows:

	Serum-free T_4	Serum TSH
Overt hypothyroidism	Low	Elevated
Subclinical hypothyroidism	Normal	Elevated
Overt hyperthyroidism	High	Suppressed
Subclinical hyperthyroidism	Normal	Suppressed

Subclinical thyroid disease probably represents a milder form of overt thyroid disease, with the assumption that the pituitary gland senses changes in circulating TH levels that diverge from the individual's intrinsic set point, even when the levels are within the broad range of normal for the population. Thus, the individual's TSH level is an earlier and more sensitive marker for thyroid disease than the free T_4 level. In the following subheadings, overt and subclinical thyroid disease in the elderly will be considered separately.

There are a number of caveats to keep in mind when reviewing data on the prevalence of both overt and subclinical thyroid disease in elderly populations: The prevalence of thyroid disease varies with ethnic group, dietary I intake, and prevalence of antithyroid antibodies; as discussed, studies that did not exclude hospitalized or chronically ill patients may include patients with abnormal TH levels caused by nonthyroidal illness or medication use; the definition of "elderly" in various studies ranges from 55 to 100 yr old; and some studies include subjects with known thyroid disease who are receiving therapy, but other studies exclude such subjects.

HYPOTHYROIDISM

Depending on the population studied, the prevalence of overt hypothyroidism in the elderly ranges between 0.6 and 3%, with a higher prevalence among women than men *(72–83)*. Subclinical hypothyroidism is more prevalent, occurring in 1.4–7.8% of the elderly population, and is also more common in women (range 7–18% for women vs 2–15% for men) *(72–85)*. In longitudinal studies, elderly subjects with initial normal TSH levels, but with the presence of antithyroid antibodies, have at least a 2% annualized rate of developing overt or subclinical hypothyroidism (*see* Causes of Thyroid Dysfunction regarding the significance of antithyroid antibodies in the elderly) *(79,86–88)*. Elderly subjects with initial isolated elevations in TSH (subclinical hypothyroidism) have at least a 2–3% annualized rate of progression to overt hypothyroidism. This rate increases to 4–5% per year, if antithyroid antibodies are present *(73,88–90)*. Thus, subclinical hypothyroidism is quite prevalent in the elderly population, especially in women, and often progresses to overt hypothyroidism.

HYPERTHYROIDISM

Compared to data on hypothyroidism, there are fewer studies on the prevalence of hyperthyroidism in the elderly. Overt hyperthyroidism has been reported in 0.2–2% of the elderly population, with some (but not all) studies suggesting higher rates in elderly women, compared to elderly men *(74,78,80,82,83,91,92)*. Subclinical hyperthyroidism occurs in less than 2% of elderly subjects, and may also be more common in women *(61,73,74,82,91,92)*. To date, there are no longitudinal studies on the development of overt or subclinical hyperthyroidism in elderly subjects with initial normal TSH levels. Elderly subjects with initial isolated suppression of TSH have high rates of developing overt hyperthyroidism on subsequent evaluation, but also have high rates of reverting to detectable or normal TSH levels *(73,91,93,94)*. These data are in contrast to the more predictable progression from subclinical to overt hypothyroidism, and suggest that other factors (such as nonthyroidal illness or medications) may cause transient TSH suppression in these subjects.

Causes of Thyroid Dysfunction in the Elderly

HYPOTHYROIDISM

In general, the causes of overt and subclinical hypothyroidism in the elderly are similar to the causes of hypothyroidism in the general population *(54–57)*. Based on antithyroid antibody studies, most hypothyroidism in the elderly is caused by autoimmune (Hashimoto's) thyroiditis *(82,83,86,95,96)*. There is an age-dependent increase in the prevalence of antithyroid antibodies in the ambulatory population, with up to 16% of older women and up to 9% of older men having antimicrosomal (antithyroid peroxidase) antibodies. Forty–70% of older subjects with elevated TSH levels have positive antithyroid antibodies, but only a minority of older subjects with positive antithyroid antibodies have elevated TSH levels. Euthyroid subjects with positive antithyroid antibody titers have increased rates of development of elevated TSH levels, and the rate of progression from subclinical to overt hypothyroidism is also much higher in subjects who have antithyroid antibodies. These data suggest that there is a significant correlation between the presence of antithyroid antibodies (and hence autoimmune thyroiditis) and hypothyroidism in the older population. However, screening elderly subjects for thyroid disease with antibody titers alone is not recommended, because this strategy will miss 30–50% of subjects with elevated TSH levels.

Aside from Hashimoto's thyroiditis, other causes of hypothyroidism in the elderly include neck surgery or radiation therapy, late sequella of treatment for Graves' disease, recovery from subacute or silent thyroiditis, and underreplacement of I-T_4 in subjects with known hypothyroidism. In addition, drugs, such as lithium, I-containing compounds (for example, radiocontrast agents or amiodarone), and cytokines, can lead to hypothyroidism in the elderly (60).

HYPERTHYROIDISM

The causes of overt and subclinical hyperthyroidism in the elderly are similar to the causes of hyperthyroidism in young subjects, and include Graves' disease, toxic multinodular goiter, toxic adenoma, subacute or silent thyroiditis, or overreplacement with levthyroxine L-T_4 for hypothyroidism (88,97). However, Graves' disease tends to be less common in the elderly, and toxic multinodular goiter is more common (68). In addition, the development of hyperthyroidism in an elderly patient often occurs after administration of amiodarone or an I-containing radiocontrast agent, because older patients with underlying thyroid abnormalities are more likely to receive these agents (89).

Risks of Thyroid Disease in the Elderly

HYPOTHYROIDISM

In general, the risks of overt hypothyroidism in the elderly parallel those of hypothyroidism in younger subjects, and include decreased quality of life, hypertension, hyperlipidemia, and decreased cardiac function (98–100). However, few studies have addressed risks of hypothyroidism specifically in the elderly population. One could conjecture that the cardiovascular risks of hypothyroidism may be of greater import in older subjects, because they are more likely to have underlying organic heart disease, but this has not been studied. The same adverse effects that occur in overt hypothyroidism are present in at least some patients with subclinical hypothyroidism, including impaired cardiac function, hyperlipidemia, and neuropsychiatric derangements, although to a lesser degree (82,101–109).

HYPERTHYROIDISM

In addition to the clinical effects of hyperthyroidism, there are two specific risks associated with TH excess that are particularly important in elderly patients.

Cardiovascular Risks. Overt hyperthyroidism leads to marked effects on the cardiovascular system, including enhanced myocardial contractility, accelerated heart rate, increased cardiac output, and peripheral vasodilatation. This may lead to increased myocardial oxygen demand, cardiac hypertrophy, or angina, in older patients with underlying structural cardiac disease (110). Similar, although less pronounced, changes in myocardial function may occur in subclinical hyperthyroidism, although the data are variable (111,112). In addition, the risk of atrial fibrillation is increased by overt or subclinical hyperthyroidism, especially in older subjects (93,113). Results from the Framingham study showed that 28% of subjects with subclinical hyperthyroidism developed atrial fibrillation over 10 yr, compared to 11% of age-matched euthyroid subjects (113). These data clearly suggest that elderly subjects with suppressed TSH levels should be carefully evaluated for cardiac sequella.

Risks of Osteoporosis. Overt hyperthyroidism leads to excess bone resorption and the development of osteoporosis, especially in women *(114)*. The effects of subclinical hyperthyroidism on bone are less pronounced, but even such mild abnormalities in thyroid function may lead to bone loss in postmenopausal women with estrogen deficiency *(115–120)*. For this reason, measurement of bone density may be indicated in older women with subclinical hyperthyroidism, to assist with treatment decisions.

Treatment of Thyroid Disease in the Elderly

HYPOTHYROIDISM

Overt hypothyroidism in an elderly patient should be treated with synthetic L-T$_4$, rather than other TH preparations such as desiccated thyroid extract or combinations of L-T$_4$ and L-T$_3$. The goal of treatment is attainment of a normal serum TSH level. The target dose of L-T$_4$ is lower than the typical replacement dose used in young subjects, because the elderly have decreased metabolism of T$_4$ *(121,122)*. In most cases, it is prudent to begin with a low starting dose of L-T$_4$ (25 µg/d or less), especially in a patient with long-standing hypothyroidism and/or known cardiac disease. The dose may be gradually increased every 4–8 wk, until the TSH is normalized. In rare cases, the development of angina precludes the use of full replacement doses of L-T$_4$. In these cases, it is appropriate to consider surgical therapy or angioplasty for coronary artery disease while the patient is still hypothyroid *(123)*, to be followed by attempts to achieve euthyroidism, once the angina is well-controlled. If possible, patients with cardiac disease should not remain permanently hypothyroid, because this can contribute to further decrements in cardiac function.

It is unclear whether all elderly patients with subclinical hypothyroidism should be treated. Such treatment would prevent progression to overt hypothyroidism and treat the subtle tissue effects of mild hypothyroidism, including neuropsychiatric symptoms, cardiovascular effects, and hyperlipidemia. However, this approach has not been tested in an elderly population. If one decides not to treat all older patients with subclinical hypothyroidism, then risk stratification should be performed for the projected rate of progression to overt disease, as well as the presence of symptoms, cardiac disease, and/or hyperlipidemia. Patients with suggestive symptoms, abnormal cardiac function, or hyperlipidemia may benefit most from therapy for subclinical hypothyroidism, as recently shown by a cost-effectiveness analysis of screening for thyroid disease in the general population *(124)*.

HYPERTHYROIDISM

The treatment of overt hyperthyroidism in the elderly depends to some extent on the cause of the disease. Graves' disease is best treated by radioactive ^{131}I, although a course of thionamide therapy may be used initially to stabilize an elderly patient with cardiac disease, severe wasting, or an acute illness. Toxic multinodular goiters and toxic adenomas may be treated with radioactive I (at higher doses than those used to treat Graves' disease) or surgery, with the choice depending on the patient's suitability for surgery, and the presence of any worrisome nodules that would warrant excision. The therapy for I-induced hyperthyroidism caused by administration of radiocontrast agents or amiodarone is more difficult, because radioactive I is unlikely to be effective in the face of a high total body burden of I. In these cases, thionamides have some role, although they may also be relatively ineffective *(125)*. Treatment of patients receiving inappropriately high doses of L-T$_4$ consists simply of reducing the dose of L-T$_4$ until the TSH becomes normal (note that there may be a 1–3 mo lag in recovery of suppressed TSH levels once the dose of L-T$_4$ has been decreased).

The decision to treat subclinical hyperthyroidism is difficult, because treatment options are complicated and carry some risks, and because the overall risk of subclinical hyperthyroidism has not been well quantified. The first step in deciding to treat subclinical hyperthyroidism is to repeat the TSH measurement, because there is a high rate of normalization of suppressed TSH levels over time. In addition, care must be taken that the patient does not have altered TSH levels caused by nonthyroidal illness or medication use. A T$_3$ level should also be obtained, to rule out T$_3$-toxicosis. Once these issues have been settled, one should decide whether to treat based on the presence of symptoms (remembering that hyperthyroidism may be masked in elderly patients), risks for osteoporosis, and risks for atrial fibrillation or other cardiac events. In some cases, it may be prudent to initiate a trial of antithyroid drug therapy prior to therapy with radioiodine. This affords the physician and the patient a chance to see if symptoms and other parameters improve with treatment of the subclinical hyperthyroidism.

Thyroid Nodules

PREVALENCE

Thyroid nodules, either solitary or multiple, increase in frequency with aging. Studies show that 90% of women over age 60 yr and 60% of men over age 80 yr have a nodular thyroid gland (126). The prevalence of thyroid nodules is fivefold higher in women than in men (127). Thyroid nodules in asymptomatic individuals (incidentalomas) have been identified frequently by ultrasonography, which is much more sensitive than palpation. The prevalence of incidentalomas was 67% by high-resolution ultrasonography, and only 21% by neck palpation (128). A large autopsy series showed that 50% of the population with no known history of thyroid disease had discrete nodules, and in 35% the nodules were greater than 2 cm in diameter (129).

CLINICAL EVALUATION

Evaluation of the thyroid nodule focuses on the detection of malignancy. The age and gender of the patient are important risk factors for malignancy. Although thyroid nodules are more frequent in women, the likelihood of malignancy is somewhat higher in men. Radiation exposure during childhood predisposes to thyroid nodules and thyroid carcinoma, but the latency period probably does not exceed 50 yr, so that the chance of radiation-induced thyroid cancer from childhood exposure is low in the elderly. A family history of thyroid cancer suggests familial medullary thyroid cancer as a component of multiple endocrine neoplasia (MEN) type 2A or familial papillary cancer. Multinodular goiter is also prevalent in many families.

Most thyroid nodules are asymptomatic. Hemorrhage into a thyroid nodule or cyst may cause rapid enlargement and pain. Rapid growth of a nodule over a period of several weeks is suspicious of malignancy. Persistent hoarseness may result from recurrent laryngeal nerve involvement by cancer or a large multinodular goiter.

On physical examination, a firm fixed nodule is more likely to be malignant, but many differentiated carcinomas are soft. Lymphadenopathy suggests malignancy. The distinction between a solitary nodule and multinodular goiter by neck palpation is limited. In approx 50% of cases of a clinically solitary nodule on palpation, the lesion was subsequently found to be a dominant nodule in a multinodular goiter, on histological examination *(130)*. The relative risk of cancer in solitary vs multinodular thyroid glands is controversial. Many studies have reported lower rates of thyroid carcinoma in palpable multinodular glands (5–13%), compared to solitary nodules (9–25%), but other studies have found a similar incidence of cancer in solitary nodules and in multinodular glands.

DIAGNOSTIC TESTS

A low serum TSH concentration suggests the presence of either an autonomously functioning adenoma, or a toxic multinodular goiter. Elevated antiperoxidase and anti-thyroglobulin antibody titers indicate lymphocytic thyroiditis, which may present as a nodule. The serum thyroglobulin level is not a useful test to distinguish benign from malignant nodules, because it is increased with any goitrous process.

Thyroid ultrasound is a noninvasive test that discriminates cystic from solid lesions. It has proven useful to differentiate thyroid from nonthyroid neck masses, and to localize nodules deep within the gland. In such cases, it can be used to guide fine-needle aspiration biopsy (FNA). Thyroid ultrasound is capable of identifying impalpable solid nodules as small as 0.3 mm in diameter, and cystic nodules of 0.2 mm *(128)*. The clinical significance of small nodules detected by ultrasonography remains uncertain. Ultrasonography does not help in the overall diagnosis of malignancy. Cystic nodules constitute 15–25% of all thyroid nodules, and a significant fraction may harbor papillary carcinomas *(131)*.

FNA provides reliable information, and is the most effective method to diagnose the cause of the nodule. Utilization of FNA has dramatically reduced the need for surgery to diagnose benign thyroid nodules. Results of FNAs are divided into four general categories: benign, suspicious (includes aspirates with some features of thyroid carcinoma, but not conclusive), malignant, and insufficient. In a large series of patients with FNA biopsy of the thyroid, benign cytology was found in 69% (mostly colloid goiter), malignant cytology in 3.5%, and suspicious cytology in 10% *(132)*. The suspicious category consists of variants of follicular neoplasm, but follicular adenomas are about 10-fold more common than follicular carcinomas. Those patients with a nondiagnostic or insufficient cytologic diagnosis should have a repeat biopsy, because an adequate specimen is obtained in 30–50% of repeat aspiration of nodules *(133)*. Ultrasound-guided FNA is used for sampling of impalpable nodules larger than 1.5 cm and for the solid component of cystic nodules. In patients with nodules that are follicular lesions, radioiodine scan should be performed. Hot or functional nodules are rarely malignant.

MANAGEMENT

Treatment of the thyroid nodule depends on the functional state of the nodule and the cytologic diagnosis of the FNA biopsy. The hyperfunctioning hot nodule is treated with radioiodine ablation or surgery. The vast majority of thyroid nodules are benign and can be managed medically. Medical management with TH-suppressive therapy is based on the assumption that growth of the nodule is TSH-dependent. Spontaneous regression of thyroid nodules may occur. L-thyroxine-suppressive therapy is useful for nodules that do not decrease in size over several months of initial observation. The suppressive therapy in treatment of benign thyroid nodules has been challenged in the past few years, by failure of some studies to show a significant decrease of nodule size *(134)*, and by concern about reducing bone mineral density *(118–120)*. However, several recent studies showed greater than 50% reduction in nodule size in 40% of patients with a single nodule *(135,136)*. Generally, patients are followed by palpation at intervals of 3–4 mo. Ultrasound examination can be performed to assess growth or shrinkage of a nodule, if more objective documentation is required.

If the cytologic diagnosis indicates malignancy, or is strongly suspicious for malignancy, the nodule should be removed surgically. About one-fourth of patients who go to surgery because of suspicious cytologic findings are found to have a malignant lesion. Altogether, only about 6% of thyroid nodules are malignant *(132)*.

Thyroid Cancer

Thyroid cancer accounts for 0.6–1.6% of all cancers in the United States, and mortality from thyroid cancer is less than 0.5% of all cancer deaths *(137)*. Thyroid cancer is classified into five major types: papillary, follicular, medullary, and anaplastic and thyroid lymphoma.

PAPILLARY THYROID CARCINOMA

Papillary carcinoma is the most common type of thyroid cancer, and accounts for 80% of all thyroid cancers. In autopsy studies, the prevalence of occult papillary carcinoma (less than 1 cm) was found to be 7% in patients over 80 yr old *(138)*. Papillary carcinoma usually grows slowly. The tumor tends to invade lymphatics and metastasize to the regional lymph nodes and the lungs. Distant spread may occur to bone and the central nervous system. The disease is more aggressive in older patients. Thyroid tumors smaller than 1.5 cm rarely metastasize to distant sites; larger tumors are associated with higher mortality rates. Extension of the tumor through the thyroid capsule, and into the surrounding structures, is associated with poorer prognosis. Cervical lymph node metastases occur in about 50% of patients with papillary carcinoma, and carries only a slightly higher rate of recurrence and mortality.

Surgery, either near-total or total thyroidectomy, is the initial treatment of choice for papillary carcinoma. The chief disadvantage of total thyroidectomy is the higher incidence of hypoparathyroidism. Radioiodine therapy is used as an adjunct to surgery, to treat patients with residual or recurrent papillary cancer in the neck *(139)*. The prophylactic use of radioactive iodine after surgery reduces the mortality rate and increases survival: It is generally given to any older person with papillary cancer.

TH in a suppressive dose is prescribed after thyroidectomy, in order to reduce recurrence. TSH stimulates thyroid tumors that contain TSH receptors. The dose of T_4 should be adjusted to keep the TSH suppressed without causing clinical thyrotoxicosis. The degree of suppression should be based on the staging of the patient. In patients with a good prognosis, TSH should be suppressed to the slightly subnormal range. In patients with worse prognosis, which includes many of the elderly, TSH should be suppressed to <0.05 mU/L without causing clinical thyrotoxicosis.

FOLLICULAR THYROID CARCINOMA

Follicular thyroid carcinoma accounts for about 5–10% of all thyroid cancers in the United States, and occurs more frequently in the elderly. Hurthle cell carcinoma is a variant of follicular thyroid carcinoma, and carries a poorer prognosis. Follicular carcinoma also metastasizes to the lungs, bone, central nervous system, and other soft tissues, with higher frequency than papillary carcinoma. Tumor recurrence in distant sites is more frequently seen with follicular than papillary carcinoma, and occurs with higher prevalence in highly invasive tumors.

Treatment includes total thyroidectomy, and ^{131}I therapy to ablate residual tumor. Radioiodine is the principal treatment of metastatic tumors. If the tumor does not concentrate the isotope, external radiation may be effective. As with papillary carcinoma, thyroxine therapy should be given to suppress serum TSH levels to the subnormal range.

MEDULLARY THYROID CARCINOMA

Medullary carcinoma accounts for 2–4% of thyroid cancers, and is derived from the calcitonin-secreting cells or parafollicular cells. Elevated serum calcitonin levels establish the diagnosis, and correlate with tumor mass. About 20% are familial tumors, and are associated with other endocrine neoplasias (MEN 2A or 2B). The recognition of point mutations in RET proto-oncogene on chromosome 10 has enhanced the ability to detect these neoplasms at an early and potentially curable stage in suspected family members. Approximately 80% of medullary carcinoma is sporadic and diagnosed later in life, mostly after age 50 (140). The preferred treatment consists of total thyroidectomy and a modified radical neck dissection on the side of the tumor.

ANAPLASTIC THYROID CARCINOMA

Anaplastic thyroid carcinoma is the most aggressive and lethal cancer. It accounts for 5% of thyroid cancer. In 28–70% of patients, there is a previous differentiated thyroid carcinoma (141). The peak occurrence is in the seventh decade: 90% of patients are 60 yr or older. Patients present with a rapidly growing thyroid mass. In 80%, the tumor is more than 5 cm, and, in 30%, vocal cord paralysis is present at the onset. Treatment includes surgery followed by external radiation and chemotherapy, but only a small percentage survive more than 1 yr.

THYROID LYMPHOMA

Thyroid lymphoma accounts for about 5% of thyroid malignancies, and is almost always accompanied by chronic lymphocytic thyroiditis. The patients are usually over 60 yr of age, and there is a female preponderance. This tumor nearly always arises from B-cell lymphocytes. It usually invades the walls of blood vessels, and extends outside the thyroid gland. It presents as a rapidly enlarging thyroid mass in a patient with long history of a goiter or diagnosis of Hashimoto's thyroiditus. The patient may complain of neck pressure, local swelling of the thyroid gland, hoarseness, or dysphagia. FNA may suggest the diagnosis, but definitive diagnosis usually requires an open biopsy. Surgical removal of the lymphoma by total thyroidectomy is unwise. Treatment with external radiation and 4–6 courses of chemotherapy nearly always produces a permanent remission (142).

REFERENCES

1. Scott DE, Sladek JR Jr. Age related changes in the endocrine hypothalalmus. I. Tanycytes and the blood-brain-cerebrospinal fluid barrier. Neurobiol Aging 1981;2:89–94.
2. Feden G, Baldinger A, Miller-Soule D, Blumenthal HT. An in vivo and in vitro study of an aging-related neuron cytoplasmic-binding antibody in male Fischer rats. J Gerontol 1979;34:651–660.
3. Zoli M, Ferragut F, Frasoldati A, Biagini G, Agnati LF. Age-related alterations in tanycytes of the mediobasal hypothalamus of the male rat. Neurobiol Aging 1995;16:77–83.
4. Lin KH, Peng YM, Peng MT, Tseng TM. Changes in the nuclear volume of rat hypothalamic neurons in old age. Neuroendocrinology 1976;21:247–254.
5. Verbitskaia LB, Bogolepov NN. Changes in the hypothalamic ultrastructure during aging. Zh Nevropatol Psikhiatr 1984;84:987–993.
6. Sartin JL, Lamperti AA. Neuron numbers in hypothalamic nuclei of young, middle-aged and aged male rats. Experientia 1985;41:109–111.

7. Pekary AE, Mirell CJ, Turner LF, Jr, Walfish PG, Hershman JM. Hypothalamic secretion of thyrotropin releasing hormone declines in aging rats. J Gerontol 1987;42:447–450.

8. Donda A, Reymond MJ, Lemarchand-Beraud T. Influence of age on the control of thyrotropin secretion by thyrotropin-releasing hormone in the male rats. Neuroendocrinology 1989;49:389–394.

9. Szabo M, Kovathana N, Gordon K, Frohman LA. Effect of passive immunization with antiserum to thyrotropin-releasing hormone on plasma levels in thyroidectomized rats. Endocrinology 1978;102: 799–805.

10. Mori M, Kobayayashi I, Wakabayashi I. Suppression of serum thyrotropin (TSH) concentrations following thyroidectomy and cold exposure by passive immunization with antiserum to thyrotropin-releasing hormone (TRH) in rats. Metabolism 1978;27:1485–1490.

11. Roubein IF, Embree LJ, Jackson DW. Changes in catecholamine levels in discrete regions of rat brain during aging. Exp Aging Res 1986;12:193–196.

12. Ferguson AV, Turner SL, Cooper KE, Veale WL. Neurotransmitter effects on body temperature are modified with increasing age. Physiol Behav 1985;34:977–981.

13. Simpkins JW, Millard WJ. Influence of age on neurotransmitter function. Endocrinol Metab Clin North Am 1987;16:893–917.

14. Shaposhnikov VM. The ultrastructural features of secretory cells of some endocrine glands in aging. Mech Ageing Dev 1985;30:123–142.

15. Console GM, Gomez Dumm CL, Goya RG. Immunohistochemical and radioimmunological assessment of thyrotrophs in the pituitary of aging rats. Acta Anat 1995;152:28–32.

16. Parker DC, Pekary AE, Hershman JM. Effect of normal and reversed sleep-wake cycles upon nyctohemeral rhythmicity of plasma thyrotropin: evidence suggestive of an inhibitory influence in sleep. J Clin Endocrinol Metab 1976;43:318–329.

17. Greenspan SL, Klibanski A, Rowe JW, Elahi D. Age-related alterations in pulsatile secretion of TSH: role of dopaminergic regulation. Am J Physiol 1991;260:E486–E491.

18. van Coevorden A, Mockel J, Laurent E, Kerkhofs M, L'Hermite-Baleriaux M, Decoster C, Neve P, Van Cauter E. Neuroendocrine rhythms and sleep in aging men. Am J Physiol 1991;260:E651–E661.

19. Amir SM, Kubota K, Tramontano D, Ingbar SH, Keutmann HT. The carbohydrate moiety of bovine thyrotropin is essential for full bioactivity but not for receptor recognition. Endocrinology 1987;120: 345–351.

20. Beck-Peccoz P, Bersani L. Variable biological activity of thyroid-stimulating hormone. Eur J Endocrinol 1994;131:331–340.

21. Choy VJ, Klemme WR, Timiras PS. Variant forms of immunoreactive thyrotropin in aged rats. Mech Ageing Dev 1982;19:273–278.

22. Klug TL, Adelman RC. Altered hypothalamic-pituitary regulation of thyrotropin in male rats during aging. Endocrinology 1979;104:1136–1142.

23. Azukizawa M, Pekary AE, Hershman JM. Plasma thyrotropin, thyroxine, and triiodothyronine relationships in man. J Clin Endocrinol Metab 1976;43:533–542.

24. Jordan D, Veisseire M, Borson-Chazot F, Mornex R. Postnatal development of TRH and TSH rhythms in the rat. Horm Res 1987;27:216–224.

25. Yamada M, Saga Y, Shibusawa N, Hirato J, Murakami M, Iwasaki T, et al. Tertiary hypothyroidism and hyperglycemia in mice with targeted disruption of the thyrotropin-releasing hormone gene. Proc Natl Acad Sci USA 1997;94:10,862–10,867.

26. Cizza G, Brady LS, Calogero AE, Bagdy G, Lynn AB, Kling MA, et al. Central hypothyroidism is associated with advanced age in male Fischer 344/N rats: in vivo and in vitro studies. Endocrinology 1992;131:2672–2680.

27. Valueva GV, Verzhikovskaya NV. Thyrotropin activity of hypophysis in rats of different ages. Neurosci Behav Physiol 1979;9:366–369.

28. Pekary AE, Hershman JM, Sugawara M, Gieschen KI, Sogol PB, Reed AW, Pardridge WM, Walfish PG. Preferential release of triiodothyronine: an intrathyroidal adaptation to reduced serum thyroxine in aging rats. J Gerontol 1983;38:653–659.

29. Correa da Costa VM, Rosenthal D. Effect of aging on thyroidal and pituitary T4-5'-deiodinase activity in female rats. Life Sci 1996;59:1515–1520.

30. Kunitake J, Pekary AE, Hershman JM. Aging and the hypothalamic-pituitary-thyroid axis. In: Morley JE, Korenman SG, eds. Endocrinology and Metabolism in the Elderly. Blackwell, Boston, 1992, pp. 92–100.

31. Kurihara H, Uchida K, Fujita H. Distribution of microtubules and microfilaments in thyroid follicular epithelial cells of normal, TSH-treated, aged, and hypophysectomized rats. Histochemistry 1990;93: 335–345.

32. Melander A, Sundler F, Westgren U. Sympathetic innervation of the thyroid: variation with species and with age. Endocrinology 1975;96:102–106.
33. Kakudo K, Uematsu K, Sakurai K, Suehiro M, Fukuchi M. Somatostatin-like immunoreactivity in rat thyroid. Age-associated S-cell hyperplasia. Cell Tissue Res 1984;238:661–663.
34. Hotta H, Ooka H, Sato A. Changes in basal secretion rates of thyroxine and 3,3',5-triiodothyronine from the thyroid gland during aging of the rat. Jpn J Physiol 1991;41:75–84.
35. Segal J, Troen BR, Ingbar SH. Influence of age and sex on the concentrations of thyroid hormone in serum in the rat. J Endocrinol 1982;93:177–181.
36. Chen HJ, Walfish PG. Effect of age and ovarian function on the pituitary-thyroid system in female rats. J Endocrinol 1978;78:225–232.
37. Reymond F, Denereaz N, Lemarchand-Beraud T. Thyrotropin action is impaired in the thyroid gland of old rats. Acta Endocrinol 1992;126:55–63.
38. Ambesi-Impiombato FS, Perrild H. FRTL-5 Today. Int Congr Ser 818, Excerpta Medica, Amsterdam, 1989, p. 1.
39. Cowin AJ, Davis JRE, Bidey SP. Transforming growth factor-β_1 production in porcine thyroid follicular cells: regulation by intrathyroidal organic iodine. J Mol Endocrinol 1992;9:197–205.
40. Cowin AJ, Heaton EL, Cheshire SH, Bidey SP. The proliferative responses of procine thyroid follicular cells to epidermal growth factor and thyrotrophin reflect the autocrine production of transforming growth factor-β1. J Endocrinol 1996;148:87–94.
41. Derwahl M, Seto P, Rapoport B. An abnormal splice donor site in one allele of the thyroid peroxidase gene in FRTL-5 rat thyroid cells introduces a premature stop codon: association with the absence of functional enzymatic activity. Mol Endocrinol 1990;4:793–799.
42. Beere HM, Soden J, Tomlinson S, Bidey SP. Insulin-like growth factor-I production and action in porcine thyroid follicular cells in monolayer: regulation by transforming growth factor-β. J Endocrinol 1991;130:3–9.
43. Tsushima T, Arai M, Saji M, Ohba Y, Murakami H, Ohmura E, Sato K, Shizume K. Effects of transforming growth factor-β on deoxyribonucleic acid synthesis and iodide metabolism in porcine thyroid cells in culture. Endocrinology 1988;123:1187–1194.
44. Bellur S, Tahara K, Saji M, Grollman EF, Kohn LD. Repeatedly passed FRTL-5 rat thyroid cells can develop insulin and insulin-like growth factor-I-sensitive cyclooxygenase and prostaglandin E_2 isomerase-like activities together with altered basal and thyrotropin-responsive thymidine incorporation into DNA. Endocrinology 1990;127:1526–1540.
45. Taton M, Lamy F, Roger PP, Dumont JE. General inhibition by transforming growth factor β_1 of thyrotropin and cAMP responses in human thyroid cells in primary culture. Mol Cell Endocrinol 1993; 95:13–21.
46. Coppa A, Mincione G, Mammarella S, Ranieri A, Colletta G. Epithelial rat thyroid cell clones, escaping from transforming growth factor beta negative growth control, are still inhibited by this factor in the ability to trap iodide. Cell Growth Diff 1995;6:281–290.
47. Yuasa R, Eggo MC, Meinkoth J, Dillmann WH, Burrow GN. Iodide induces transforming growth factor beta1 (TGF-β_1) mRNA in sheep thyroid cells. Thyroid 1992;2:141–145.
48. Grubeck-Loebenstein B, Buchan G, Sadeghi R, Kissonerghis M, Londei M, Turner M, et al. Transforming growth factor beta regulates thyroid growth. Role in the pathogenesis of nontoxic goiter. J Clin Invest 1989;83:764–770.
49. Pekary AE, Hershman JM. Tumor necrosis factor, ceramide, Transforming growth factor-β_1 and aging reduce Na$^+$/I$^-$ symporter messenger ribonucleic acid levels in FRTL-5 cells. Endocrinology 1998;139: 703–712.
50. Pekary AE, Berg L, Wang J, Lee P, Dubinett SM, Hershman JM. TNF-α, TSH and aging regulate TGF-β_1 synthesis and secretion in FRTL-5 rat thyroid cells. Am J Physiol 1995;268:R808–R815.
51. Pekary AE, Levin SR, Johnson DG, Berg L, Hershman JM. Tumor necrosis factor-α (TNF-α) and transforming growth factor-β_1 (TGF-β_1) inhibit the expression and activity of Na$^+$/K$^+$-ATPase in FRTL-5 rat thyroid cells. J Interferon Cytokine Res 1997;17:185–195.
52. Sporn MB, Roberts AB, ed. Peptide Growth Factors and Their Receptors, Vols 1 and 2, Springer-Verlag, New York, 1990.
53. Bassing CH, Howe DJ, Segarini PR, Donahoe PK, Wang X-F. A single heteromeric receptor complex is sufficient to mediate biological effects of transforming growth factor-β ligands. J Biol Chem 1994;269:14,861–14,864.
54. Robuschi G, Safran M, Braverman LE, Gnudi A, Roti E. Hypothyroidism in the elderly. Endocr Rev 1987;8:142–152.

55. Griffin JE. Hypothyroidism in the elderly. Am J Med Sci 1990;299:334–345.
56. Levy EG. Thyroid disease in the elderly. Med Clin N Am 1991;75:151–167.
57. Mokshagundam S, Barzel US. Thyroid disease in the elderly. J Am Geriatrics Soc 41: 1993;1361–1369.
58. Chopra IJ. Euthyroid sick syndrome: is it a misnomer? J Clin Endocrinol Metab 1997;82:329–334.
59. Martin FIR, Tress B, Colman PG, Ream DR. Iodine-induced hyperthyroidism due to nonionic contrast radiography in the elderly. Am J Med 1993;95:78–82.
60. Surks MI, Sievert R. Drugs and thyroid function. N Engl J Med 1995;333:1688–1694.
61. Hershman JM, Pekary AE, Berg L, Solomon DH, Sawin CT. Serum thyrotropin and thyroid hormone levels in elderly and middle-aged euthyroid persons. J Am Geriatrics Soc 1993;41:823–828.
62. Barreca T, Franceschini R, Messina V, Bottaro L, Rolandi E. 24-hour thyroid-stimulating hormone secretory pattern in elderly men. Gerontology 1985;31:119–123.
63. Doucet J, Trivalle Ch, Chassagne PH, Perol MB, Vuillermet P, Manchon ND, Menard JF, Bercoff E. Does age play a role in the clinical presentation of hypothyroidism? J Am Geriatr Soc 1994;42:984–986.
64. Davis PJ, Davis FB. Hyperthyroidism in patients over the age of 60 years. Clinical features in 85 patients. Medicine 1974;53:161–179.
65. Tibaldi JM, Barzel US, Albin J, Surks M. Thyrotoxicosis in the very old. Am J Med 1986;81:619–622.
66. Nordyke RA, Gilbert FI, Harada ASM. Graves' Disease. Influence of age on clinical findings. Arch Intern Med 1988;148:626–631.
67. Martin FIR, Deam DR. Hyperthyroidism in elderly hospitalised patients. Clinical features and treatment outcomes. Med J Aust 1996;164:200–203.
68. Trivalle C, Doucet J, Chassagne P, Landrin I, Kadri N, Menard JF, Bercoff E. Differences in the signs and symptoms of hyperthyroidism in older and younger patients. J Am Geriatr Soc 1996;44:50–53.
69. Lahey FH. Apathetic thyroidism. Ann Surg 1931;94:1026–1030.
70. Surks MI, Ocampo E. Subclinical thyroid disease. Am J Med 1996;100:217–223.
71. Ayala AR, Wartofsky L. Minimally symptomatic (subclinical) hypothyroidism. Endocrinologist 1997; 7:44–50.
72. Sawin CT, Castelli WP, Hershman JM, McNamara P, Bacharach P. The aging thyroid. Thyroid deficiency in the Framingham Study. Arch Intern Med 1985;145:1386–1388.
73. Parle JV, Franklyn JA, Cross KW, Jones SC, Sheppard MC. Prevalence and follow-up of abnormal thyrotrophin (TSH) concentrations in the elderly in the United Kingdom. Clin Endocrinol 1991;34: 77–83.
74. Bagchi N, Brown TR, Parish RF. Thyroid dysfunction in adults over age 55 years. A study in an urban US community. Arch Intern Med 1990;150:785–787.
75. Falkenberg M, Kagedal B, Norr A. Screening of an elderly female population for hypo- and hyperthyroidism by use of a thyroid hormone panel. Acta Med Scand 1983;214:361–365.
76. Bemben D, Winn P, Hamm RM, Morgan L, Davis A, Barton E. Thyroid disease in the elderly. Part 1. Prevalence of undiagnosed hypothyroidism. J Fam Pract 1994;38:577–582.
77. Drinka PJ, Nolten WE. Prevalence of previously undiagnosed hypothyroidism in residents of a midwestern nursing home. South Med J 1990;83:1259–1265.
78. Brochmann H, Bjoro T, Baarder PI, Hanson F, Frey HM. Prevalence of thyroid dysfunction in elderly subjects. A randomized study in a Norwegian community (Naeroy). Acta Endocrinol 1988;117:7–12.
79. Rosenthal MJ, Hunt WC, Garry PJ, Goodwin JS. Thyroid failure in the elderly. Microsomal antibodies as discriminant for therapy. JAMA 1987;258:209–213.
80. Livingston EH, Hershman JM, Sawin CT, Yoshikawa TT. Prevalence of thyroid disease and abnormal thyroid tests in older hospitalized and ambulatory persons. J Am Geriatrics Soc 1987;35:109–114.
81. Sawin CT, Chopra D, Azizi F, Mannix JE, Bacharach P. The aging thyroid. Increased prevalence of elevated serum thyrotropin levels in the elderly. JAMA 1979;242:247–250.
82. Manciet G, Dartigues JF, Decamps A, Barberger-Gateau P, Letenneur L, Latapie MJ, Latapie JL. The PAQUID survey and correlates of subclinical hypothyroidism in elderly community residents in the southwest of France. Age Aging 1995;24:235–241.
83. Tunbridge WMG, Evered DC, Hall R, Appleton D, Brewis M, Clark F, et al. The spectrum of thyroid disease in a community: the Whickham survey. Clin Endocrinol 1977;7:481–493.
84. Mariotti S, Barbesino G, Caturegli P, Bartalena L, Sansoni P, Fagnoni F, et al. Complex alteration of thyroid function in healthy centenarians. J Clin Endocrinol Metab 1993;77:1130–1134.
85. Luboshitzky R, Oberman AS, Kaufman N, Reichman N, Flatau E. Prevalence of cognitive dysfunction and hypothyroidism in an elderly community population. Isr J Med Sci 1996;32:60–65.

86. Hawkins BR, Dawkins RL, Burger HG, Mackay IR, Cheah PS, Whittingham S, Patel Y, Welcorn TA. Diagnostic significance of thyroid microsomal antibodies in randomly selected population. Lancet 1980;ii:1057–1059.

87. Geul KW, van Sluisveld ILL, Grobbee DE, Docter R, deBruyn AM, Hooykaas H, et al. The importance of thyroid microsomal antibodies in the development of elevated serum TSH in middle-aged women: associations with serum lipids. Clin Endocrinol 1993;39:275–280.

88. Vanderpump MPJ, Tunbridge WMG, French JM, Appleton D, Bates D, Clark F, et al. The incidence of thyroid disorders in the community: a twenty-year follow-up of the Whickham survey. Clin Endocrinol 1995;43:55–68.

89. Gordin A, Lamberg BA. Spontaneous hypothyroidism in symptomless autoimmune thyroiditis. A long-term follow-up study. Clin Endocrinol 1981;15:537–543.

90. Huber G, Mitrache C, Guglielmetti M, Huber P, Staub JJ. Predictors of overt hypothyroidism and natural course: a long-term follow-up study in impending thyroid failure. Thyroid 1997;7(Suppl 1): S-2 (abstract).

91. Sawin CT, Geller A, Kaplan MM, Bacharach P, Wilson PWF, Hershman JM. Low serum thyrotropin (thyroid stimulating hormone) in older persons without hyperthyroidism. Arch Intern Med 1991;151: 165–168.

92. Sundbeck G, Jagenburg R, Johansson PM, Eden S, Lindstedt G. Clinical significance of low serum thyrotropin concentration by chemiluminometric assay in 85-year old women and men. Arch Intern Med 1991;151:549–556.

93. Tenerz A, Forberg R, Jansson RJ. Is a more active attitude warranted in patients with subclinical thyrotoxicosis? J Int Med 1990;228:229–233.

94. Stott DJ, McLellan AR, Finlayson J, Chu P, Alexander WD. Elderly patients with suppressed serum TSH but normal free thyroid hormone levels usually have mild thyroid overactivity and are at increased risk of developing overt hyperthyroidism. Quart J Med 1991;285:77–84.

95. Sawin CT, Bigos ST, Land S, Bacharach P. The aging thyroid. Relationship between elevated serum thyrotropin level and thyroid antibodies in elderly patients. Am J Med 1985;79:591–594.

96. Sundbeck G, Eden S, Jagenburg R, Lundberg PA, Lindstedt G. Prevalence of serum antithyroid peroxidase antibodies in 85-year-old women and men. Clin Chem 1995;41:707–712.

97. Charkes ND. The many causes of subclinical hyperthyroidism. Thyroid 1996;6:391–396.

98. Crowley WF, Ridgway EC, Bough EW. Noninvasive evaluation of cardiac function in hypothyroidism. N Engl J Med 1977;296:1–6.

99. Franels GS, Daniel GH, Kourides IA, Myers GS, Maloof F, Kinlaw WB. Thyroid disorders and cholesterol: identifying the realm of clinical relevance. The Endocrinologist 1995;5:147–155.

100. Arem R, Escalante DA, Arem N, Morrisett JD, Patsch W. Effect of I-thyroxine therapy on lipoprotein fractions in overt and subclinical hypothyroidism, with special reference to lipoprotein(a). Metabolism 1995;44:1159–1163.

101. Ridgway EC, Ladenson PW, Cooper DS, Daniels GH, Francis GS, Maloof F. Cardiac function in mild and severe primary hypothyroidism. Life Sci 1982;30:651–659.

102. Nystrom E, Caidahl K, Fager G, Wikkelso C, Lundberg PA, Lindstedt G. A double-blind crossover 12-month study of L-thyroxine treatment of women with subclinical hypothyroidism. Clin Endocrinol 29:1988;63–76.

103. Arem R, Rokey R, Kiefe C, Escalante DA, Rodriquez A. Cardiac systolic and diastolic function at rest and exercise in subclinical hypothyroidism: effect of thyroid hormone therapy. Thyroid 1996;6:397–402.

104. Bogner U, Arntz HR, Peters H, Schleusener H. Subclinical hypothyroidism and hyperlipoproteinaemia: indiscriminate L-thyroxine treatment not justified. Acta Endocrinol 1993;128:202–206.

105. Arem R, Ratsch W. Lipoprotein and apolipoprotein levels in subclinical hypothyroidism. Effect of levothyroxine therapy. Arch Intern Met 1990;150:2097–2100.

106. Franklyn JA, Daykin J, Betteridge J, Hughes EA, Holder R, Jones SR, Sheppard MC. Thyroxine replacement therapy and circulating lipid concentrations. Clin Endocrinol 1993;38:453–459.

107. Staub JJ, Althaus BU, Engler H, Ryff AS, Trabucco P, Marquardt K, et al. Spectrum of subclinical and overt hypothyroidism: effect on thyrotropin, prolactin, and thyroid reserve, and metabolic impact on peripheral target tissues. Am J Med 1992;92:631–642.

108. Ridgway EC, Cooper DS, Walker H, Rodbard D, Maloof F. Peripheral responses to thyroid hormone before and after I-thyroxine therapy in patients with subclinical hypothyroidism. J Clin Endocrinol Metab 1981;53:1238–1242.

109. Monzani F, Del Guerra P, Caraccio N, Pruneti CA, Pucci E, Luisi M, Baschieri L. Subclinical hypothyroidism: neurobehavioral features and beneficial effect of I-thyroxine treatment. Clin Invest 1993;71: 367–371.

110. Klein I, Ojamaa K. Editorial: thyroid hormone and the cardiovascular system: from theory to practice. J Clin Endocrinol Metab 1994;78:1026–1027.

111. Biondi B, Fazio S, Carella C, Amato G, Cittadini A, Lupoli G, et al. Cardiac effects of long term thyrotropin-suppressive therapy with levothyroxine. J Clin Endocrinol Metab 1993;77:334–338.

112. Shapiro LE, Sievert R, Ong L, Ocampo EL, Chance RA, Lee M, et al. Minimal cardiac effects in asymptomatic athyreotic patients chronically treated with thyrotropin-suppressive doses of I-thyroxine. J Clin Endocrinol Metab 1997;82:2592–2595.

113. Sawin CT, Geller A, Wolf PA, Belanger AJ, Baker E, Bacharach P, et al. Low serum thyrotropin concentrations as a risk factor for atrial fibrillation in older persons. N Engl J Med 1994;331:1249–1252.

114. Lee MS, Kim SY, Lee MC, et al. Negative correlation between the change in bone mineral density and serum osteocalcin in patients with hyperthyroidism. J Clin Endocrinol Metab 1990;70:766–770.

115. Mudde AH, Reijinders FJL, Nieuwenhuijzen Kruseman AC. Peripheral bone density in women with untreated multinodular goitre. Clin Endocrinol 1992;37:35–39.

116. Foldes J, Tarjan G, Szathmari M, Varga F, Krasznai I, Horvath C. Bone mineral density in patients with endogenous subclinical hyperthyroidism: is this thyroid status a risk factor for osteoporosis? Clin Endocrinol 1993;39:521–527.

117. Faber J, Galloe AM. Changes in bone mass during prolonged subclinical hyperthyroidism due to I-thyroxine treatment: a meta-analysis. Eur J Endocrinol 1994;130:350–356.

118. Uzzan B, Campos J, Cucherat M, Nony P, Boissel JP, Perret GY. Effects on bone mass of long-term treatment with thyroid hormones: a meta-analysis. J Clin Endocrinol Metab 1996;81:4278–4289.

119. Stall GM, Harris S, Sokoll LJ, Dawson-Hughes B. Accelerated bone loss in hypothyroid patients overtreated with I-thyroxine. Ann Int Med 1990;113:265–269.

120. Pioli G, Pedrazzoni M, Palummeri E, Sianesi M, Del Frate R, Vescove PP, et al. Longitudinal study of bone loss after thyroidectomy and suppressive thyroxine therapy in premenopausal women. Acta Endocrinol 1992;126:238–242.

121. Rosenbaum RL, Barzel US. Levothyroxine replacement dose for primary hypothyroidism decreases with age. Ann Int Med 1982;96:53–55.

122. Sawin CT, Herman T, Molitch ME, London MH, Kramer SM. Aging and the thyroid. Decreased requirement for thyroid hormone in older hypothyroid patients. Am J Med 1983;75:206–209.

123. Ladenson PW, Levin AA, Ridgway EC, Daniels GH. Complications of surgery in hypothyroid patients. AM J Med 1984;77:261–266.

124. Danese M, Ladenson P, Powe N. Effect of L-thyroxine on serum lipids in mild thyroid failure: a meta-analysis. American Thyroid Association 1997;179:(S-90) (Abstract).

125. Rotti E, Colzani R, Braverman LE. Adverse effects of iodine on the thyroid. Endocrinologist 1997;7: 245–254.

126. Morley JE. The aging endocrine system: evaluation and treatment of age-related disorders. Postgrad Med 1983;73:107–120.

127. Vander JB, Gaston EA, Dawber TR. The significance of nontoxic thyroid nodules: final report of a 15-year study of the incidence of thyroid malignancy. Ann Intern Med 1968;69:537–540.

128. Ezzat S, Sarti DA, Cain DR, Braunstein GD. Thyroid incidentalomas. Prevalence by palpation and ultrasonography. Arch Intern Med 1994;154:1838–1840.

129. Mortensen JD, Woolner LB, Bennett WA. Gross and microscopic findings in clinically normal thyroid glands. J Clin Endocrinol Metab 1955;15:1270–1276.

130. Wheeler MH. Investigation of the solitary thyroid nodule. Clin Endocrinol 1996;44: 245–247.

131. Mazzaferri EL. Management of a solitary thyroid nodule. N Engl J Med 1993;328:553–559.

132. Gharib H, Goellner JR. Fine needle aspiration biopsy of the thyroid: an appraisal: Ann Int Med 1993; 118:282–289.

133. Gharib H. Fine-needle asiration biopsy of thyroid nodules: advantages, limitations, and effect. Mayo Clin Proc 1994;69:44–49.

134. Gharib H, Mazzaferri EL. Thyroxine suppressive therapy in patients with nodular thyroid disease. Ann Intern Med 1998;128:386–394.

135. La Rosa GL, Lupo L, Giuffrida D, Gullo D, Vigneri R, Bellfiore A. Levothyroxine and potassium iodide are both effective in treating benign solitary solid cold nodules of the thyroid. Ann Intern Med 1995;122:1–8.

136. Celani MF, Mariani M, Mariani G. On the usefulness of levothyroxine suppressive therapy in the medical treatment of benign solitary solid, or predominantly solid, thyroid nodules. Acta Endocrinol 1990;123:603–608.

137. Boring CC, Squires TS, Tong T. Cancer statistics. CA Cancer J Clin 1993;43:7–26.

138. Bondeson L, Ljungberg O. Occult papillary thyroid carcinoma in the young and the aged. Cancer 1984; 53:1790–1792.

139. Dulgeroff AJ, Hershman JM. Medical therapy for differentiated thyroid carcinoma. Endocr Rev 1994; 15:500–515.

140. Sizemore GW. Medullary carcinoma of the thyroid gland. Semin Oncol 1987;14:306–314.

141. Ain K. Anaplastic thyroid cancer. Behavior, biology, and therapeutic approaches. Thyroid 1998;8: 715–726.

142. Matsuzuka F, Miyauchi A, Katayama S, Narabayashi I, Ikeda H, Kuma K, Sugawara M. Clinical aspects of primary thyroid lymphoma: diagnosis and treatment based on our experience of 119 cases. Thyroid 1993;3:93–99.

5

Stress, Hormones, and Aging

Scott P. Van Sant, MD,
Emile D. Risby, MD,
and Charles B. Nemeroff, MD, PHD

CONTENTS

INTRODUCTION

The relationship among stress, hormones, and aging is complex and involves the interplay between three major physiological levels: molecular, cellular, and neuroendocrine *(1)*. In this context, the molecular level refers to those intracellular biochemical processes directly related to the genome, such as transcription, and how gene expression is modified by age, stress, or a combination of the two. The cellular level refers to the heterogeneous cell populations within complex tissues that proliferate and/or die off during the life-span. A loss or gain of a particular cell type, or a change in the ratio of responsive to nonresponsive cells, would likely alter the organism's response to a stressor, as a direct result of the natural aging process. The neuroendocrine level refers to the various neurotransmitter and hormonal systems that modulate a host of biological functions, including those systems preeminently involved in the organism's response to stress. Stress can be defined as any force that changes the organism's baseline equilibrium or homeostasis *(2)*. Environmental factors can generically be described as "stress." An organism's adaptive response to stress is generally aimed at minimizing dysequilibrium and reestablishing homeostasis. If the adaptive responses to stress are inadequate for the reestablishment of homeostasis, or are prolonged or excessive, the organism will acquire negative stress-induced consequences. Stress and changes in the stress response system can either protect against or facilitate aging. Thus, many genetic factors are responsible for the aging process, but the interplay between the organism and its external environment is clearly of paramount importance *(1)*.

From: *Contemporary Endocrinology: Endocrinology of Aging*
Edited by: J. E. Morley and L. van den Berg © Humana Press Inc., Totowa, NJ

MOLECULAR AND CELLULAR LEVELS

There are several molecular-based conceptualizations of the aging process. Programmed senescence encompasses the concept of a genetically predetermined maximum life-span. However, stress can induce hormonal and biochemical changes in the organism that can modify the genetically predetermined programmed senescence and the rate at which an organism ages *(3)*. Another genetically determined concept of the aging process is the "life maintenance reserve," which describes the organism's functional potential. Two key components of the life maintenance reserve are the organism's maximum metabolic capacity, which is genetically predetermined, and its stress responses. Stress can stimulate numerous pathways that increase the production of oxidants and free radicals. Oxidative damage occurs when the highly reactive free radicals form indiscriminant bonds with a variety of molecules, such as cellular enzymes, membranes, and the cellular genome, damaging them in the process. Mitochondrial DNAs are particularly susceptible to this damage, because of their proximity to the respiratory centers of the cell. The oxidative-induced DNA damage may modify gene expression at the transcriptional level, producing changes in cytokines, growth factors, and/or hormonal regulators. This damage compromises the cell's metabolic and recuperative abilities to further stress challenges, and thus decreases the life maintenance reserve. Subsequent stressors will have more deleterious effects on the cell, because of the decreased ability of the cell to remove oxidative toxins, and because of altered biochemical regulators. This can lead to metabolic derangement and cell death, particularly in times of physical or biologic stress *(4)*. Therefore, stress-induced changes at the cellular level, and in the cellular genome, contribute to the aging process *(4,5)*.

NEUROENDOCRINE LEVEL

Physiologic Stress Response

An animal's physiologic response to stress involves activation of multiple biochemical and hormonal cascades. In general, however, central and peripheral stress response systems are designed to preserve the organism when stressed. In times of stress, pathways are activated in the central nervous system (CNS) that mediate arousal, alertness, vigilance, cognition, attention, and aggression. There is an adaptive redirection of energy in the periphery, with an increase in cardiovascular tone, respiratory rate, gluconeogenesis, and lipolysis. Pathways that subserve vegetative functions, such as feeding and reproduction, are inhibited *(6)*.

The brainstem locus coeruleus–norepinephrine (LC–NE) system plays a key role in the acute stress response. The LC–NE system contributes to activating the mesocortical and mesolimbic dopamine (DA) systems. The mesocortical system innervates the prefrontal cortex, which is thought to be involved in anticipatory phenomena and cognitive function. The mesolimbic DA system includes the nucleus accumbens, which is thought to play a principal role in motivational/reinforcement phenomena. Noradrenergic neurons originating from the LC–NE system also stimulate the amygdala–hippocampus complex. Emotional stressors originating from memory-storing subcortical and cortical areas of the brain can also activate this complex. Activation of the amygdala is important for retrieval and emotional analysis of information pertinent to the stressor (Fig. 1). The LC–NE system also innervates and activates the paraventricular nucleus–corticotropin-

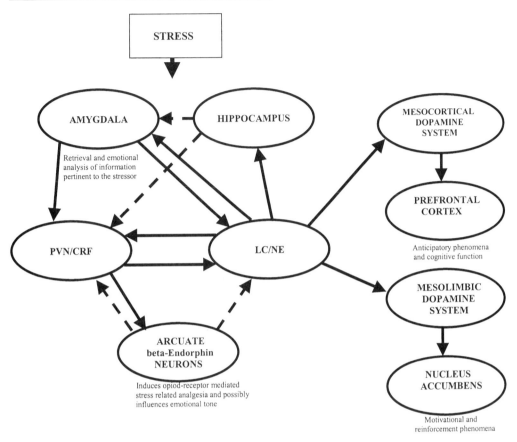

Fig. 1. Brain systems tied into the stress response. PVN=paraventricular nucleus. CRF=corticotropin releasing factor. LC=locus coeruleus. NE=norepinephrine. POMC=proopiomelanocortin. Dotted lines indicate inhibitory influence; solid lines indicate stimulatory influence.

releasing factor (PVN–CRF) system. In addition to its primary role in releasing CRF from nerve terminals in the median eminence, which activates the hypothalamic–pituitary–thyroid (HPA) axis by releasing adrenocorticotrophic hormone (ACTH) from the anterior pituitary, CRF neurons in the PVN also project to and stimulate β-endorphin neurons in the arcuate nucleus. These pro-opiomelanocortin-containing neurons project back to the PVN and brainstem to inhibit the activity of CRF neurons and the LC–NE system, respectively. β-endorphin inhibition of sympathomimetic activation may be one mechanism of stress-related analgesia via endogenous opioid receptors, and may indirectly influence emotional tone (Fig. 1; *6*). The hippocampus appears to exert an inhibitory influence on the activity of the amygdala and the PVN–CRF system.

The LC–NE and CRF systems are interconnected via a positive feedback loop, so that activation of one system tends to activate the other system as well (Fig. 2). Anatomically, this involves noradrenergic projections from the LC–NE system to the PVN, and projections of CRF-secreting neurons from the PVN back to the LC. Furthermore, the same neurochemical modulators also affect the PVN–CRF and LC–NE system. Serotonin and acetylcholine activate both systems; γ-aminobutyric acid, opioids, and glucocorticoids inhibit them (Fig. 1; *6*).

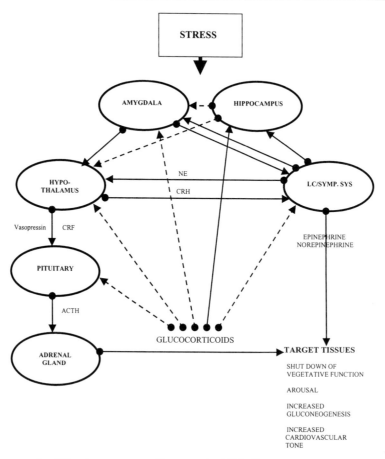

Fig. 2. Components of the stress system. Glucocorticoid binding to receptors in the Hippocampus is transmitted as an inhibitory neural signal to the HPA axis. NE=norepinephrine. CRF=corticotropin-releasing factor. ACTH=adrenocorticotropic hormone. LC/symp. sys.=Locus Coeruleus/sympathetic system. Solid lines indicate stimulatory effect, dotted lines a negative effect.

As noted above, activation of CRF neurons ultimately results in an increase in HPA axis activity, with increased release and production of glucocorticoids. It is believed that the physiological function of stress-induced increases in glucocorticoids is to help protect the organism from the damaging effects of the acute stress response. Glucocorticoids have an inhibitory effect on the entire LC–NE system, as well as feedback inhibition of the HPA axis, thereby acting as a safety buffer against extreme or prolonged stress responses. If there are defects in this buffer system, or if the buffer system is overwhelmed, the organism can suffer negative physiologic consequences of prolonged stress. The available research data suggest that glucocorticoid receptors are involved in the feedback inhibition of the LC–NE system and the HPA axis. Short-term elevations in glucocorticoid levels activate glucocorticoid receptors in the PVN and LC. These activated glucocorticoid receptors mediate the inhibition of both LC and HPA axis activity (Fig. 2). However, in the presence of long-term elevations of glucocorticoid levels, downregulation of glucocorticoid receptors occur, decreasing the central inhibitory effects of the glucocorticoids, which results in an increase in the activity of both the LC–NE and HPA systems. Thus, although the secretion of glucocorticoids is the final stage in the neuroendocrine response to stress, prolonged periods of stress lead to persistent downregulation of glucocorticoid receptors, and thereby disrupt negative feedback (2).

Glucocorticoids themselves inhibit numerous intracellular processes associated with growth, repair, immune function, and metabolism. Therefore, glucocorticoids impair the capacity of cells to recover from injury (7). Furthermore, glucocorticoids enhance the excitatory amino acid (EAA)-induced increases in intracellular calcium (Ca), thereby exacerbating the physiologic effects of these endogenous neurotoxins. Intracellular calcium activates membrane-bound phospholipase A_2 which results in the formation of arachidonic acid and free radicals. Both arachidonic acid and free radicals enhance the release of glutamate, thus perpetuating a vicious cycle. Ca^{2+} also activates proteases, lipases, and nucleases that cause enzymatic damage to the cell's regenerating machinery, thereby producing more free radicals. Finally, the combination of free radical damage and Ca-induced enzymatic damage eventually overcomes the cell's recuperative abilities, resulting in permanent cellular degeneration. Therefore, glucocorticoids increase the vulnerability of cells, especially neurons, to metabolic insults, and potentate the deleterious actions of EAAs and oxidative stress (8).

Glucocorticoids and catecholamines are both critical to surviving an acute stressor, but they are capable of causing end organ damage, if persistently elevated. This may lead to many of the disease states associated with aging, such as muscle atrophy, hypertension, insulin resistance, amenorrhea, elevated cholesterol and triglyceride levels, an increase in atherosclerosis and osteoporosis, and a decreased immune function and tissue repair. Chronic increases in glucocorticoids may contribute to the cognitive disturbances reported in both depression and aging. Glucocorticoid-induced memory disturbances in humans appear to be secondary to their effects on hippocampal-dependent memory processes. The administration of glucocorticoids decreases declarative memory performance in all healthy adults, but the elderly appear to be more sensitive to this glucocorticoid effect (9,10).

Therefore, chronic stress can induce disease, aging, and even death (11). The neuroendocrine stress response system can effect numerous other hormonal systems. Figure 3 outlines some of the various interactions between the stress system and other biological systems. Collectively, the function of these stress-induced hormonal reactions appear to be the conservation of energy during periods of prolonged stress (6).

Psychological Aspects

Activation of the stress response system can occur in times of distress or pleasure. Adaptive and controlled activation of the stress system is often associated with pleasure; maladaptive activation is often associated with dysphoria (12). An individual's psychological makeup, coping style, and subjective experience of the stress all influence the response to the stressor. The supposition is that individuals with emotional instability, significant psychological conflicts, and limited coping abilities will have a less adaptive stress response, and suffer more negative consequences from stress, including an increase in stress-mediated illnesses and the aging process (13). Because of different coping abilities, individuals may have different responses to the same stressor (6). For the purposes of this discussion, coping may be defined as the individual's ability to avoid being stressed. In a study of parents whose children were dying of leukemia, there were differences found in the excretion of urinary corticosteroids (a measure of the HPA axis stress response) among parents with different personalities and coping styles (14). Those parents exhibiting

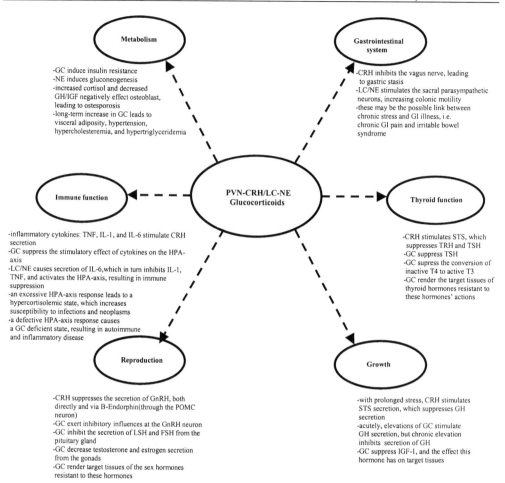

Fig. 3. Effect of the stress system on other endocrine systems. GC=glucocorticoids. NE=norepine-phrine. CRF=corticotropin-releasing-factor. STS=somatostatin. IGF-1=insulin-like-growth factor. IL-1=interleukin-1. IL-6=interleukin-6. TNF=tumor necrosis factor. HPA-axis=hypothalamic-pituitary-adrenal axis. LC/NE=locus coeruleus/norepinephrine. T4=thyroxine. T3=triodothyronine. TRH=thryoid releasing hormone. TSH=thyroid stimulating hormone. (Chrousos and Gold, 1992)

significant levels of hysteria demonstrated relatively normal levels of corticosteroid secretion, rather than the expected elevated levels. Those parents who used denial as a defense only showed elevated levels when forced to face their child's impending death *(14)*.

The individual's perception of the stress is also clearly important. The perception of the stress may result in sensitization or attenuation of future stress responses. These sensitized or attenuated responses may be pathological, or they may be adaptive. For example, large increases in peripheral stress hormones are observed in first-time para-chutists, yet, with subsequent jumps, there is a blunting in this hormonal response *(14)*. Therefore, expectations and psychological defense mechanisms can modify one's response to a stressor. These modifications may be healthy or unhealthy, depending on the circum-stances. Unfortunately, chronic activation of the stress response system generally has detri-mental effects *(15)*.

There is evidence that exposure to stress in early development can alter physiologic responses to subsequent stress on permanent basis. Shalyapina et al. *(16)* demonstrated that external stress or the administration of corticosteroids during certain critical periods of a rat's development had permanent effects on stress responsiveness later in life. In this study, corticosteroid levels were used as an indicator of HPA axis activity. They linked the evolution of the HPA system with critical periods in the rat's development, which included when the rat's ears and eyes opened (orientative/investigative), when they developed the ability to move (adaptive), and when they were weaned from their mothers (exaltation). When stress was introduced at these critical periods of development, these adult rats differed from controls in having an increased sensitivity of the HPA axis to stress. In addition, rats given corticosteroids (an artificial induction of the stress response) in early neonatal ontogenesis, also demonstrated hypersensitivity in the HPA axis, and weakening of the HPA negative feedback mechanism later in life *(16)*. This data supports the theory that an acute stress response can have long-term effects on an organism. As reviewed by Chrousos and Gold *(6)*, there is an association between dysregulation of the HPA axis and several psychiatric conditions, including depression, anorexia nervosa, panic/anxiety, obsessive-compulsive disorder, and chronic active alcoholism. It is unclear whether this dysregulation is a primary or secondary effect.

Many factors are involved in an individuals response to stress, including the magnitude and duration of the stressor, the timing of the event, the genetic makeup of the individual, and the influences of the social environment *(6)*. Therefore, in man, the physiological stress response cannot be viewed purely from a biochemical or hormonal perspective, but as the interplay between the psychological aspects of stress with the biological response to stress.

AGING

Depending on the duration of the stressor, the stress response can either protect against, or facilitate, the aging process. Furthermore, aged organisms might have a decreased ability to return to homeostasis once a stress has occurred. For example, in the classic rat-immobilization stress paradigm, postimmobilization corticosterone secretion ceases promptly within 1 h, and quickly returns to basal levels in young rats. In contrast, in aged rats, the increased secretion of corticosterone persists for several hours after the immobilization. Therefore, the senescent animal is quite capable of mounting a robust stress response, but has a decreased ability to terminate it. In the rat, the cause of this defect is believed to be age-related degeneration of the hippocampus, which is an important mediator of glucocorticoid feedback regulation. Activation of glucocorticoid receptors in the hippocampus results in inhibition of CRF release from the PVN, thereby decreasing activity of the HPA axis. The aged hippocampus loses glucocorticoid receptors, primarily because of the death of the pyramidal neurons that contain them. This decreases the ability of the hippocampus to detect the glucocorticoid signal and transmit the inhibitory glucocorticoid signal to the HPA axis (Fig. 1). Although the aging human hippocampus does appear to sustain neuronal loss *(11)*, hippocampal dysfunction is not typically found in the normal elderly human. However, because of normal hippocampal cell death, dysregulation of systems that are mediated by the hippocampus is more likely to occur in aged humans with co-morbid conditions. Wilkinson et al. (17) demonstrated, in healthy elderly subjects, compared to healthy young subjects, that there is a reduced responsiveness to glucocorticoid feedback inhibition by cortisol on the HPA axis. Thus, the elderly are more vulnerable to develop adrenocortical dysfunction, particularly HPA axis hyperactivity. For example, age is positively correlated with hypercortisolism in depressed patients. Thus, the older the depressed patient, the more likely the patient will exhibit elevated basal and postdexamethasone levels of cortisol. In aged rats, both the basal and poststress hypersecretion of corticosterone appear to be secondary to a defect in the normal feedback inhibition of the HPA axis. The defect appears to be at a suprapituitary level, because there are also elevations in basal levels of ACTH, a decrease in adrenal sensitivity to ACTH, and a decrease in pituitary sensitivity to CRF. As in aged rats, hypercortisolemia in depressed humans appears to be secondary to a defect at the level of the hypothalamus, because of elevated ACTH concentrations and decreased pituitary responsiveness to CRF. An elegant example of the interaction of stress, aging, and the HPA axis was the demonstration by Stein-Behrans and Sapolsky *(7)* that tumor growth in rats was associated with stress-induced HPA axis activity. Aged rats had the greatest HPA axis response to stress, and exhibited the greatest tumor growth.

What is the connection among stress, hormones, and aging? The neuroendocrine responses to stress may ultimately induce cell damage and/or accelerate normal cell loss. One major determinant of hippocampal neuron loss appears to be the cumulative exposure of hippocampal neurons to glucocorticoids. Prolonged glucocorticoid exposure produces hippocampal degeneration similar to that observed during normal aging. The concatenation of studies reveals that prolonged exposure to glucocorticoids, whether because of exogenous hormone administration or repeated stressors, accelerates hippocampal aging. The loss of hippocampal inhibition of glucocorticoid secretion perpetuates a feed-forward cascade of senescent degeneration *(7)*. Elevated glucocorticoid levels secondary to stress, and hippocampal neuronal loss associated with normal aging, both result in a decrease in the inhibiting/buffering effects of brain glucocorticoid receptors. This may lead to a reduced brake function, so that each stress response is amplified in magnitude and protracted in time *(13)*. Consequently, the negative effects of a prolonged stress response is cellular damage, cell death, and aging. Cell damage results in a decreased ability to deal with further stress, setting off a vicious dysregulatory cascade.

SUMMARY

Stress is associated with the activation of both the LC–NE system and the HPA axis (via the PVN–CRF pathway). These systems are anatomically and functionally interconnected. The stress response of an organism is usually protective in nature, but, with prolonged stress, or when there is dysregulatory cascade, the stress response can produce detrimental effects. An appropriate adaptational response to stress requires the acute stress response system to respond quickly, followed by the activation of counterregulatory elements that protect the organism from the negative consequences of the acute stress response *(6)*. Although glucocorticoid secretion is vital to surviving short-term stress, overexposure to glucocorticoids or repeated stress can be deleterious, causing a variety of stress-related diseases. In humans, perception of the stressor may have more to do with the subsequent physiological response to the stressor than the specific characteristics of the stressor itself. Moreover, the individual biological responses to a specific stress, and the effects of that stress on the aging process, can be quite variable. The aging process itself is quite complex, and is at least partly determined by genetic influences, and partly by environmental effects on cellular and neuroendocrine processes. Taken together, however, it is clear that the HPA axis response is altered in the elderly in a variety of species, particularly by persistence of the glucocorticoid response to stress as well as hypersecretion. This has been hypothesized to be associated hippocampal neuronal degeneration, depression, impaired immune function, and cognitive impairment.

REFERENCES

1. Roth GS. Hormone action during aging: alterations and mechanisms. Mech Aging Dev 1979;9:497–514.
2. Chrousos GP. Stressors, stress, and neuroendocrine integration of the adaptive response. The 1997 Hans Selye memorial lecture. Ann NY Acad Sci 1997;851:311–335.
3. Parsons PA. Rapid development and a long life: an association expected under a stress theory of aging. Experientia 1996;52:643–646.
4. Mann DMA. Molecular biology's impact our understanding of aging. Br Med J 1997;315:1078–1081.
5. Jazwinski SM. Longevity, genes, and aging. Science 1996;273:54–59.
6. Chrousos GP, Gold PW. The concepts of stress and stress system disorders: overview of physical and behavioral homeostasis. JAMA 1992;267:1244–1252.
7. Stein-Behrens BA, Sapolsky RM. Stress, glucocorticoids, and aging. Aging 1992;4:197–210.
8. Busciglio J, Anderson JK, Schipper HM, Gilad GD, McCarty R, Marzatico F, Toussaint O. Stress, aging, and neurodegenerative disorders. Molecular mechanisms. Ann NY Acad Sci 1998;851:429–443.
9. Keenan PA, Jacobson MW, Soleymani RM, Newcomer JW. Commonly used therapeutic doses of glucocorticoids impair explicit memory. Ann NY Acad Sci 1995;761:400–402.
10. Newcomer JW, Craft S, Hershey T, Askins K, Bardgett ME. Glucocorticoid-induced impairment in declarative memory performance in adult humans. J Neurosci 1994;14:2047–2053.
11. Sapolsky R, Armanimi MS, Packan D, Tombaugh G. Stress and glucocorticoids and aging. Endocrinol Metab Clin 1987;16:965–980.
12. Stratakis CA, Chrousos GP. Neuroendocrinology and pathophysiology of the stress system. Ann NY Acad Sci 1995;771:1–18.
13. Bjornthorp P. Neuroendocrine ageing. J Intern Med 1995;238:401–404.
14. Rose RM. Overview of endocrinology of stress. In: Brown GM, ed. Neuroendocrinology and Psychiatric Disorder. Raven, New York, 1984, pp. 95–122.
15. Murburg MM. The psychobiology of posttraumatic stress disorder: an overview. Ann NY Acad Sci 1997;821:352–358.
16. Shalyapina VG, Ordyan NE, Pinvina SG, Rakitskaya VV. Neuroendocrine mechanisms of the formation of adaptive behavior. Neurosci Behav Physiol 1997;27:275–279.
17. Wilkinson CW, Peskind ER, Raskind MA. Decreased hypothalamic-pituitary-adrenal axis sensitivity to cortisol feedback inhibition in human aging. Neuroendocrinology 1997;65:79–90.

6

Water Balance in Older Persons

Myron Miller, MD

CONTENTS

INTRODUCTION

The normal regulation of water and electrolyte balance involves the interplay of many homeostatic systems that operate to maintain the composition of fluid and electrolyte compartments within a narrow range. In association with the normal aging process, the homeostatic systems involved may be compromised *(1)*. The key regulatory components of fluid balance include thirst perception, which governs fluid intake, and the kidney, which is governed by hemodynamic and hormonal influences through the actions of arginine vasopressin (AVP) or antidiuretic hormone (ADH), atrial natriuretic hormone (ANH), and aldosterone. Clinicians who are involved in the care of the elderly recognize that disturbances of water and electrolyte balance are common in this age group, especially when older persons are challenged by disease, drugs, or extrinsic factors, such as access to fluids or control of diet composition.

The confluence of normal aging changes, diseases common in the elderly, and the administration of many classes of drugs can lead to water retention or loss, and to hyponatremia or hypernatremia, with resultant symptomatic consequences. In some individuals, an impaired ability to conserve water may underlie the development of nocturnal urinary frequency, as well as urinary incontinence.

NORMAL AGING EFFECTS ON FLUID REGULATORY SYSTEMS
(TABLE 1)

Body Composition

Aging effects on body composition have the potential to contribute to derangements in fluid balance. Normal aging is accompanied by a decrease in lean body mass, an increase in fat, and a decrease in total body water *(2)*. Thus, total body water declines from the approximate values of 60% of body wt in young men and 52% in young women to 54 and 46%, respectively, in individuals over the age of 65 yr, primarily through a

From: *Contemporary Endocrinology: Endocrinology of Aging*
Edited by: J. E. Morley and L. van den Berg © Humana Press Inc., Totowa, NJ

Table 1
Aging Effects on Sodium and Water Regulatory Systems

Body composition
  Decreased total body water
  Decreased intracellular fluid compartment
Fluid intake
  Decreased thirst perception
Renal function
  Decreased kidney mass
  Decline in renal blood flow
  Decline in glomerular filtration rate
  Impaired distal renal tubular diluting capacity
  Impaired renal concentrating capacity
  Impaired sodium conservation
  Impaired renal response to vasopressin
Hormonal systems
  Vasopressin
    Normal or increased basal secretion
    Increased response to osmotic stimulation
    Decreased nocturnal secretion
  Atrial natriuretic hormone
    Increased basal secretion
    Increased response to stimulation
  Decreased plasma renin activity
  Decreased aldosterone production

decrease in the intracellular fluid compartment *(3)*. The decrease in total body water may place the older person at increased risk for dehydration when challanged by fluid loss or decreased fluid intake, and at increased risk for fluid overload and hyponatremia when exposed to excessive oral or parenteral fluid intake.

Aging and Fluid Intake

The ingestion of a sufficient volume of fluid to maintain a normal state of fluid balance requires that thirst perception be present, that a suitable source of fluid be available, and that the individual be physically capable of obtaining and consuming the fluid. In healthy young individuals, thirst becomes evident when plasma osmolality rises to values greater than 292 mosM/kg *(4)*. Healthy older persons (aged 67–75 yr), subjected to prolonged water deprivation capable of raising plasma osmolality to greater than 296 mosM/kg, have shown diminished subjective awareness of thirst. Thus, when these individuals are subsequently presented with water, they consume significantly less than young subjects whose plasma osmolality rose to a lesser level (mean 290 mosM/kg) following the same period of water deprivation *(5)*. Other studies of elderly patients with cerebrovascular accidents have similarly documented impaired thirst perception in the face of volume depletion and hyperosmolality, both normally being potent stimuli for thirst *(6)*. Elderly patients with Alzheimer's disease fail to drink adequately when exposed to water deprivation, in spite of the accompanying elevation of blood osmolality to levels above the usual thirst threshold *(7)*. Further confounding the ability of the elderly to ingest adequate amounts of fluid is the frequent presence of physical disability (e.g., blindness, arthritis, stroke) and impaired mobility, thus limiting the capacity of the patient to gain access to fluids.

Renal Changes of Normal Aging

STRUCTURAL AND FUNCTIONAL CHANGES

Normal aging is accompanied by changes in renal anatomy and in renal function. Kidney mass undergoes progressive decline, from a normal weight of approx 250–340 g in young adults to between 180 and 200 g by age 80–90 yr *(8)*. Histologically, the number of glomeruli decline with increasing age, and the percent of glomeruli that are hyalinized or sclerotic increase *(9)*. This process accelerates after the age of 40 yr, and the residual glomeruli also undergo changes with age *(10)*. Thus, there is a decrease in effective filtering surface, and an increase in number of mesangial cells, a decrease in number of epithelial cells, and thickening of the glomerular basement membrane *(11)*.

As part of the normal aging process, there are changes in the renal vasculature that lead to obliteration of the arteriolar lumen and loss of the glomerular capillary tuft. These changes take place primarily in the cortical glomeruli *(12,13)*. In the juxtamedullary area, glomerular sclerosis may lead to anastomosis between afferent and efferent arterioles, with direct shunting of blood between these vessels. Blood flow to the medulla, through the arteria rectae, is maintained in old age.

The anatomical changes of the aging kidney are paralleled by alterations in renal function, although a direct relationship between anatomical and functional changes is not firmly established. Renal blood flow declines during the course of normal aging by approx 10% per decade after young adulthood, so that, by the age of 90 yr, the renal plasma flow is approx 300 mL/min, a 50% reduction of the value found at 30 yr of age *(14)*. The decrease in renal perfusion is most extensive in the outer cortex, with lesser impairment of inner cortex and minimal effect on the medulla.

Glomerular filtration rate (GFR) remains relatively stable until age 40, after which it undergoes decline at an annual rate of approx $0.8 \text{ mL/min}/1.73 \text{ M}^2$ *(15)*. There is considerable variability of this renal alteration within the elderly population, so that decline in GFR is not seen in all aged individuals *(16)*.

WATER REGULATORY CAPACITY

Renal Water Retention. The aging kidney exhibits a modest age-related impairment in the ability to dilute the urine and excrete a water load. The ability to generate free water is dependent on several factors, including adequate delivery of solute to the diluting region (sufficient renal perfusion and glomerular filtration rate); a functional, intact distal diluting site (ascending limb of Henle's loop and the distal tubule); and suppression of ADH, in order to escape water reabsorption in the collecting duct *(17)*. The age-related decline in GFR is the most important factor in the aged kidney's diluting capacity. The presence of an age-related diluting defect that is independent of changes in GFR remains controversial.

The diluting capacity of the aging kidney has been evaluated in men by determining the minimum urine osmolality and maximum free water clearance after water loading *(18)*. The minimal urine osmolality in young men (mean age 31 yr) was 52 mosM/kg; in middle-aged men (mean age 60 yr), 74 mosM/kg; and in older men (mean age 84 yr), 92 mosM/kg. The free water clearance was lowest in the older group. However, when these results were expressed as free water clearance per mL of GFR, the values were not different, suggesting that the defect in diluting capacity was the result of an age-related reduction in GFR. Crowe et al. *(19)* carried out a similar study, in which healthy elderly subjects aged 63–80 yr (mean 72 yr) and healthy young subjects aged 21–26 yr (mean 22 yr) were administered a water load. The peak free water clearance was 5.7 mL/min in the older group and 8.4 mL/min in the younger group. However, when adjustments were made for changes in creatinine clearance, the difference in these indices was not statistically significant.

Dontas et al. *(20)* reported a significantly lower free water clearance:creatinine ratio in elderly subjects from an institutional setting, compared with healthy younger subjects. The maximal urinary dilution (urinary/plasma osmolality) declined from 0.247 in younger subjects to 0.418 in the elderly. The authors concluded that the free water clearance defects persist following correction for a lower GFR. A smaller study in healthy elderly subjects came to a similar conclusion *(21)*.

In addition to impaired diluting capacity, the age-related decrease in renal plasma flow and glomerular filtration rate can lead to passive reabsorption of fluid, thereby increasing the risk of water overload and hyponatremia. This effect is clinically evident in elderly patients who have congestive heart failure, extracellular volume depletion, and hypoalbuminemia. The ability of diuretics, especially thiazides, to decrease renal diluting capacity is well known *(22)*. In the elderly, this effect becomes especially important, because it is superimposed on the already diminished diluting capacity of the aged kidney. Thus, the many changes in the kidney that occur with aging can increase the risk in the elderly of developing water intoxication by impairing their ability to excrete excess water promptly.

Renal Water Loss. It has been known for many years that there is an age-related change in renal concentrating capacity. In a study of healthy men aged 40–101 yr who underwent 24 h of water deprivation, maximum attainable urine specific gravity declined from 1.030 at 40 yr to 1.023 at 89 yr *(23)*. Hospitalized men aged 23–72 yr, who underwent 24 h of dehydration, demonstrated a progressive decline in maximum urine osmolality with increasing age *(24)*. Rowe et al. *(25)* examined urine concentrating ability in healthy, active community-dwelling volunteers who were participating in the Baltimore Longitudinal Study of Aging. Young subjects responded to 12 h of water deprivation with a marked decrease in urine flow (1.02 ± 0.10 to 0.49 ± 0.03 mL/min) and a moderate increase in urine osmolality (969 ± 41 to 1109 ± 22 mosM/kg); elderly subjects were unable to significantly alter urine flow (1.05 ± 0.15 to 1.03 ± 0.13 mL/min) or osmolality (852 ± 64 to 882 ± 49 mosM/kg). This effect of age persisted after correction for the age-related decrease in GFR.

The effect of age on renal tubular response to vasopressin was studied by Miller and Shock *(26)*, who measured the urine:plasma inulin concentration ratio in men who ranged in age from 26–86 yr, and who were free of clinically demonstrable cardiovascular and renal disease. The ratio fell from 118 in young men (mean age 35 yr) to 77 in the middle-aged group (mean age 55 yr), and to 45 in the older men (mean age 73 yr).

The decreased renal sensitivity to vasopressin with age may be a result of an age-related increase in vasopressin secretion. Rats aged 8–9 mo were injected daily for 28 d with vasopressin to produce a twofold increase in plasma AVP concentration *(27)*. Response to water deprivation or intraperitoneal desmopressin acetate (DDAVP,® Rhone-Poulenc Rorer, Collegeville, PA) in these animals was decreased, compared with controls. Cyclic adenosine monophosphate content of renal medullary slices from control animals doubled in response to exposure to DDAVP, but no change was observed in the group that had received chronic vasopressin injections. These data suggest that chronic exposure of the kidney to increased vasopressin results in diminished renal responsiveness to the hormone.

Rats heterozygous for hypothalamic diabetes insipidus have half the vasopressin secretory capacity of normal rats, and a reduced plasma AVP concentration. The decreased AVP secretion in these animals was found to be associated with maintenance of maximal urine concentrating capacity with age, in contrast to the decline noted in aging of normal rats (27). Thus, an age-related increase in vasopressin secretion may result in decreased hormone responsiveness, perhaps through downregulation of renal AVP receptors, and may be the basis for decreased renal concentrating capacity in the elderly.

SODIUM REGULATORY CAPACITY

Renal Sodium Retention. Several situations may lead to sodium (Na) retention and accompanying water overload in the elderly. The previously described age-related decrease in renal blood flow and glomerular filtration rate favors enhanced conservation of Na. Disease states resulting in secondary hyperaldosteronism, such as congestive heart failure, cirrhosis, or nephrotic syndrome, are common in the elderly. In addition, drugs such as nonsteroidal antiinflammatory agents, which are frequently used in the elderly, may promote Na retention.

Renal Sodium Loss. Elderly individuals are more likely to have exaggerated natriuresis after a water load than are younger subjects (28). In a study of patients with benign hypertension, Schalekamp et al. (17) described an excess of Na excretion related to increased patient age. Epstein and Hollenberg (29) have shown that the aged kidney's response to salt restriction is sluggish. Restriction in Na intake to 10 mEq/d was followed by a half-life for reduction of urinary Na excretion of 17.6 h in young individuals and 30.9 h in old subjects. These data suggest that the aging kidney is more prone to Na wasting. Mechanisms underlying this tendency may be multifactorial and are related to the effects of age on ANH, the renin–angiotensin–aldosterone system, and renal tubular function.

Vasopressin System in Normal Aging (Table 2)

NEUROHYPOPHYSEAL SYSTEM

The magnocellular neurons of the hypothalamus, where AVP is synthesized, do not appear to undergo age-related degenerative changes (30). There is no evidence of the cell destruction, neuronal dropout, or loss of dendritic arborization found in other segments of the aged brain. Moreover, neurosecretory material in supraoptic nuclei (SON) and paraventricular (PVN) nuclei does not appear to differ in amount from that in younger subjects (31,32).

Morphologic data provide evidence that these nuclei, in fact, become more active with age. Fliers et al. (33) investigated age-related changes in the human hypothalamic neurohypophyseal system in subjects ranging from 10–93 yr of age. A gradual increase in the size of the SON and PVN was observed after 60 yr of age, suggesting that AVP production increases in senescence. In a subsequent study, Hoogendijk et al. (34) observed similar changes in the nuclear size of AVP neurons. Fliers and Swaab (35) estimated the functional properties of the magnocellular nuclei by staining for the enzyme, thiamine pyrophosphate. The distribution of this marker enzyme in the Golgi apparatus in old, compared with young, rats was found to be similar in the SON, but increased in the PVN. Possibly contributing to the maintenance of normal or increased amounts of AVP in the magnocellular neurons is the observation of a 25% reduction in the rate of axonal transport of AVP and its associated neurophysin with advancing age (36). Thus, it appears that neurosecretory activity of hypothalamic AVP neurons does not decrease, but, in fact, remains constant, or is elevated with age.

Table 2
Aging Effects on the Vasopressin System

Morphology of the neurohypophyseal system
  Normal or increased supraoptic nucleus cell number/AVP content
  Normal or increased paraventricular nucleus cell number/AVP content
  Decreased suprachiasmatic nucleus cell number/AVP content
  Normal extrahypothalamic nucleus cell number/AVP content
Hypothalamic vasopressin content
  Normal or increased
Cerebrospinal fluid vasopressin concentration
  Normal
Blood vasopressin concentration
  Normal or increased basal
  Increased after osmotic and pharmacologic stimulation
  Decreased response to volume/pressure stimulation
  Decreased nocturnal secretion
Renal response to vasopressin
  Decreased

Changes are in comparison to values observed in the young.

BASAL PLASMA VASOPRESSIN LEVELS

Conflicting data have been gathered regarding basal concentration of AVP in the blood during normal aging. In young normal individuals, there is a diurnal rhythm of vasopressin secretion, with increased AVP secretion occurring at night (37). This rhythm appears to be linked to the wake–sleep cycle, rather than to time of day (38). The sleep-associated peak is absent in the majority of healthy elderly persons (39,40). Low AVP levels and the lack of definite diurnal rhythm may, to some extent, explain increased diuresis during the night in some elderly individuals (39,40). In a study by Faull et al. (41), healthy elderly subjects were found to have basal plasma AVP levels that were significantly lower than in young subjects. In association with the reduced AVP concentration, plasma osmolality was elevated, suggesting that the elderly subjects had a water-losing state similar to that in partial diabetes insipidus. Clark et al. (42) also found lower plasma AVP levels in healthy elderly males.

Helderman et al. (43) studied older individuals with a mean age of 59 yr (range, 52–66 yr) and younger individuals with a mean age of 37 yr, and demonstrated that, under basal conditions, plasma vasopressin levels did not change with advancing age. Likewise, Chiodera et al. (44) found similar basal AVP levels in normal men aged 22–81 yr, who were divided into three age groups, with mean ages of 30.6, 52.1, and 72.5 yr. Duggan et al. (45) found that basal plasma levels of AVP did not differ among young, middle-aged, and elderly healthy individuals, who were studied under both supine and ambulatory conditions. Furthermore, there were no differences in plasma osmolality among the groups.

Other studies, however, have reported elevated basal vasopressin levels in healthy elderly persons, compared with younger individuals. Frolkis et al. (32) studied healthy human subjects aged 20–80 yr, and observed a progressive rise in plasma AVP concentration with age, which become most evident in subjects older than 60 yr. Similar findings were also reported by Crawford et al. (46). In a study by Rondeau et al. (47), plasma AVP levels, both in normals and in patients with heart failure, rose steadily with increasing age, and the patients with cardiac insufficiency as a group always had higher values. Kirkland et al. *(48)* demonstrated that healthy older persons (aged 61–82 yr) have higher basal levels of AVP than do younger subjects under identical conditions. Johnson et al. *(49)* also demonstrated a higher basal plasma AVP concentration in healthy elderly subjects (age 78.6 ± 3.1 yr), compared with younger adults (age 35.1 ± 9.4 yr). Baseline plasma AVP was strongly correlated with serum osmolality in the younger adults, but not in the elderly subjects.

Debate exists regarding a sex-related difference in plasma AVP levels in the elderly. Aspund and Aberg *(39)* reported a twofold higher plasma AVP concentration in elderly men, compared to women. Other studies, however, have failed to identify an effect of gender on basal plasma AVP *(49,50)*.

A rise in basal plasma AVP with age cannot be attributed to age-related changes in vasopressin pharmacokinetics. Engel et al. *(51)* showed that no differences existed between young and old subjects in vasopressin half-life, volume of distribution, or clearance. Thus, evidence of increased basal plasma vasopressin probably reflects age-related changes in central control systems for vasopressin release.

VASOPRESSIN STIMULATION

Secretion of AVP normally varies in response to changes in blood tonicity, blood volume, and blood pressure. Hormone release is also affected by other variables, such as nausea, pain, emotional stress, a variety of drugs, cigaret smoking, and glucopenia *(52, 53)*. In recent years, a growing body of information has suggested that normal aging affects the way these stimuli act and interact to influence AVP release.

The major physiologic stimulus for vasopressin secretion in humans, plasma osmolality, is regulated by hypothalamic osmoreceptors *(54)*. Helderman et al. *(43)* tested osmoreceptor sensitivity in the elderly by comparing the AVP response to hypertonic saline infusion in healthy elderly persons (aged 34–92 yr) to the response in younger individuals (aged 21–49 yr). Hypertonic saline raised plasma osmolality, with a consequent increase in plasma AVP in both groups, but the hormone concentrations in the older subjects were almost double those in the younger subjects. Thus, for any given level of osmotic stimulus, there was a greater release of AVP in the elderly, suggesting that aging resulted in osmoreceptor hypersensitivity.

Studies using water deprivation as a stimulus for vasopressin secretion have supported the concept of an age-related enhancement in vasopressin secretion. Phillips et al. *(5)* water-deprived young healthy individuals (20–31 yr) and healthy elderly men (67–75 yr) for a period of 24 h. The older persons responded to water deprivation and hyperosmolality with higher serum concentrations of AVP than in the younger individuals. Only one study has produced results that conflict with these findings. In this study, by Li et al. *(55)*, water deprivation for 14 h in healthy subjects, aged 63–87 yr, was reported to result in mean AVP concentrations significantly lower than those in the young control group.

The sensitivity of the hypothalamic–neurohypophyseal axis to volume/pressure stimuli was studied by Rowe et al. *(56)*. Acute upright posture was assumed by younger (aged 19–31 yr) and older (aged 62–80 yr) subjects after overnight dehydration. In the older subjects, the expected change in pulse and blood pressure did not uniformly lead to increased vasopressin secretion, with only eight of 15 older individuals experiencing increased plasma vasopressin. A subsequent study by Bevilacqua et al. *(57)* produced similar findings, suggesting the presence of an aged-related failure of volume/pressure-mediated vasopressin release.

Helderman et al. *(43)* evaluated the ability of iv ethanol infusion to inhibit AVP secretion in young (aged 21–49 yr) and old (aged 54–92 yr) subjects. The younger subjects demonstrated a sustained inhibition of AVP secretion during the infusion of ethanol; there was a paradoxical response in the older group, with initial AVP inhibition followed by breakthrough secretion and rebound to twice basal levels. Not only was ethanol less effective in inhibiting AVP release in the elderly, but it eventually lost its suppressive effect entirely, because of the introduction of a hyperosmotic stimulus resulting from the ethanol-induced constriction in plasma volume.

Metoclopramide can stimulate vasopressin secretion in man through cholinergic mechanisms *(58,59)*. Intravenous metoclopramide injection in normal elderly subjects aged 65–80 yr, and in normal young subjects aged 16–35 yr, produced significantly higher plasma AVP concentrations in the older group, with no significant changes in plasma osmolality, blood pressure, or heart rate *(58)*. Responses of AVP to cigaret smoking and insulin-induced hypoglycemia, as well as to metoclopramide, were evaluated by Chiodera et al. *(44)* in male subjects aged 22–81 yr. Corroborating the prior findings of Norbiato et al. *(58)*, the AVP response to metoclopramide was significantly higher in the older group, compared to two younger groups. The AVP response to cigaret smoking was similar; plasma AVP concentration increased 3.25× after smoking in the older group, compared with 2.5× in the two younger groups. In contrast, the AVP response during the insulin hypoglycemia test was identical in pattern and magnitude in all age groups.

The results of stimulation studies indicate that, in aging, AVP response to osmotic stimuli is increased because of a hyperresponsive osmoreceptor, the AVP response to upright posture is reduced as a result of impaired baroreceptor function. Input from the baroreceptor to the osmoreceptor is usually inhibitory, and a defect in this reflex arc would result in a lesser dampening, and consequent heightening, of osmotically stimulated ADH release.

Anatomical studies showing an increased size of the SON and PVN support the clinical data of increased basal secretion of vasopressin, as well as enhanced release of AVP in response to osmotic stimuli. When coupled with the many alterations in renal function that occur with aging, these changes can increase the risk in elderly persons for hyponatremia, by impairing their ability to excrete excess water promptly.

Age-related Changes in Atrial Natriuretic
Hormone Secretion, Regulation, and Action

ANH is synthesized, stored, and released in the atria of the heart in humans and animals. Through its action on the kidney, ANH produces a pronounced natriuresis and diuresis; through its action on blood vessels, it produces vasodilation, and has been shown to decrease blood pressure in both normal and hypertensive individuals *(60)*. As an important regulator of Na excretion, ANH may be a significant factor in mediating the altered renal Na handling of age.

Ohashi et al. *(61)* compared young normal men and elderly male nursing home residents, and noted a fivefold increase in mean basal ANH levels, and an exaggerated ANH response to the stimulus of saline infusion in the elderly group. McKnight et al. *(62)* also reported an age-related increase in basal ANH levels, but no changes with age in the response to saline infusion. Tajima et al. *(63)* compared ANH levels in young (aged 21–28 yr) and healthy old individuals (aged 62–73 yr). Baseline ANH levels were twice as high in the old subjects as in the young, and ANH response to the stimulus of head-out water immersion was greater in the elderly. The author has studied healthy male and female subjects, aged 22–64 yr, to determine the influence of age on circulating levels of ANH, both under basal conditions and after physiologic stimulation of ANH release by controlled exercise. Supine exercise, using a bicycle ergometer to 80% of maximum predicted heart rate, resulted in marked increases in ANH. Subjects aged more than 50 yr had higher baseline levels and a greater response to exercise, compared with subjects younger than 50 yr. Thus, increasing age results in increased ANH basal levels, and an increased ANH response to both physiologic and pharmacologic stimuli.

Heim et al. *(64)* suggest that the renal effects of ANH may be exaggerated in elderly vs young individuals. In their study, natriuretic response to a bolus injection of ANH was higher in older individuals (mean age 52.3 yr), compared with younger subjects (mean age 26 yr). These findings require confirmation, because rapid iv infusion of ANH results in higher ANH levels in the elderly, as a result of diminished ANH clearance *(65)*. Jansen et al. *(66)* did not measure the renal action of ANH, but noted no change with age in the blood pressure response to ANH iv infusion after correction for higher ANH levels in the elderly.

ANH is known to interact with the renin–angiotensin–aldosterone system. Increases of ANH result in suppression of renal renin secretion, plasma renin activity, plasma angiotensin II, and aldosterone levels, suggesting indirect inhibition of aldosterone secretion by ANH *(67)*. Cuneo et al. *(68)* found that minimal increases in ANH within physiological levels, produced by slow-rate ANH infusion, can inhibit angiotensin-II-induced aldosterone secretion in normal men, thus suggesting a direct inhibitory effect of ANH on aldosterone release. Clinkingbeard et al. *(69)* have confirmed that ANH can suppress aldosterone in man through both direct and indirect actions. Thus, ANH may further promote renal Na loss through inhibition of aldosterone release.

AHN may be an important mediator of age-related renal Na loss. This effect may be the consequence of increased basal ANH levels, increased ANH response to stimuli, increased renal sensitivity to ANH, and ANH-induced suppression of adrenal Na-retaining hormones.

RENIN–ANGIOTENSIN–ALDOSTERONE

A substantial body of evidence indicates that the normal aging process affects the renin–angiotensin–aldosterone system *(70)*. Healthy older individuals (62–70 yr) have lower plasma renin activity and aldosterone concentration, while in the supine position and consuming a normal Na intake, than young healthy persons (20–30 yr) *(71)*. Under the stimuli of upright posture and Na depletion, there were significant increases in circulating renin and aldosterone in both age groups, but mean values achieved were always significantly lower in the elderly group. The decrease in plasma renin activity in the elderly is not caused by changes in plasma renin substrate concentration, but rather by a decrease in active renin concentration *(72)*. Decreased conversion of inactive to active renin might be at least partially responsible for the reduced active renin concentration in the elderly. The decrease in plasma renin activity may also be related to the inhibitory effect of increased amounts of ANH on renin secretion (*see* Atrial Natriuretic Hormone Secretion Regulation). Decreased aldosterone concentration with age appears to be a direct result of age-related decrease of plasma renin activity, and not of aging changes in the adrenal gland, because aldosterone and cortisol responses to corticotropin infusion are not altered in the elderly *(72)*. It is likely that the age-related decrease in aldosterone concentration is a predisposing factor to renal salt wasting in the elderly.

Intrinsic renal tubular changes may also play a role in Na wasting. An impaired capacity to reabsorb Na has been described, along with decreased tubular responsiveness to aldosterone administration *(73,74)*. However, a subsequent study failed to find an effect of age on renal tubular sensitivity to aldosterone *(75)*.

The age-associated decline in the renin–angiotensin–aldosterone system may also be linked to alterations in potassium regulation. Hyporeninemic hypoaldosteronism occurs most commonly in elderly persons, especially those with diabetes mellitus *(76,77)*. The hyperkalemia characteristic of the disorder responds to treatment with mineralocorticoid, and may be the consequence of interaction of changes from chronic renal disease with the hormonal changes of normal aging. The risk of angiotensin-converting enzyme inhibitors in producing hyperkalemia is especially high in elderly persons, and may also be related to the interplay between drug action and physiologic alterations caused by aging *(78)*.

DISORDERS OF FLUID REGULATION

Hyponatremia

Hyponatremia, usually defined as a serum Na concentration of less than 136 mEq/L, appears when there is an alteration in the relationship between the amount of Na and water in the extracellular body fluid compartment, and can be the consequence of either a decrease in extracellular Na content (i.e., Na depletion) or an increase in extracellular water (i.e., dilutional hyponatremia). In the elderly person, dilutional hyponatremia is the more common mechanism.

EPIDEMIOLOGY

Hyponatremia is a common finding in elderly persons. Analysis of plasma Na values in healthy individuals has shown an age-related decrease of approx 1 mEq/L per decade from a mean value of 141 ± 4 mEq/L in young subjects *(79)*. In a population of individuals aged more than 65 yr, who were living at home and who were without acute illness, a 7% incidence of serum Na concentration of 137 mEq/L or less was observed *(80)*. Similarly, an 11% incidence of hyponatremia was found in the population of a geriatric medicine outpatient practice *(81)*. In hospitalized patients, hyponatremia is even more common. An analysis of 5000 consecutive sets of plasma electrolytes, from a hospital population with a mean age 54 yr, revealed a mean serum Na of 134 ± 6 mEq/L, with the values skewed toward the hyponatremic end of the distribution curve *(79)*. A high prevalence of hyponatremia has been found in patients hospitalized for a variety of acute illnesses, with the risk being greater with increasing age of the patient *(82,83)*.

Elderly residents of long-term care institutions appear to be especially prone to hyponatremia. In a study of patients with a mean age of 72 yr, who resided in a chronic disease hospital, 22.5% had repeated serum Na determinations of less than 135 mEq/L *(84)*. Of patients admitted to an acute geriatric unit, 11.3% were found to have serum Na concentrations of 130 mEq/L or less *(85)*. A survey of nursing home residents, aged more than 60 yr, revealed a cross-sectional incidence of 18% with serum Na less than 136 mEq/L. When this population was observed on a longitudinal basis over a 12-mo period, 53% were observed to experience one or more episodes of hyponatremia *(86)*. Persons with

Table 3
Risk Factors for Hyponatremia in the Elderly

Physiologic changes of normal aging
 Decreased renal sodium conserving ability
  Altered renal tubular function
  Increased atrial natriuretic hormone secretion
  Decreased renin–angiotensin–aldosterone secretion
 Decreased renal water excretion ability
  Decreased renal blood flow and glomerular filtration rate
  Decreased distal renal tubular diluting capacity
  Increased renal passive reabsorption of water
  Increased vasopressin secretion
Diseases accompanied by SIADH (see Table 4)
Drugs accompanied by sodium loss or SIADH (see Table 5)
Increased water intake
 Oral fluids
 Intravenous hypotonic fluids
Decreased sodium intake
 Low sodium diet
 Tube feeding
Increased sodium loss
 Renal disease
 Gastrointestinal tract
  Vomiting
  Diarrhea
  Gastric suctioning
Idiopathic SIADH of the elderly
 Age >80 yr
 Race other than black

SIADH, Syndrome of Inappropriate Antidiuretic Hormone Secretion.

central nervous system (CNS) and spinal cord disease were at highest risk, and water load testing indicated that most patients had features consistent with the syndrome of inappropriate antidiuretic hormone secretion (SIADH).

Risk Factors (Table 3)

Hyponatremia often is a marker for severe underlying disease with poor prognosis and high mortality (87,88). A major risk for the development or worsening of hyponatremia is the administration of hypotonic fluid, either as an increase in oral water intake or as iv 0.45% saline solution or 5% glucose in water, a finding in 78% of nursing home residents with hyponatremia (86). Low Na intake, coupled with age-associated impaired renal Na-conserving ability, can, over time, lead to Na depletion with hyponatremia. Many patients whose nutritional support is primarily or entirely provided by tube feeding will develop either intermittent or persistent hyponatremia. The underlying cause appears to be Na depletion caused by the low Na content of most tube-feeding diets (86,89). The hyponatremia will usually resolve in response to increasing the dietary Na intake.

Advanced age itself may be a risk factor for hyponatremia. SIADH has been described in elderly individuals, generally over the age of 80 yr, in whom no identifiable cause for hyponatremia could be found, suggesting that there is an idiopathic form of SIADH that

Table 4
Diseases Associated with Hyponatremia in the Elderly

Central nervous system disorders
  Vascular diseases
  Trauma (subdural hematoma, intracranial hemmorhage)
  Tumor
  Infectious disease
Malignancy with ectopic AVP production
  Pulmonary (small-cell carcinoma)
  Pancreatic carcinoma
  Thymoma
  Lymphosarcoma, reticulum cell sarcoma, Hodgkin's disease
Pulmonary disease
  Pneumonia
  Tuberculosis
  Lung abscess
  Bronchiectasis
Endocrine disease
  Hypothyroidism
  Diabetes mellitus with hyperglycemia
  Adrenal insufficiency

may represent the clinical expression of physiologic changes that take place in the regulation of water balance during aging *(81,90–92)*. Race may play a role, because Blacks appear to be at lower risk than Whites or Hispanics *(81)*.

Disease States Causing the Syndrome of Inappropriate Antidiuretic Hormone Secretion (SIADH)

Many diseases common in the elderly can cause SIADH (Table 4). Almost all CNS disorders can lead to dysfunction of the hypothalamic system involved in the normal regulation of AVP secretion, with resultant increased secretion of the hormone, and consequent risk for water retention and hyponatremia *(93)*. Such CNS disorders include vascular injury (thrombosis, embolism, hemorrhage), trauma with subdural hematoma, vasculitis, tumor, and infection. Malignancies can cause SIADH, as a result of autonomous release of AVP from the cancer tissue where it is synthesized, stored, and discharged in the absence of known stimuli. The malignancy most commonly associated with SIADH in the elderly is small-cell carcinoma of the lung, in which as many as 68% of patients have been found to have evidence of impaired water excretion and elevated blood AVP concentration *(94)*. Other malignancies include pancreatic carcinoma, thymoma, pharyngeal carcinoma, lymphosarcoma, and Hodgkin's disease. Many inflammatory lung diseases can also cause SIADH, perhaps as a result of AVP production by diseased pulmonary tissue, and include such entities as bronchiectasis, pneumonia, lung abscess, and tuberculosis.

Drugs and Fluid Regulation

Numerous drugs taken by elderly persons can affect water balance by direct action on the kidney, or by altering AVP release from the neurohypophyseal system or its action on the kidney (Table 5) *(95,96)*. In particular, many drugs increase the risk for SIADH.

Table 5
Drug-Induced Changes in Sodium and Water Regulation

Sodium retention
    Nonsteroidal anti-inflamatory agents
Sodium loss
    Thiazide and loop diuretics
Impaired diluting capacity
    Thiazide diuretics
Impaired concentrating capacity
    Lithium
    Demeclocycline
    Potassium-losing diuretics
Syndrome of inappropriate antidiuretic hormone secretion
    Central nervous system agents
        Tricyclic antidepressants
        Selective serotonin reuptake inhibitor antidepressants
        Phenothiazine antipsychotics
        Carbamazepine anticonvulsant
    Angiotensin-converting enzyme (ACE) inhibitors
    Antineoplastic drugs
        Vincristine
        Vinblastine
        Cyclophosphamide
    Chlorpropamide
    Clofibrate
    Narcotics

Hyponatremia with the characteristics of SIADH is recognized as a side effect of several older antipsychotic agents, i.e., fluphenazine, thiothixene, and phenothiazine, as well as the tricyclic antidepressants. There is evidence that the newer selective serotonin reuptake inhibitor antidepressants (SSRIs) can also induce SIADH (97,98). Although fluoxetine is the SSRI most commonly reported to produce hyponatremia, other SSRIs, including paroxetine, sertraline, and fluvoxamine, have also been involved (99–101). Individuals at highest risk for SSRI-induced hyponatremia are those over the age of 65 yr in whom the onset of hyponatremia typically occurs within 2 wk after initiation of drug therapy.

Angiotensin-converting enzyme (ACE) inhibitors, used in the elderly for the management of hypertension and congestive heart failure, have been associated with the development of hyponatremia (102). In most cases, the level of hyponatremia has been clinically significant, with serum Na concentrations as low as 101 mEq/L, and with symptoms ranging from confusion to seizures and coma. Although initial reports indicated that the risk was greatest when ACE inhibitors were used in combination with thiazide diuretics, it now appears that the ACE inhibitors alone can precipitate hyponatremia. The hyponatremia appears to be dilutional, with features of SIADH, and may be mediated by potentiation of plasma renin activity, with subsequent increase in brain angiotensin levels, which in turn stimulate both a release of AVP from the hypothalamus and an increase in thirst. Discontinuing the ACE inhibitor is associated with rapid resolution of the hyponatremia.

Diuretics, both of the loop and thiazide types, can produce hyponatremia (103). Loop diuretics appear to have a greater natriuretic effect in older persons than in the young (104). Hyponatremia can occur when diuretic-induced Na and water loss is replaced by

Table 6
Risk Factors for Hypernatremia in the Elderly

Increased water loss
  Renal
    Age-associated impaired concentrating capacity
    Resistance to vasopressin action
      Age-associated
      Acquired (drugs, hypokalemia, hypercalcemia)
    Osmotic diuresis (glycosuria, diuretic-induced natriuresis)
    Renal tubular disease
  Gastrointestinal tract
    Vomiting
    Diarrhea
  Skin (sweating)
  Lung (tachypnea)
Decreased water intake
  Impaired thirst perception
  Impaired cognition (delerium, dementia)
  Impaired access to fluids

hypotonic fluids, resulting in a combined depletional and dilutional hyponatremia. With thiazide diuretics, the induced Na loss is often accompanied by loss of total body potassium, with consequent decrease in intracellular solute content and decreased cell volume. This circumstance can activate hypothalamic pathways, leading to increased AVP discharge, water retention, and SIADH. This form of thiazide-induced hyponatremia occurs almost entirely in the elderly, and can be reversed by correcting the underlying potassium depletion (105).

Other drugs associated with development of hyponatremia in the elderly include the sulfonylurea, chlorpropamide; the anticonvulsant, carbamazepine; and the antineoplastic agents, vincristine, vinblastine, and cyclophosphamide. Analgesics, particularly the narcotics, may be responsible for the occurrence of hyponatremia in the elderly postoperative patient.

Hypernatremia

The renal and hormonal alterations of aging described thus far are among the factors associated with an increased risk for hypernatremia (Table 6). In a study of 15,187 hospitalized patients aged more than 60 yr, a 1% incidence of hypernatremia was reported, with a mean serum Na concentration of 154 mEq/L (106). Similarly, a study of elderly residents in a long-term care institution revealed a 1% incidence of hypernatremia, which increased to 18% when the patients were monitored over a 12-mo period (107). Of 264 nursing home patients in whom acute illness developed requiring hospitalization, 34% became markedly hypernatremic, with serum Na concentration greater than 150 mEq/L (108).

Most commonly, hypernatremia is the result of loss of body water in excess of Na losses, in association with inadequate fluid intake. Frequent causes are febrile illness with increased insensible fluid loss, tachypnea with increased water loss from the lungs, diarrhea and osmotic-induced polyuria from poorly controlled diabetes mellitus or use

Table 7
Alzheimer's Disease and Disordered Water Regulation

Alterations in water regulation
    Impaired thirst perception
    Decreased vasopressin secretion
       Basal
       Response to stimulation
       Diurnal pattern
Clinical consequences
    Increased risk of dehydration
    Hypertonicity (increased serum sodium and osmolality)
    Reversal of day/night urine flow rate
    Nocturnal polyuria and incontinence

of loop diuretics (106,109). There is a high morbidity and mortality in elderly patients who develop serum Na concentrations above 148 mEq/L, and such elevations of serum Na are often a consequence of a severe underlying disease process (106,109).

Water Balance in Alzheimer's Disease

Persons with Alzheimer's disease are at increased risk for disturbed water regulation (Table 7). The secretion of vasopressin may be lower in those with Alzheimer's disease than in comparably aged persons with normal cognitive function (33,34,110–112). Following dehydration, individuals with Alzheimer's disease had a lesser rise in plasma vasopressin than age-matched normal subjects (113). Similarly, pharmacologic stimulation with metoclopramide (114) or physostigmine (115) is accompanied by marked blunting of plasma vasopressin response.

Clinically, patients with Alzheimer's disease appear to be at increased risk for dehydration. Overnight fluid restriction results in greater rise in plasma osmolality, greater water loss, and, in spite of these stimuli for thirst, a marked reduction in spontaneous water intake (7). There appears to be a direct correlation between mini mental status examination score and impairment of water intake (7).

Urinary Incontinence

In normal young persons, there is a diurnal pattern of vasopressin secretion, with highest levels occuring during sleep (37). This is reflected by a lower rate of urine flow at night than during the daytime, so that daytime urine volume is approx twice that produced at night (116). In many older persons, as well as in patients with Alzheimer's disease, there is loss of nocturnal vasopressin secretion, and an accompanying reversal of day–night urine production, so that nighttime urine flow rate exceeds the daytime flow rate (40,117,118). This alteration in renal function leads to a diabetes insipidus-like nocturnal polyuria, and, when coupled with diminished bladder capacity and detrusor hyperreflexia, may be a contributing factor to the nocturnal urinary frequency seen so commonly in older persons. In patients with Alzheimer's disease, the cognitive impairment can cause the nighttime polyuria to be clinically expressed as urinary incontinence (117). The vasopressin analog, DDAVP, may be helpful in treating both nocturnal frequency and nocturnal urinary incontinence (118–120).

CONCLUSION

Normal aging is accompanied by many changes in the various regulatory systems involved in the control of Na and water balance. As a consequence of these alterations, the elderly person has a diminished capacity to withstand the challenges of illness, drugs, and physiologic stresses, and, thus, has an increased risk for the development of clinically significant alterations in Na and water balance. Awareness of these limitations of homeostasis ability allows the physician to anticipate the impact of illnesses and drugs on volume and electrolyte status of the elderly patient, and will lead to a more rational approach to therapeutic intervention and management.

REFERENCES

1. Miller M, Gold GC, Friedlander DA. Physiological changes of aging affecting salt and water balance. Rev Clin Gerontol 1991;1:215–230.
2. Mitchell CO, Lipschitz DA. Detection of protein calorie malnutrition in the elderly. Am J Clin Nutr 1982;35:398–406.
3. Norris AH, Lundy T, Shock NW. Tends in selected indices of body composition in men between the ages of 30 and 80 years. Ann NY Acad Sci 1963;110:623–639.
4. Robertson GL. Thirst and vasopressin function in normal and disordered states of water balance. J Lab Clin Med 1983;101:351–371.
5. Phillips PA, Rolls BJ, Ledingham JGG, Forsling ML, Morton JJ, Crowe MJ, Wollner L. Reduced thirst after water deprivation in healthy elderly men. N Engl J Med 1984;311:753–759.
6. Miller PD, Krebs RA, Neal BJ, McIntyre DO. Hypodipsia in geriatric patients. Am J Med 1982;73: 354–356.
7. Albert SG, Nakra BRS, Grossberg GT, Caminal ER. Drinking behavior and vasopressin responses to hyperosmolality in Alzheimer's disease. Int Psychogeriatr 1994;6:78–86.
8. McLachlan M, Wasserman P. Changes in size and distensibility of the aging kidney. Br J Radiol 1981; 54:488–491.
9. Kaplan C, Pasternack B, Shah H, Gallo G. Age-related incidence of sclerotic glomeruli in human kidneys. Am J Pathol 1975;80:227–234.
10. Kappel B, Olsen S. Cortical interstitial tissue and sclerosed gloeruli in the normal human kidney, related to age and sex. Virchows Arch (A) 1980;387:271–277.
11. Taylor SA, Price RG. Age-related changes in rat glomerular basement membrane. Int J Biochem 1982; 14:201–206.
12. Ljungvist A, Lagergren C. Normal intrarenal arterial pattern in adult and aging human kidney. J Anat 1962;96:285–298.
13. Takazakura E, Sawabu N, Handa A, Takada A, Shinoda A, Takeuch J. Intrarenal vascular changes with age and disease. Kidney Int 1972;2:224–230.
14. Davies DF, Shock NW. Age changes in glomerular filtration, effective renal plasma flow and tubular excretory capacity in adult males. J Clin Invest 1950;29:496–506.
15. Rowe JW, Andres RA, Tobin JD, Norris AH, Shock NW. The effect of age on creatinine clearance in man: a cross-sectional and longitudinal study. J Gerontol 1976;311:155–163.
16. Lindeman RD, Tobin JD, Shock NW. Longitudinal studies on the rate of decline in renal function with age. J Am Geriatr Soc 1985;33:278–285.
17. Schalekamp MA, Krauss XH, Schalekamp-Kuyken MP, Klosters G, Birkenhager WH. Studies on the mechanism of hypernatriuresis in essential hypertension in relation to measurements of plasma renin concentration, body fluid compartments and renal function. Clin Sci 1971;41:219–231.
18. Lindeman RD, Lee DT, Yiengst MJ, Shock NW. Influence of age, renal disease, hypertension, diuretics and calcium on the antidiuretic responses to suboptimal infusions of vasopressin. J Lab Clin Med 1966;68:202–223.
19. Crowe MJ, Forsling ML, Rolls BJ, Philips PA, Ledingham JG, Smith RF. Altered water excretion in healthy elderly men. Age Aging 1987;16:285–293.
20. Dontas AS, Karkenos S, Papanayioutou P. Mechanisms of renal tubular defects in old age. Postgrad Med J 1972;48:295–303.

21. Lye M. Electrolyte disorders in the elderly. In: Morgan DB, ed. Clinics in Endocrinology and Metabolism. WB Saunders, Philadelphia, 1984, pp. 377–398.
22. Januszewicz W, Heinemann HO, Demartini FE,Laragh JH. A clinical study of effects of hydrochloro-thiazide on renal excretion of electrolyte and free water. N Engl J Med 1959;261:264–269.
23. Lewis WH, Alving AS. Changes with age in the renal function in adult men. Am J Physiol 1938;123: 500–515.
24. Lindeman RD, Van Buren C, Raisz LG. Osmolar renal concentrating ability in healthy young men and hospitalized patients without renal disease. N Engl J Med 1960;262:1306–1309.
25. Rowe JW, Shock NW, DeFronzo RA. The influence of age on the renal response to water deprivation in man. Nephron 1976;17:270–278.
26. Miller JH, Shock NW. Age differences in the renal tubular response to antidiuretic hormone. J Gerontol 1953;8:446–450.
27. Miller M. Influence of aging on vasopressin secretion and water regulation. In: Schrier RW, ed. Vasopressin. Raven, New York, 1985, pp. 249–258.
28. Lindeman RD, Adler, S, Yiengst MJ, Beard ES. Natriuresis and carbohydrate-induced antinatriuresis after overnight fast and hydration. Nephron 1970;7:289–300.
29. Epstein M, Hollenberg NK. Age as a determinant of renal sodium conservation in normal man. J Lab Clin Med 1976;87:411–417.
30. Hsou HK, Peng MT. Hypothalamic neuron number of old female rats. Gerontology 1978;24:434–440.
31. Currie AR, Adamson H, VanDyke HB. Vasopressin and oxytocin in the posterior lobe of the pituitary in man. J Clin Endocrinol Metab 1960;20:947–951.
32. Frolkis VV, Golovchenko SF, Medved VI, Frolkis RA. Vasopressin and cardiovascular system in aging. Gerontology 1982;28:290–302.
33. Fliers E, Swaab DF, Pool Ch W, Verwer RW. The vasopressin and oxytocin neurons in the human supraoptic and paraventricular nucleus: change with aging and in senile dementia. Brain Res 1985; 342:45–53.
34. Hoogendijk JE, Fliers E, Swaab DF, Verwer RW. Activation of vasopressin neurons in the human supraoptic and paraventricular nucleus in senescence and senile dementia. J Neurol Sci 1985;69:291–299.
35. Fliers E, Swaab DF. Activation of vasopressinergic and oxytocinergic neurons during aging in the Wistar rat. Peptides 1983;4:165–170.
36. Fotheringham AP, Davidson YS, Davies I, Morris JA. Age-associated changes in neuroaxonal trans-port in the hypothalamo-neurohypophyseal system of the mouse. Mech Aging Dev 1991;60:113–121.
37. George CPL, Messerli FH, Genest J, Nowaczynski W, Boucher R, Kuchel Orofo-Ortega M. Diurnal variation of plasma vasopressin in man. J Clin Endocrinol Metab 1975;41:332–338.
38. Nadal M. Secretory rhythm of vasopressin in healthy subjects with inversed sleep-wake cycle: evidence for the existance of an intrinsic regulation. Eur J Endocrinol 1996;134:174–176.
39. Asplund R, Aberg H. Diurnal variation in the levels of antidiuretic hormone in the elderly. J Intern Med 1991;299:131–134.
40. Kikuchi Y. Participation of atrial natriuretic peptide (hANP) levels and arginine vasopressin (AVP) in aged persons with nocturia. Jap J Urol 1995;86:1651–1659.
41. Faull CM, Holmes C, Baylis PH. Water balance in elderly people: is there a deficiency of vasopressin? Age Aging 1993;22:114–120.
42. Clark BA, Elahi D, Fish L, McAloon-Dyke M, Davis F, Minaker KL, Epstein FH. Atrial natriuretic peptide suppresses osmostimulated vasopresin release in young and elderly humans. Am J Physiol 1991;261:E252–E256.
43. Helderman JH, Vestal RE, Rowe JW, Tobin JD, Andres R, Robertson GL. The response of arginine vasopressin to intravenous ethanol and hypertonic saline in man. The impact of aging. J Gerontol 1978; 33:39–47.
44. Chiodera P, Capretti L, Marches M. Abnormal arginine vasopressin response to cigarette smoking and metoclopramide (but not to insulin-induced hypoglycemia) in elderly subjects. J Gerontol 1991;46: M6–M10.
45. Duggan J, Kilfeather S, Lightman SL, O'Malley K. The association of age with plasma arginine vasopressin and plasma osmolality. Age Aging 1993;22:332–336.
46. Crawford GA, Johnson AG, Gyory AZ, Kelly D. Change in arginine vasopressin concentration with age. Clin Chem 1993;39:2023.
47. Rondeau E, Delima J, Caillens H, Ardaillau R, Vahanian A, Acar J. High plasma anti-diuretic hormone in patients with cardiac failure. influence of age. Min Electrolyte Metab 1982;8;267–274.

48. Kirkland J, Lye M, Goddard C, Vargas E, Davies I. Plasma arginine vasopressin in dehydrated elderly patients. Clin Endocrinol 1984;20:451–456.
49. Johnson AG, Crawford GA, Kelly D, Nguyen TV, Gyory AZ. Arginine vasopressin and osmolality in the elderly. J Am Geriatr Soc 1994;42:399–404.
50. Bursztyn M, Bresnahan M, Gavras I, Gavras H. Pressor hormones in elderly hypertensive persons: racial differences. Hypertension 1990;15(Suppl 2):I88–I92.
51. Engel PA, Rowe JW, Minaker KL, Robertson GL. Stimulation of vasopressin release by exogenous vasopressin: effect of sodium intake and age. Am J Physiol 1984;246:E202–E207.
52. Baylis PH, Zerbe RL, Robertson GL. Arginine-vasopressin response to insulin induced hypoglycemia in man. J Clin Endocrinol Metab 1981;53:935–940.
53. Robertson GL, Rowe JW. The effect of aging on neurohypophysial function. Peptides 1980;1(Suppl 1): 159–162.
54. Robertson GL, Shelton RL, Athar J. The osmoregulation of vasopressin. Kidney Int 1976;10:25–37.
55. Li CH, Hsieh SM, Nagai I. The response of plasma arginine vasopressin to 14 h. water deprivation in the elderly. Acta Endocrinol 1984;150:314–317.
56. Rowe JW, Minaker KL, Robertson GL. Age-related failure of volume pressure mediated vasopressin release in man. J Clin Endocrinol Metab 1982;54:661–664.
57. Bevilacqua M, Norbiato G, Chebat E, Raggi U, Cavaiani P, Guzzetti R, Bertora P. Osmotic and nonosmotic control of vasopressin release in the elderly: effect of metoclopramide. J Clin Endocrinol Metab 1987;54:1243–1247.
58. Norbiato G, Bevilacqua M, Chebat E, Bertora P, Cavaiani P, Baruto C, Fumagallis S, Raggi U. Metoclopramide increases vasopressin secretion. J Clin Endocrinol Metab 1986;63:747–750.
59. Steardo L, Iovino M, Monteleone P, Bevilacqua M, Norbiato G. Evidence that cholinergic receptors of muscarinic type may modulate vasopressin release induced by metoclopramide. J Neurol Transm 1990;82:213–217.
60. Espiner EA, Richards AM, Yandle TG, Nicholls MG. Natriuretic hormones. Endocrinol Metab Clin N Am 1995;24:481–509.
61. Ohashi M, Fujio N, Nawata H, Kato K, Ibayashi H, Kangawa K, Matsuo H. High plasma concentrations of human atrial natriuretic polypepetide in aged men. J Clin Endocrinol Metab 1987;64:81–85.
62. McKnight JA, Roberts G, Sheridan B, Brew Atkinson A. Relationship between basal and sodium stimulated plasma atrial natriuretic factor, age, sex and blood pressure in normal man. Human Hypertens 1989;3:157–163.
63. Tajima F, Sagawa S, Iwamoto J, Miki K, Claybaugh JR, Shiraki K. Renal and endocrine responses in the elderly during headout water immersion. Am J Physiol 1988;254:R977–R983.
64. Heim JM, Gottmann JW, Strom TM, Gerzer R. Effects of a bolus dose of atrial natriuretic factor in young and elderly volunteers. Eur J Clin Invest 1989;19:265–271.
65. Ohashi M, Fujio N, Nawata H, Kato K, Matsuo H, Ibayashi H. Pharmacokinetics of synthetic alpha-human atrial natriuretic polypeptide in normal men: effect of aging. Regul Pept 1987;19:265–271.
66. Jansen TL, Tan AC, Smits P, deBoo T, Benraad TJ, Thien T. Hemodynamic effects of atrial natriuretic factor in young and elderly subjects. Clin Pharmacol Ther 1990;48:179–188.
67. Genest J, Larochelle P, Cusson JR, Gutkowska J, Cantin M. The atrial natriuretic factor in hypertension: state of the art lecture. Hypertension 1988;11(Suppl 1):13–17.
68. Cuneo RC, Espiner EA, Nicholls MG, Yandle TC, Livessey JH. Effect of physiological levels of atrial natriuretic peptide on hormone secretion: inhibition of angiotensin-induced aldosterone secretion and renin release in normal man. J Clin Endocrinol Metab 1987;65:765–772.
69. Clinkingbeard C, Sessions C, Shenker Y. The physiological role of atrial natriuretic hormone in the regulation of salt and water metabolism. J Clin Endocrinol Metab 1990;70:582–589.
70. Bauer JH. Age-related changes in the renin-aldosterone system. Physiological effects and clinical implications. Drugs Aging 1993;3:238–245.
71. Weidmann P, DeMyttenaere-Bursztein S, Maxwell MH, DeLima J. Effect of aging on plasma renin and aldosterone in normal man. Kidney Int 1975;8:325–333.
72. Tsunoda K, Abe K, Goto T, Yasujima M, Sato M, Omata K, Seino M, Yoshinaga K. Effect of age on the renin-angiotensin-aldosterone system in normal subjects: simultaneous measurement of active and inactive renin, renin substrate, and aldosterone in plasma. J Clin Endocrinol Metab 1986;62:384–389.
73. Macias Nunez JF, Garcia Iglesias C, Bondia Roman A, Rodriguez Commes JL, Corbacho Becerra L, Tabernero Romo JM, Decastro del Pozo S. Renal handling of sodium in old people. A functional study. Age Aging 1978;7:178–182.

74. Ceruso D, Squadrito G, Quartarone M, Rarisi M. Comportamente della funzionalita renale e degli elettroliti ematici ed urinari dopo aldosterone in soggietti anziani. G Geronol 1970;18:862–867.

75. Macias Nunez JF, Garcia Iglesias C, Tabernero Romo JM, Rodriguez Commes JL, Corbacho Becerra L, Sanchez Tomero JA. Renal management of sodium under indomethacin and aldosterone in the elderly. Age Aging 1980;9:165–172.

76. Perez GO, Lespier L, Jacobi J. Hyporeninemia and hypoaldosteronism in diabetes mellitus. Arch Intern Med 1977;137:852–855.

77. Phelps KR, Lieberman RL, Oh MS, Carroll HJ. Pathophysiology of the syndrome of hyporeninemic hypoaldosteronism. Metabolism 1980;29:186–199.

78. Ponce SP, Jennings AE, Madias, NE, Harrington JT. Drug-induced hyperkalemia. Medicine 1985;64: 357–370.

79. Owen JA, Campbell DG. A comparison of plasma electrolyte and urea values in healthy persons and in hospital patients. Clin Chem Acta 1968;22:611–618.

80. Caird FI, Andrews GR, Kennedy RD. Effect of posture on blood pressure in the elderly. Br Heart J 1973;35:527–530.

81. Miller M, Hecker MS, Friedlander DA, Carter JM. Apparent idiopathic hyponatremia in an ambulatory geriatric population. J Am Geriatr Soc 1996;44:404–408.

82. Anderson RJ, Chung H, Kluge R, Schrier RW. Hyponatremia: a prospective analysis of its epidemiology and the pathogenetic role of vasopressin. Ann Intern Med 1985;102:164–168.

83. Hochman I, Cabili S, Peer G. Hyponatremia in internal medicine ward patients: causes, treatment and prognosis. Isr J Med Sci 1989;25:73–76.

84. Kleinfeld M, Casimir M, Borra S. Hyponatremia as observed in a chronic disease facility. J Am Geriatr Soc 1979;27:156–161.

85. Sunderam SG, Mankikar GD. Hyponatremia in the elderly. Age Aging 1983;12:77–80.

86. Miller M, Morley JE, Rubenstein LZ. Hyponatremia in a nursing home population. J Am Geriatr Soc 1995;43:1410–1413.

87. Kennedy PGE, Mitchell DM, Hoffbrand BI. Severe hyponatremia in hospital inpatients. Br Med J 1978;2:1251–1253.

88. Tierney WM, Martin DK, Greenlee MC, Zerbe RL, McDonald CJ. The prognosis of hyponatremia at hospital admission. J Genl Int Med 1986;1:380–385.

89. Rudman D, Racette D, Rudman IW, Mattson DE, Erve PR. Hyponatremia in tube-fed elderly men. J Chronic Dis 1986;39:73–80.

90. Crowe M. Hyponatremia due to syndrome of inappropriate antidiuretic hormone secretion in the elderly. Irish Med J 1980;73:482–483.

91. Ditzel J. Hyponatremia in an elderly woman and inappropriate secretion of antidiuretic hormone. Acta Med Scand 1966;179:407–416.

92. Goldstein CS, Braunstein S, Goldfarb S. Idiopathic syndrome of inappropriate antidiuretic hormone secretion possibly related to advanced age. Ann Intern Med 1983;99:185–188.

93. Bartter FC, Schwartz WB. The syndrome of inappropriate secretion of antidiuretic hormone. Am J Med 1967;42:790–806.

94. Comis RL, Miller M, Ginsberg SJ. Abnormalities in water homeostasis in small cell anaplastic lung cancer. Cancer 1980;45:2414–2421.

95. Miller M, Moses AM. Drug-induced states of impaired water excretion. Kidney Int 1976;10:96–103.

96. Moses A M, Miller M, Streeten DHP. Pathophysiologic and pharmacologic alterations in the release and action of ADH. Metabolism 1976;25:697–721.

97. Liu BA, Mittmann N, Knowles SR, Shear NH. Hyponatremia and the syndrome of inappropriate secretion of antidiuretic hormone associated with the use of selective serotonin reuptake inhibitors: a review of spontaneous reports. Can Med Assoc J 1996;155:519–527.

98. Sharma H, Pompei P. Antidepressant-induced hyponatremia in the aged. Avoidance and management strategies. Drugs Aging 1996;8:430–435.

99. Cohen BJ, Mahelsky M, Adler L. More cases of SIADH with fluoxetine. Am J Psychiatry 1990;147: 948–949.

100. Gommans JG, Edwards RA. Fluoxetine and hyponatremia. N Z Med J 1990;103:106.

101. Hwang AS, Magraw RM. Syndrome of inappropriate secretion of antidiuretic hormone due to fluoxetine. Am J Psychiatry 1989;146:399.

102. Subramanian D, Ayus JC. Case report: severe symptomatic hyponatremia associated with lisinopril therapy. Am J Med Sci 1992;303:177–179.

103. Sonnenblick M, Freidlander Y, Rosin AJ. Diuretic-induced severe hyponatremia. Review and analysis of 129 reported patients. Chest 1993;103:601–606.
104. Andreasen F, Hansen U, Husted SE, Mogensen CE, Pedersen EB. The influence of age on renal and extrarenal effects of furosemide. Br J Clin Pharmacol 1984;18:65–74.
105. Fichman MP, Vorherr H, Kleeman CR, Telfer N. Diuretic-induced hyponatremia. Ann Intern Med 1971;75:853–863.
106. Snyder NA, Feigel DW, Arieff AI. Hypernatremia in elderly patients. A heterogeneous, morbid, and iatrogenic entity. Ann Intern Med 1987;107:309–319.
107. Miller M, Morley JE, Rubenstein LA, Ouslander J, Strome S. Hyponatremia in a nursing home population. Gerontologist 1985;25:11.
108. Lavizo-Mourey R, Johnson J, Stolley P. Risk factors for dehydration among elderly nursing home residents. J Am Geriatr Soc 1988;36:213–218.
109. Palevsky PM, Bhagrath R, Greenberg A. Hypernatremia in hospitalized patients. Ann Intern Med 1996;124:197–203.
110. Goudsmit E, Neijmeijer-Leloux A, Swaab DF. The human hypothalamo-neurhypophysial system in relation to development, aging and Alzheimer's disease. Progr Brain Res 1992;93:237–248.
111. Miller M. Hormonal aspects of fluid and sodium balance in the elderly. Endocrinol Metab Clin N Am 1995;24:233–253.
112. Sorensen PS, Hammer M, Vorstrup S, Gjerris F. CSF and plasma vasopressin concentration in dementia. J Neurol Neurosurg Psychiatry 1983;46:911–916.
113. Albert SG, Nakra BRS, Grossberg, Caminal ER. Vasopressin response to dehydration in Alzheimer's disease. J Am Geriatr Soc 1989;37:843–847.
114. Lipponi G, Cadeddu G, Antonicelli R, Compagnucci M, Spazzafumo L, Foschi F, Gaetti R. Vasopressin, prolactin and growth hormone in Alzheimer's disease: their evaluation after metoclopramide stimulation. Arch Gerontol Geriatr 1990;10:269–278.
115. Raskind MA, Peskind ER, Veith RC, Risse SC, Lampe TH, Borson S, Gumbrecht G, Dorsa DM. Neuroendocrine responses to physostigmine in Alzheimer's disease. Arch Gen Psychiatry 1989;46:535–540.
116. Kirkland JL, Lye M, Levy DW, Banerjee AK. Patterns of urine flow and electrolyte excretion in healthy elderly people. Br Med J 1983;287:1665–1667.
117. Ouslander JG, Schnelle JF. Incontinence in the nursing home. Ann Intern Med 1995;122:438–449.
118. Seiler WO, Stahelin HB, Hefti U. Desmopressin reduces night urine volume in geriatric patients: implications for treatment of the nocturnal incontinence. Clin Invest 1992;70:619.
119. Asplund R. The nocturnal polyuria syndrome (NPS). Gen Pharmacol 1995;26:1203–1209.
120. Asplund R, Aberg H. Desmopressin in elderly subjects with increased nocturnal diuresis. a two-month treatment study. Scand J Urol Nephrol 1993;27:77–82.

7

Bone Disease and Aging

B. E. Christopher Nordin, MD, DSC,
Allan G. Need, MD, Howard A. Morris, PHD,
and Michael Horowitz, PHD

CONTENTS

INTRODUCTION
BACKGROUND
DEFINITION
PRESENTATION
BONE DENSITOMETRY
CLINICAL GUIDELINES
CONCLUSIONS
REFERENCES

INTRODUCTION

There must be few fields of clinical medicine that are subject to as much confusion as osteoporosis. The diagnosis in any particular case is frequently uncertain, and may vary from specialist to specialist. There are no agreed investigation protocols, for diagnosing osteoporosis and the treatment tends to be arbitrary and stereotyped. There have been many excellent trials, but their clinical application is slow, and clinical results are seldom published.

The causes of this troubled state of affairs are both conceptual and practical. As long as disagreement about the pathogenesis of osteoporosis continues, there is bound to be uncertainty about management. But even if and when a particular working model is adopted, the difficulty of fitting a case into the appropriate place within the model remains almost insuperable, unless some very obvious pathogenetic factor like hyperthyroidism can be identified. It is therefore often necessary to return to first principles, and attempt to categorize patients in a way that can justify rational therapy.

BACKGROUND

Both men and women lose bone with age, starting at the menopause in women and at about age 50 in men (Fig. 1). The decline in bone mass is associated with a rise in bone resorption in women *(1,2)*, but not, it seems, in men *(3)*, in whom the cause may be a decline in bone formation, possibly secondary to a declining testosterone level *(3)*. However,

From: *Contemporary Endocrinology: Endocrinology of Aging*
Edited by: J. E. Morley and L. van den Berg © Humana Press Inc., Totowa, NJ

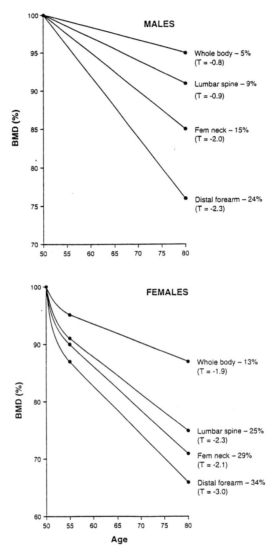

Fig. 1. BMD (% of young mean) as a function of age in men and women at four different sites.

there is evidence of increased bone resorption in at least some osteoporotic men *(4)*, just as there is evidence of impaired bone formation in some osteoporotic women *(5)*.

It is well established that calcium (Ca) deficiency causes osteoporosis in experimental animals *(6,7)*, but the contribution of primary negative Ca balance to age- and meno-pause-related bone loss remains uncertain. There is little doubt that Ca absorption falls and obligatory urinary Ca rises at the menopause *(8,9)*, but there must also be some increase in sensitivity of bone to resorbing stimuli, to explain all the known facts *(10,11)*. Whatever the truth may be, there can be no disagreement that treatment that improves Ca balance must also benefit the skeleton, where 99% of the body Ca resides.

DEFINITION

Osteoporosis is a descriptive term that means low bone (organ) density, in the same way as hypertension means high blood pressure. It is no more logical to include fracture

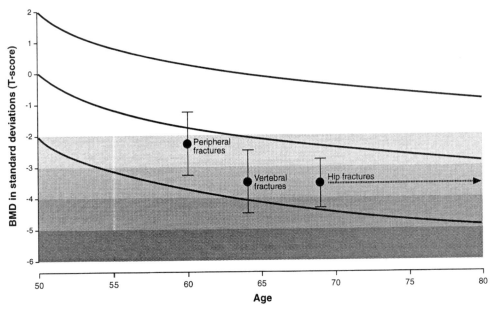

Fig. 2. Diagrammatic representation of mean BMD (±1 SD) in women with three types of fracture.

in the definition of osteoporosis *(12)* than it is to include stroke in the definition of hypertension. Osteoporosis simply increases the risk of fracture, in the way that hypertension increases the risk of stroke. Bone density is a continuous variable, but there is a practical need to define the density level below which a bone is classed as porotic. With most biochemical variables, values more than two standard deviations (SDs) from the normal mean are regarded as abnormal, and there is no particular reason why this should not apply to bone density *(13)*, but a cutoff point of −2.5 SD has been suggested by a World Health Organization committee *(12)*.

PRESENTATION

The patient, whether man or woman, generally presents in one of two ways: with fracture or with low bone mineral density (BMD). The fracture is either a peripheral fracture, such as the Colles' fracture (median age about 60 yr in women), a vertebral fracture (median age about 65 yr in women), or a hip fracture (generally over age 70 yr in women). In peripheral fractures, the mean BMD is about 2 SDs below the young normal mean, but well within the normal range for age. In vertebral fracture cases, the mean BMD is about 3 SDs below the young mean, and is also low for age. In hip fractures, the mean BMD is similar to that in vertebral fractures, but, because the patients are older, it is more likely to fall within the normal range for age (Fig. 2; *14*). Thus, by any definition, only about 50% of nonhip peripheral fracture cases have osteoporosis, but most vertebral and hip fracture patients are osteoporotic.

BONE DENSITOMETRY

Technical Aspects

BMD may be measured at one or more of at least four sites: total body, lumbar spine, proximal femur, or forearm. Each of them is generally related to reference lines provided

Table 1
Regression Equation of BMD (g/cm^2) on Height (cm)
at Four Sites in Postmenopausal Women Without Known Vertebral Fractures

Site	Intercept	Slope	P	T-score/10 cm
Forearm	0.22	0.00087	<0.001	0.18
Femoral neck	0.41	0.0020	0.001	0.15
Lumbar 2–4	0.031	0.0054	<0.001	0.33
Total body	0.041	0.0052	<0.001	0.60

by the manufacturers of the instruments and expressed as T-scores (number of SDs above or below the young mean) and Z-scores (age-related T-scores). Unfortunately, these reference lines are of variable quality, and not necessarily internally compatible, because different populations may have been used for different sites. This is one reason why BMD measurements on the same individual in different makes of densitometer do not agree well, although there is good agreement when a subject is measured in different instruments of the same brand.

The discrepancies between T-scores at different sites are not only the result of discordant reference lines; some represent a biological reality. Although there are very significant correlations between BMDs at the principal sites, even after correction for age (coefficients around 0.7 [15]), peripheral BMD may be disproportionately low in such conditions as primary hyperparathyroidism (16) and rheumatoid arthritis; spinal BMD tends to be selectively reduced in patients on corticosteroids (17), and perhaps in the first years after menopause (18). Conversely, vertebral density may be spuriously high because of degenerative disease and/or compression fractures.

In addition to these problems with BMD, there is the added weakness that current bone densitomtery (other than computerized tomography) yields results in areal density terms (g/cm^2), rather than in volume density terms (g/cm^3). Bone mass (BMC in grams of bone mineral) must be size-corrected, because large people have large bones and small people small bones; without size correction, none of the former and all the latter would appear to be osteoporotic. Unfortunately, areal density constitutes only an incomplete correction for bone size; this is unimportant in subjects of average height, but becomes important in subjects significantly below or above average height. This is shown in Table 1, which gives BMD as a function of height in postmenopausal women without vertebral fractures. The slopes are such that every 10-cm reduction in height lowers BMD quite substantially, at least in the lumbar spine and total body; small subjects are therefore liable to be labeled as osteoporotic, when their bone mass is in fact normal for their height.

It is clear from these considerations that clinicians need to interpret BMD results with some caution, and pay particular attention to the origin and validity of the reference lines. Osteoporosis is generally a disorder of the whole skeleton; most sites are affected by the osteoporotic process, even if at somewhat different rates. Between the ages of 50 and 80 yr, there is proportionately more loss of bone from the distal forearm than from the femoral neck, spine, or whole skeleton (Fig. 1), but all these sites lose bone.

Thus, the BMD is not always easy to interpret, yet it is the essential basis for the diagnosis of osteoporosis, unless bone biospy is undertaken, and even then the outcome may be equivocal unless osteomalacia or some other pathology is found. Vertebral compression strongly suggests a diagnosis of osteoporosis, particularly if more than one

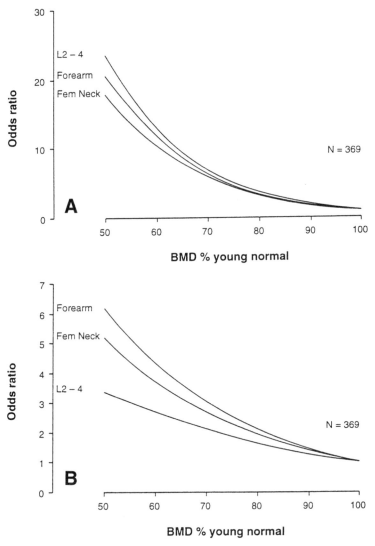

Fig. 3. Fracture odds ratios as a function of BMD at three different sites.

vertebra is involved, but even vertebral fractures may be traumatic in origin, and peripheral fractures (other than hip) are only pointers. However, although densitometry has its weaknesses, they can be minimized by measuring at more than one site; two sites are better than one, and measuring at three sites is marginally even more useful *(19)*. It has been claimed that prediction of fracture risk from BMD is site specific, i.e., that femoral neck BMD predicts hip-fracture risk, spine BMD predicts vertebral-fracture risk, and so on *(20)*, but this is probably too simplistic an approach. As Fig. 3 shows, femoral neck is almost as good as lumbar spine in discriminating between vertebral fracture cases and controls, and distal forearm and femoral neck are better than lumbar spine in discriminating between peripheral fracture cases and controls. In fact, if only one site can be measured, the distal forearm is probably the most cost effective for both cross-sectional and longitudinal purposes. If multiple sites can be measured, then the sites of choice are distal forearm, spine, and hip.

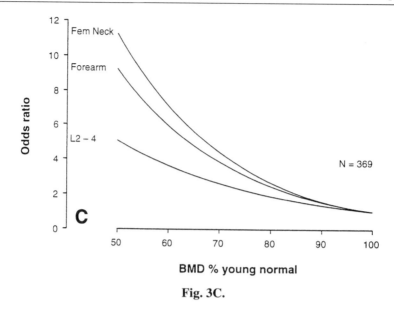

Fig. 3C.

Interpretation

In interpreting BMD, the clinician must appreciate the large genetic component in BMD *(21,22)*. Inheritance is the chief determinant of BMD in children and adolescents *(23)*, and of peak bone density in young adults *(24)*. Genes remain dominant even after bone loss commences in midlife, because the population variance of BMD (SD 10–15%) is large, relative to the rate of bone loss (0.5–1.5%/yr). Until about age 65 yr, therefore, peak bone density is the chief determinant of BMD, but, after that, BMD is increasingly determined by the rate of bone loss *(25,26)*. The older the patient, therefore, the more confidently can it be assumed that low BMD has a proximate cause. This is particularly true in patients with low Z-scores, i.e., those whose BMD is not only low in absolute terms, but also low for age. Very broadly speaking, a low BMD that is normal for age can be attributed to genetic makeup and normal aging processes (whatever they may be), but a BMD that is low for age suggests other risk factors than normal aging. But here, too, there is a caveat. Rapid loss from a high peak value may yield the same result, at age 65, as normal loss from a midnormal peak value or slow loss from a low peak value. This is an important caveat, because it emphasizes the point that knowing the rate of bone loss is at least as important as knowing the BMD. Even subjects with absolutely normal BMD and low apparent fracture risk may be in trouble in a relatively short time if they are fast bone-losers *(27)*, not only because they reach a low BMD prematurely, but also perhaps because high bone turnover itself increases fracture risk, as can be inferred from the fact that the effects of treatment on fracture rates are greater than can be accounted for by their effects on BMD *(28–30)*. The rate of bone loss can be calculated from successive BMD measurements, but, even with the most meticulous care, this cannot be done with any confidence in less than 6–12 mo (some would say 2 yr), unless bone loss is very rapid. An alternative is therefore to measure one or more of the markers of bone turnover in the urine (hydroxyproline, pyridinoline) or serum ([bone] alkaline phosphatase, osteocalcin), all of which tend to be raised in fast bone-losers *(27,31,32)*. It could be argued that these markers should be measured in all patients under review, but it is particularly important to do so if the BMD is low. An example of the predictive power of a bone resorption marker is shown in Fig. 4 *(33)*.

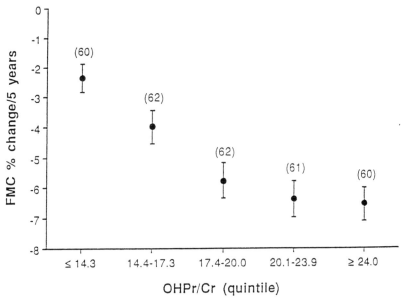

Fig. 4. Rates of forearm bone mineral content as a function of initial urinary hydroxyproline in 307 postmenopausal women followed-up for 5 yr *(33).*

CLINICAL GUIDELINES

Acting on Bone Mineral Density

The clinician, now armed with a knowledge of the patient's fracture history and BMD, may wish to follow the guidelines in Fig. 5. If BMD is in the high normal range (T-score >1), the risk of osteoporosis is very low and no action is required other than to suggest remeasurement in 5 yr or so.

If the T-score falls between 1 and −1, all that may be required is dietary advice and a BMD measurement in about 2 yr, but serum $25(OH)D_3$ (calcidiol) should be measured in any patient who is at risk of inadequate sunlight exposure. By dietary advice, we imply restricting dietary salt and animal protein, and increasing Ca (*see* Table 2).

If the T-score lies between −1 and −2, the patient is at definite risk of osteoporosis because any signficant bone loss will take him/her into the osteoporotic range and greatly increase the fracture risk because of the exponential relation between BMD and fracture risk shown in Fig. 3. Two courses of action are open. One is to take preventive action by giving dietary advice and nonspecific treatment (Ca and/or hormones in women). The second is to use bone markers to select the rapid bone-losers, and actively to treat only those with evidence of high bone turnover. Whichever course is followed, BMD should be measured regularly, and fuller investigation undertaken if bone is lost or a fracture occurs.

If the T-score is below −2 but the Z-score is normal, major risk factors should be excluded, essential investigations performed, dietary advice given, active treatment commenced, the response monitored with bone markers, and the BMD remeasured in 12 mo.

If the T-score is below −2 and the Z-score below −1, or if there is vertebral fracture, full investigation is required (*see* Investigations), and active treatment should be tailored to the results. All these patients should also have lateral spine radiography and be given standard dietary advice. Their progress should be monitored by turnover markers, 6-mo

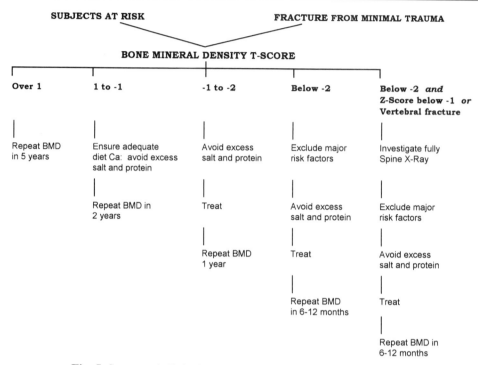

Fig. 5. Suggested clinical guidelines based on bone densitometry.

high-precision forearm BMD (if available), and spinal and, perhaps, femoral neck BMD every year. But the treatment selected should depend on risk factors and the results of investigation, as indicated below.

Risk Factors

The above account has made several references to risk factors because it is seldom possible to identify a single cause of osteoporosis; the condition usually results from a combination of risk factors, which are difficult to classify, because only some of them, such as thyroid hormone, act directly on bone; others have more than one effect, or act indirectly through Ca absorption or excretion. Thus, for instance, estrogens have a direct action on bone but also modulate Ca absorption and excretion (11). Corticosteroids depress bone formation but also impair Ca absorption and promote Ca excretion (34).

However, the prinicipal known risk factors, and the way in which they appear to act, are shown in Table 2. The more severe the osteoporosis and the more abnormal the bone markers, the more energetically should the clinician look for risk factors, by history, physical examination, and investigation, and then seek to eliminate them.

Investigations

PROTOCOL

The investigational protocol for osteoporosis varies from center to center. The one described below has been in use in Adelaide for some 15 yr (35), and is subject to the outcome of history-taking and physical examination. After the consultation, the patient is provided with a clean polyethylene container in which to collect urine for 24 h (usually

Table 2
Principal Risk Factors for Osteoporosis

Independent variable	Nature of effect on bone	Dependent variable and direction of effect		Effect on BMD
Genetic makeup	Direct	Peak bone density	–	–
Oestrogens	Direct[a]	Bone resorption	−ve	Positive
Androgens	Direct[a]	Bone formation	+ve	Positive
Aging	Direct[a]	Bone formation	−ve	Negative
Body weight	Direct	Bone formation	+ve	Positive
Exercise	Direct	Bone formation	+ve	Positive
Immobilization	Direct	Bone resorption	+ve	Negative
Dietary Ca	Indirect	Bone resorption	−ve	Positive
Ca absorption	Indirect	Bone resorption	−ve	Positive
Ca excretion	Indirect	Bone resorption	+ve	Negative
Dietary sodium and protein	Indirect	Ca excretion	+ve	Negative
Corticosteroid hormones	Direct[a]	Bone formation	−ve	Negative
Thyroid hormone	Direct	Bone resorption	+ve	Negative
Parathyroid hormone	Direct	Bone resorption	+ve	Negative
Alcohol	Direct[a]	Bone formation	−ve	Negative
Smoking	Indirect	Ca absorption	+ve	Negative
Caffeine	Indirect	Ca excretion	−ve	Negative
Heparin and warfarin	Direct	Uncertain	?	Negative
Thiazide diuretics	Indirect	Ca excretion	−ve	Positive
Loop diuretics	Indirect	Ca excretion	+ve	Negative
Vitamin D	Direct	PTH secretion	-ve	Positive

[a]Also has an indirect effect on bone by way of Ca absorption and/or excretion.

7 AM to 7 AM), and is instructed to then take it to the clinical laboratory at about 9 AM, without breakfast, for the procedures shown in Table 3. Most of these tests are self-explanatory, but some of them, such as the bone turnover markers, require further explanation.

INTERPRETATION

Bone Turnover Markers. Acquired osteoporosis must be caused by either excessive bone resorption or impaired bone formation, or both. It might be expected, therefore, that separate markers of bone formation and resorption could be used to identify which of the variables is at fault and that appropriate treatment could then be given. In practice, because of the close link between the bone-forming and resorbing processes (coupling), any rise in bone resorption triggers a rise in bone formation. Because most bone loss (in women at least) is caused by an increase in bone breakdown, the rise in markers of resorption, e.g., at the menopause, is accompanied by a rise in the markers of bone formation. Thus, the paradox emerges that bone-losers, particularly fast bone losers, have high rates of bone formation as well as resorption. In theory, a relative deficiency in bone formation might be inferred from the ratio of formation to resorption markers, but in practice the accuracy of these markers is not good enough to draw any useful inference from the ratios. The only patients in whom relative or absolute depression of bone formation can consistently be inferred from bone formation markers appear to be those on corticosteroid therapy, in whom serum alkaline phosphatase and osteocalcin tend to be relatively low *(34)*.

Table 3
Routine Investigation of Osteoporosis

Procedure	Analyses	Calculations
Fasting venous blood	Calcium, phosphate creatinine Alkaline phosphatase Albumin, globulins Sodium, potassium Bicarbonate, chloride PTH, $25OHD_3$, $1,25(OH)_2D_3$ TSH, (Osteocalcin) (Sex hormones)	Anion gap (Na + K) - (Cl + Bic) Ionized Ca
60-min blood	Radioactivity	Radiocalcium absorption
Fasting urine	Calcium, phosphate sodium, creatinine Deoxypyridinoline (Dpyr) Pyridinoline (Pyr) Hydroxyproline (OHPr)	Ca/Cr, P/Cr, Na/Cr; OHPr/Cr; Dpyr/Cr, Pyr/Cr TmP/C_{cr} $TmCa/C_{cr}$
24-h urine	Calcium, phosphate sodium, creatinine Cortisol Deoxypyridinoline Pyridinoline	Deoxypyridinoline/Cr Pyridinoline/Cr Creatinine clearance

In practice, therefore, all bone markers tend to be used as markers of bone resorption (often called bone turnover), not only in initial investigations, but also in monitoring of response to therapy, most of which is directed toward inhibition of the resorbing process. Whether markers are measured in fasting urine (as has to be done with hydroxyproline, unless the subject is on a collagen-free diet), or in 24 h urine, is a matter of choice. They tend to be higher in fasting urine, but their diagnostic value is very similar: It is not necessary to do both. Deoxypyridinoline and hydroxyproline excretion are so closely related as to be interchangeable. Pyridinoline is less discriminatory than the deoxy derivative.

Other Analytes. It is hardly necessary to justify measurement of serum Ca, but it must be stressed that the ionized and ultrafiltrable fractions are more useful than the total. In mild hyperthyroidism and hyperparathyroidism, slight hypoalbuminemia may be sufficient to mask hypercalcemia, which may not be detected unless the ionized fraction is measured or calculated. The ultrafiltrable Ca can only be arrived at by calculation, and is needed to derive the notional tubular maximum reabsorptive capacity for calcium (TmCa). The serum phosphate is needed in its own right, and for calculation of TmP. Albumin, globulins, anion gap, and bicarbonate are needed for the calculation of the Ca fractions and may all be of value in their own right. Serum parathyroid hormone (PTH) is required in its own right and for the interpretation of hypercalcemia. Serum $25(OH)D_3$ is required to exclude nutritional deficiency of vitamin D, and serum $1,25(OH)_2D_3$ is needed to permit the distinction between malabsorption of Ca caused by calcitriol deficiency and that caused by resistance to Ca at the intestinal level. Serum alkaline phosphatase is a useful marker of bone formation, except in the presence of liver disease, when the bone-specific isoenzyme or osteocalcin needs to be determined. The fasting urine Ca is needed as a marker of the rate of obligatory Ca loss. Urine phosphate and sodium are needed in the same sample to establish whether either or both can account for a high obligatory Ca output. 24-h Ca is measured to establish whether it is high (>5 mmol) (caused by high intake, high absorption, or high obligatory loss), and, if so, whether this can be accounted for by high urine sodium or phosphate. Low 24-h Ca (below 3 mmol) suggests malabsorption of Ca or very low intake. (If radiocalcium absorption is not available, the 24-h Ca and/or its rise or failure to rise on a Ca supplement can be used as surrogates).

OUTCOMES

Underlying Diseases. The rest of the data obtained from the protocol permits calculation of Ca fractions in the serum *(35)*, the notional tubular reabsorption maxima for Ca and phosphate (TmCa and TmP) *(34)*, fractional radiocalcium absorption rate *(36)*, total and obligatory Ca excretion *(11)*, and other derived variables, such as creatinine clearance. This may allow the identification of one of a number of pathologies (in which all the markers of bone turnover are generally high).

1. Primary hyperparathyroidism, from the combination of a raised ionized Ca with a raised serum PTH. These cases may have a high TmCa, and, almost invariably, a low TmP.
2. Malignant hypercalcemia, from the combination of hypercalcemia with low PTH.
3. Secondary hyperparathyroidism, from the combination of a raised serum PTH with a low serum $25(OH)D_3$ (vitamin D deficiency) or raised serum creatinine (renal failure). In the former, serum calcitriol is generally maintained by parathyroid hormone and Ca absorption is often normal, but, in the latter, the serum calcitriol and Ca absorption are always low.
4. Hyperadrenocorticism, suspected from a raised urinary free cortisol, but requiring further investigation.
5. Myeloma, suspected from high serum globulins and possible hypercalcemia and malabsorption of Ca, but requiring further investigation.
6. Hyperthyroidism, from a low serum thyroid-stimulating hormone. There may also be marginal hypercalcemia with high serum P, low PTH, and high TmP.
7. Paget's disease, from very high bone turnover markers without other abnormality.

Allthough most patients investigated for osteoporosis will not yield such clear evidence of primary pathology, these tests may nonetheless reveal physiological abnormalities on which rational treatment decisions can be based. These are described in the next subheading.

PHYSIOLOGICAL ABNORMALITIES

Low Calcium Intake. It may not be practicable to obtain a full diet history from all patients being investigated for osteoporosis, but it is a simple matter for the clinician to ask them a few questions about the consumption of dairy products, from which it is possible to classify the dietary Ca into low, average, and high intake categories. Low intake signifies that the subject omits milk in tea and coffee, and avoids dairy products in general because of milk intolerance, on medical advice, e.g., for hypercholesterolemia, or for other reasons. (In many cases, this omission of Ca is of recent origin, and has no bearing on current bone status, but it may raise bone markers and lower urine Ca. At the other extreme, however, aversion to dairy products may have been sufficiently longstanding to lower BMD). Average intake covers the bulk of patients, e.g., those who take milk in tea and coffee and on breakfast cereal, and do not avoid cheese or other dairy products. High Ca intake comprises patients who make a point of drinking milk and eating cheese and yogurt, or who are taking a Ca supplement.

Table 4
Mean Radiocalcium Absorption (SD)
(Fraction/h) Corrected for Age and Serum Calcitriol
in Men and Women with and Without Vertebral Compression

	Men	n	Women	n
Normal	0.62 (0.039)	49	0.69 (0.011)	551
Osteoporotic	0.53 (0.027)	99	0.63 (0.025)	124
P	<0.001		<0.001	

Malabsorption of Calcium. The definition of Ca malabsorption is arbitrary, because Ca absorption is a continuous variable. With the Adelaide method *(36)*, the mean normal fractional absorption rate (α) is 0.75/h (SD 0.15) and values below 0.60 are taken to represent low absorption. (Methods using more Ca carrier *(37,38)* yield lower fractional absorption rates). Radiocalcium absorption tends to fall with age, probably before there is any significant decline in serum calcitriol, and represents a decline in the gastrointestinal responsiveness to calcitriol *(39)*, which occurs prematurely in patients with vertebral compression (Table 4; *40*).

High Obligatory Calcium Excretion. A high fasting Ca/Cr represents high obligatory Ca loss, and may be caused by high urinary sodium (resulting from high salt intake) or a high urinary phosphate (resulting from high protein intake). Alternatively, it may be caused by a raised filtered load of Ca (as in most forms of hypercalcemia), or by reduced tubular reabsorption of Ca (low TmCa). If it is a significant determinant of bone resorption, it will be associated with raised bone resorption markers. If the latter are normal, a high Ca/Cr may simply be a spillover from the previous day because of high Ca absorption or an evening Ca supplement.

Treatment

UNDERLYING DISEASES

Any underlying disease (such as hyperthyroidism) revealed by the investigations needs to be treated. This is straightforward in hyperthyroidism, the treatment of which rapidly reduces bone resorption to normal. It is more difficult in primary hyperparathyroidism because of uncertainty about the relative merits of surgical and medical measures *(41)*. There would be little disagreement that surgery is indicated in patients with a serum Ca over 3 mmol/L (ionized Ca over 1.5 mmol/L), or with kidney stones or other complications, and little dispute that a patient with a serum Ca below 2.75 mmol/L (ionized Ca below 1.38 mmol/L) can probably be kept under observation or treated medically. In the range between these limits, there is uncertainty, at least in postmenopausal women, because of the success of hormone treatment in this group *(42,43)*. Treatment of myeloma, Paget's disease, and hyperadrenocorticism are outside the scope of this chapter.

ABNORMAL PHYSIOLOGY

When underlying pathology has been excluded, bone resorption, if high,can be inhibited in patients with incipient or established osteoporosis in the following ways.

1. Supplemental Ca in a dose of 0.5 g/d in patients whose dietary Ca intake is average, and in a dose of 1.0 g/d to those whose intake is low. These relatively large doses are required, because only 5–10% of the Ca is absorbed. The immediate effect is to lower the markers of bone resorption *(44,45)*.

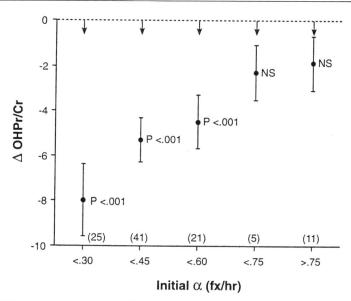

Fig. 6. The fall in urinary hydroxyproline following calcitriol treatment as a function of initial radiocalcium absorption (α). Note that the fall is significant when the initial α is low, but not when it is high.

2. Vitamin D in a dose of 500–1000 U/d (12.5–25 μg) in patients in whom the serum calcidiol is below the reference range, more particularly if the serum PTH is raised. This dose can safely be continued indefinitely. There are insufficient data to say whether this treatment has any effect on Ca absorption, unless it raises the serum calcitriol level, as it does in severe vitamin D deficiency *(46)*.

3. Calcitriol in an initial dose of 0.25 μg/d in patients whose fractional hourly rate of radio-calcium absorption (α) is below 0.60. This has the effect of improving Ca absorption within a few days and of lowering urinary hydroxyproline within a few weeks *(47)*. This treatment can safely be combined with the Ca supplement regime outlined above. If bone resorption markers do not fall, the dose of calcitriol should be raised to 0.5 μg and the Ca supplement limited to 0.5 g. Some monitoring of fasting serum Ca is advisable on higher doses but mild postprandial hypercalcemia is acceptable. Note that calcitriol only lowers bone resorption markers if initial Ca absorption is low (Fig. 6).

4. Estrogens in conventional doses for women with a high obligatory (fasting) urinary Ca that has not responded to salt and/or animal protein restriction. If the patient is asymptomatic and/or has a family history of breast cancer, then northinderone in a dose of 2.5–5.0 mg should be used, and is equally effective in the control of bone resorption *(48,49)*. However, norethindrone is also mildly androgenic (being derived from 19-nor-testosterone), and should be combined with a vaginal estrogen to prevent vaginal atrophy.

5. Bisphosphonates are also powerful inhibitors of bone resorption. Alendronate, 10 mg/d, for instance, raises BMD at all sites, and significantly reduces fracture rates *(30)*, but the indications for its use are not as well defined as are those for the other treatments described above. However, bisphosphonates should certainly be used if other treatments fail to control bone resorption, and many would use them as first line therapy.

The effects on forearm BMD of treatment on the above lines in 251 postmenopausal women is shown in Fig. 7, and compared with 157 untreated referred by outside practitioners during the same period. The untreated women have lost bone as expected; those

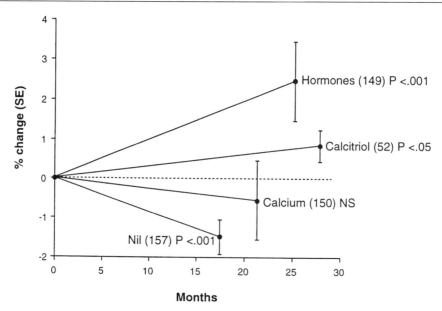

Fig. 7. Percentage change in forearm BMD as a function of duration of treatment in postmenopausal women on three different treatments, and in the untreated state.

treated with Ca or calcitriol neither gained nor lost bone; and those treated with hormones gained at a significant rate. This series does not include any cases of vitamin D deficiency treated with vitamin D, but positive effects of treatment with vitamin D in such cases has been reported from Europe *(50,51)*.

CONCLUSIONS

The term "osteoporosis" signifies a low apparent density of bone as an organ, which has the clinical effect of increasing the risk of fracture. The diagnosis is usually based on bone densitometry, but this technology suffers from systematic differences between different instruments, and inconsistencies in reference values between different manufacturers. In addition, dual-energy X-ray absorptiometry does not fully correct for body size.

Genetic factors are the chief determinants of bone status during childhood and adult life, but rates of bone loss during aging are determined by contingent risk factors. It follows that the primary task of the clinician caring for elderly subjects with incipient or established osteoporosis is to identify and eliminate or correct these risk factors.

Ca metabolism is not a black box. Its secrets can be unlocked by appropriate investigation, and its disorders managed by rational therapy. The object of this chapter has been to suggest ways in which this can be done.

REFERENCES

1. Nordin BEC, Polley KJ. Metabolic consequences of the menopause. A cross-sectional, longitudinal, and intervention study on 557 normal postmenopausal women. Calcif Tissue Int 1987;41:1–S60.
2. Kelly PJ, Pocock NA, Sambrook PN, Eisman JA. Age and menopause-related changes in indices of bone turnover. J Clin Endocrinol Metab 1989;69:1160–1165.
3. Wishart JM, Need AG, Horowitz M, Morris HA, Nordin BEC. Effect of age on bone density and bone turnover in men. Clin Endocrinol 1995;42:141–146.

 4. Need AG, Morris HA, Horowitz M, Scopacasa F, Nordin BEC. Intestinal calcium absorption in men with spinal osteoporosis. Clin Endocrinol 1998;48:163–168.
 5. Parfitt AM, Villanueva AR, Foldes J, Sudhaker-Rao D. Relations between histologic indices of bone formation: implications for the pathogenesis of spinal osteoporosis. J Bone Miner Res 1995;10:466–473.
 6. Nordin BEC. Osteomalacia, osteoporosis and calcium deficiency. Clin Orthop Rel Res 1960;17:235–258.
 7. Wu DD, Boyd RD, Fix TJ, Burr DB. Regional patterns of bone loss and altered bone remodeling in response to calcium deprivation in laboratory rabbits. Calcif Tissue Int 1990;47:18–23.
 8. Heaney RP, Recker RR, Saville PD. Menopausal changes in calcium balance performance. J Lab Clin Med 1978;92:953–963.
 9. Nordin BEC. Calcium and osteoporosis. Nutrition 1997;13:664–686.
10. Heaney RP. A unified concept of osteoporosis. Am J Med 1965;39:877–880.
11. Nordin BEC, Need AG, Morris HA, Horowitz M. Biochemical variables in pre- and postmenopausal women: reconciling the calcium and estrogen hypotheses. Osteoporosis Int 1999;9:351–357.
12. Kanis JA. Assessment of fracture risk and its application to screening for postmenopausal osteoporosis. Synopsis of a WHO Report. Osteoporosis Int 1994;4:368–381.
13. Nordin BEC. The definition and diagnosis of osteoporosis. Calcif Tissue Int 1987;40:57–58.
14. Aitken JM. Relevance of osteoporosis in women with fracture of the femoral neck. Br Med J 1984; 288:597–601.
15. Nordin BEC, Chatterton BE, Schultz CG, Need AG, Horowitz M. Regional bone mineral density inter-relationships in normal and osteoporotic postmenopausal women. J Bone Miner Res 1996;11:849–856.
16. Silverberg SJ, Shane E, De La Cruz L, Dempster DW, Feldman F, Seldin D, et al. Skeletal disease in primary hyperparathyroidism. J Bone Miner Res 1989;4:283–291.
17. Laan RFJM, Buijs WCAM, van Erning LJTO, et al. Differential effects of glucocorticoids on cortical appendicular and cortical vertebral bone mineral content. Calcif Tissue Int 1993;52:5–9.
18. Balikian P, Burbank K, Houde J, Crane G, Nairus J, Ahmadi S, Baran DT. Bone mineral density and broadband ultrasound attenuation with estrogen treatment of postmenopausal women. J Clin Densitometry 1998;1:19–26.
19. Wasnich RD, Ross PD, Davis JW, Vogel JM. A comparison of single and multi-site BMC measurements for assessment of spine fracture probability. J Nucl Med 1989;30:1166–1171.
20. Cummings SR, Black DM, Nevitt MC, Browner W, Cauley J, Ensrud K, et al. Bone density at various sites for prediction of hip fractures. Lancet 1993;341:72–75.
21. Harris M, Nguyen TV, Howard GM, Kelly PJ, Eisman JA. Genetic and environmental correlations between bone formation and bone mineral density: a twin study. Bone 1998;22:141–145.
22. Ferrari S, Rizzoli R, Sloasman D, Bonjour J-P. Familial resemblance for bone mineral mass is expressed before puberty. J Clin Endocrinol Metab 1998;83:358–361.
23. Matkovic V, Fontana D, Tominac C, Goel P, Chesnut CH. Factors that influence peak bone mass formation: a study of calcium balance and the inheritance of bone mass in adolescent females. Am J Clin Nutr 1990;52:878–888.
24. Seeman E, Hopper JL, Bach LA, Cooper ME, Parkinson E, McKay J, Jerums G. Reduced bone mass in daughters of women with osteoporosis. N Engl J Med 1989;320:554–558.
25. Slemenda CW, Christian JC, Williams CJ, Norton JA, Johnston CC. Genetic determinants of bone mass in adult women: a reevaluation of the twin model and the potential importance of gene interaction on heritability estimates. J Bone Miner Res 1991;6:561–567.
26. Nordin BEC. Keynote address. Bone mass, bone loss, bone density and fractures. Osteoporosis Int 1993;(Suppl 1):S1–S7.
27. Hansen MA, Overgaard K, Riis BJ, Christiansen C. Role of peak bone mass and bone loss in postmenopausal osteoporosis: 12 year study. Br Med J 1991;303:961–964.
28. Cumming RG, Nevitt MC. Calcium for prevention of osteoporotic fractures in postmenopausal women. J Bone Miner Res 1997;12:1321–1329.
29. Riggs BL, Melton LJ, O'Fallon WM. Drug therapy for vertebral fractures in osteoporosis: evidence that decreases in bone turnover and increases in bone mass both determine antifracture efficacy. Bone 1996; 18:197S–201S.
30. Liberman UA, Weiss SR, Broll J, Minnie HW, Quan H, Bell NH, et al. Effect of oral alendronate on bone mineral density and the incidence of fractures in postmenopausal osteoporosis. N Engl J Med 1995;333: 1437–1443.
31. Rosen CJ, Chesnut CH, Mallinak NJS. The predictive value of biochemical markers of bone turnover for bone mineral density in early postmenopausal women treated with hormone replacement or calcium supplementation. J Clin Endocrinol Metab 1997;82:1904–1910.

32. Heikkinen A-M, Parviainen M, Niskanen L, Komulainen M, Tuppurainen MJ, Kroger H, Saarikoski S. Biochemical bone markers and bone mineral density during postmenopausal hormone replacement therapy with and without vitamin D_3: a prospective, controlled, randomized study. J Clin Endocrinol Metab 1997;82:2476–2482.

33. Nordin BEC, Cleghorn DB, Chatterton BE, Morris HA, Need AG. A 5-year longitudinal study of forearm bone mass in 307 postmenopausal women. J Bone Miner Res 1993;8:1427–1432.

34. Need AG. Corticosteroid hormones. In: Nordin BEC, Need AG, Morris HA, eds. Metabolic Bone and Stone Disease, 3rd ed. Churchill Livingstone, Edinburgh, 1993, pp. 43–62.

35. Morris HA. Laboratory protocols for metabolic bone disorders. Clin Biochem Rev 1994;15:165–172.

36. Nordin BEC, Morris HA, Wishart JM, et al. Modification and validation of a single-isotope radiocalcium absorption test. J Nucl Med 1998;39:108–113.

37. Heaney RP, Weaver CM, Fitzsimmons ML. Influence of calcium load on absorption fraction. J Bone Miner Res 1990;11:1135–1138.

38. Krall EA, Dawson-Hughes B. Relation of fractional ^{47}Ca retention to season and rates of bone loss in healthy postmenopausal women. J Bone Miner Res 1991;16:1323–1329.

39. Ebeling PR, Sandgren ME, DiMagno EP, Lane AW, DeLuca HF, Riggs BL. Evidence of an age-related decrease in intestinal responsiveness to vitamin D. relationship between serum 1,25-dihydroxyvitamin D_3 and intestinal vitamin D receptor concentrations in normal women. J Clin Endocrinol Metab 1992;75: 176–182.

40. Morris HA, Need AG, Horowitz M, O'Loughlin PD, Nordin BEC. Calcium absorption in normal and osteoporotic postmenopausal women. Calcif Tissue Int 1991;49:240–243.

41. Consensus Development Panel. Diagnosis and management of asymptomatic primary hyperparathyroidism. Consensus Development Conference statement. Ann Intern Med 1991;114:593–597.

42. Marcus R, Madvig P, Crim M, Pont A, Kosek J. Conjugated estrogens in the treatment of postmenopausal women with hyperparathyroidism. Ann Intern Med 1984;100:633–640.

43. Horowitz M, Wishart J, Need AG, Morris H, Philcox J, Nordin BEC. Treatment of postmenopausal hyperparathyroidism with norethindrone: effects of biochemistry and forearm mineral density. Arch Intern Med 1987;147:681–685.

44. Horowitz M, Wishart JM, Goh D, Morris HA, Need AG, Nordin BEC Oral calcium suppresses biochemical markers of bone resorption in men. Am J Clin Nutr 1994;60:965–968.

45. Scopacasa F, Horowitz M, Wishart J, et al. Calcium supplementation suppresses bone resorption in early postmenopausal women. Calcif Tissue Int 1998;62:8–12.

46. Peacock M. Osteomalacia and rickets. In: Nordin BEC, ed. Metabolic Bone and Stone Disease, 2nd ed. Churchill Livingstone, Edinburgh, 1984, pp. 71–111.

47. Need AG, Horowitz M, Philcox JC, Nordin BEC. 1,25-dihydroxycalciferol and calcium therapy in osteoporosis with calcium malabsorption. Miner Electrolyte Metab 1985;11:35–40.

48. Horowitz M, Wishart JM, Need AG, Morris HA, Nordin BEC. Effects of norethisterone on bone related biochemical variables and forearm bone mineral in postmenopausal osteoporosis. Clin Endocrinol 1993;39:649–655.

49. Scopacasa F, Horowitz M, Need AG, Morris HA, Nordin BEC. The effects of low dose norethisterone on biochemical variables in postmenopausal women. Osteoporosis Int, in press.

50. Nordin BEC, Baker MR, Horsman A, Peacock M. A prospective trial of the effect of vitamin D supplementation on metacarpal bone loss in elderly women. Am J Clin Nutr 1985;42:470–474.

51. Chapuy MC, Arlot ME. Duboeuf F, et al. Vitamin D_3 and calcium to prevent hip fractures in elderly women. N Engl J Med 1992;327:1637–1642.

8

Paget's Disease of Bone

Dongjie Liu, MD, and Kenneth W. Lyles, MD

INTRODUCTION

Paget's disease of bone (PDB; osteitis deformans) is a chronic disorder of localized increased bone remodeling, affecting 1.2–3.0% of people over 60 yr of age in the United States. The etiology of PDB is unknown, but current studies suggest that it may be caused by a latent paramyxovirus infection. Families have also been described with a high prevalence of PDB in multiple generations. Eighty percent of these families' gene for PDB has been localized to the long arm of chromosome 18. PDB can have widely varying clinic manifestations. Symptoms of PDB depend on which part of the skeleton is involved. Bone pain, arthritic symptoms, deformity, neurological compression syndromes, fracture, and, rarely, malignant degeneration can occur in affected patients. When the diagnosis of PDB is considered, the patient should have a radioisotopic total body bone scan to localize areas of increased disease activity, then areas of increased tracer uptake should be radiographed to confirm the diagnosis. Serum markers of bone formation, such as alkaline phosphotase and bone-specific alkaline phosphotase, can be used to diagnose the disease, as well as monitor response to therapy. Urinary excretion of skeletal breakdown products (hydroxyproline, pyridinoline, N-telopeptides) are markers of bone resorption.

Safe and effective therapies are now available for PDB. Although experts agree that therapies should be initiated for disease in certain skeletal areas, it is more difficult to decide whether to treat asymptomatic patients. There are no prospective data that show that complication of the disease can be prevented by reducing or normalizing rate of abnormal bone remodeling. There are two classes of drugs that have U.S. Food and Drug Administration (FDA) approval for treatment of PDB: calcitonin and bisphosphonates. Although calcitonins are safe and effective agents to reduce bone remodeling rates,

From: *Contemporary Endocrinology: Endocrinology of Aging*
Edited by: J. E. Morley and L. van den Berg © Humana Press Inc., Totowa, NJ

bisphosphonates are currently available that can normalize bone remodeling rates. The drugs are considered to be the drugs of choice for patients with PDB.

EPIDEMIOLOGY

PDB is a focal disorder of accelerated skeletal remodeling, first described by Sir James Paget in 1877 *(1)*. In his original description, Paget described six patients with enlarged skulls, hearing loss, bowed extremities, and kyphotic spines. He called the disease "osteitis deformans," and proposed an inflammatory basis to the lesion, which he said led to the progressive deformity of the affected bones over the lifetime of an individual. Since the original description of the disorder, a clearer understanding has emerged of its pathophysiology, clinical manifestations, and how to treat it.

PDB is the second most common geriatric metabolic bone disorder, next only to osteoporosis in prevalence. In the United States, the disease occurs in 1.2–3.0% of people over 60 yr of age *(2,3)*. In England, the disease can occur in 5% of people over 55 yr. In Spain, the disease occurs in 6.3% of people over 40 yr *(4)*. The prevalence in an autopsy study has been reported to be 10–15% by the ninth decade of life. The incidence rises by approx 0.3%/yr after 55 yr *(5)*. The disorder is rarely recognized before age 40, although some cases have been reported among young adults *(6,7)*. PDB is slightly more common in men *(8)*, but a higher male:female ratio of about 3:1 is seen in familial cases *(6,9,10)*. One recent study *(11)* suggests that the incidence and severity of PDB is declining in New Zealand. Further studies will be needed to confirm this observation.

PDB may occur in families. Studies of such families suggest an autosomal dominant characteristic with low penetration *(10,12)*. As many as 25% of patients have one or more family members with the disorder. The cumulative incidence of PDB to age 90 is 4× in relatives of patients with the condition than in relatives of control subjects *(2)*. Some reports describe the risk as even higher (7× greater) in the first relative of patients with the disease than in relatives of control group *(13,14)*. Familial PDB is also associated with more severity, and involves more extensive disease than occurs in sporadic cases *(6,10, 13,15,16)*. There have been occasional case reports of PDB among identical twins *(17)*. In some families, genetic susceptibility is suggested by finding a linkage between haplotypes of the HLA-DQWI, DR1, DR2, DRW6, and HLA-DP4 *(18,19)* and the presence of PDB. Several groups have studied large kindreds with PDB and localized the disease to the long arm of chromosome 18 *(20,21,22)*. Chromosome 6 (the HLA locus) is also proposed as candidate for evidence of a genetic susceptibility to PDB *(14,23)*. However, a recent study demonstrates that there exist relatively selective robertsonian translocation in eight of 14 patients with PDB (robertsonian translocation is characterized as chromosomal translocations localized to the D and G groups). By comparison, an age- and sex-matched group of eight controls and 13 patients with osteoporosis demonstrated no robertsonian translocation. These data suggest that, in addition to genetic factors, an environment factor could affect gene replication during the development of PDB *(24)*.

There are clear geographic distributions of PDB worldwide. The disorder is most prevalent in England, western Europe, the United States, Australia, and New Zealand, but is uncommon in Scandinavia, China, Japan, and India *(25,26)*. These studies suggest a genetic predisposition as the cause of this disorder. However, there are also geographic variations within the same country. In the United States, for example, PDB is more prevalent in the northern states *(27)*. In England, the prevalence of PDB is much higher in the northwest (Lancashire) than in the rest of the country *(28)*. A focus of higher frequency also has been described in Spain *(29)*. These results suggest that environmental factors combine with genetic factors to cause this disorder.

ETIOLOGY AND PATHOLOGY

Because PDB is an idiopathic, localized disorder of accelerated bone remodeling, it is useful to briefly review the normal remodeling process. All areas of the skeleton must be remodeled throughout life to repair acquired microfractures, and to strengthen parts of the skeleton placed under new or increased mechanical loads. The process begins when osteoclasts from bone marrow colony-forming units of the macrophage lineage come to a surface that needs remodeling. They excavate a cavity 50 μ in depth over a 2–4-wk period, and then undergo apoptosis. A new series of cells, osteoblasts, derived from bone marrow colony-forming units of fibroblast lineage, appear in the resorption cavity, and fill it with layers of osteoid tissue known as lamellae. The osteoblast also forms hydroxyapatite crystals on the collagen, which provides strength to the matrix. The process of bone remodeling is tightly coupled, so that increases or decreases in rates of bone resorption are followed by an increase or decrease in bone formation. Through this coupling of the resorption and formation processes, it is possible for most people to maintain their skeleton as a serviceable, lightweight frame throughout life. The coupling process is mediated by cytokines and growth factors released by osteoblasts and osteoclasts, which serve to control the remodeling process. Factors such as interleukin-6 (IL-6), and transforming growth factor (TGF)beta play a role in modulating bone turnover.

In pagetic lesions, the primary abnormality is in the osteoclast. A major histological feature is the increased number and size of the osteoclasts and their nuclei. Normal osteoclasts have 10 nuclei, but osteoclasts from areas of the skeleton with PDB have up to 100 nuclei. The osteoclasts also contain nuclear and cytoplasmic inclusions that resemble nucleocapsids of the paramyxoviral family. There is a compensatory increase in the number and size of the osteoblasts in the areas of increased remodeling activity, which leads to large amounts of new bone formation. The increased rate of bone turnover disrupts the normal lamellar pattern of the osteiod tissue, and results in immature woven or mosaic bone. This bone has increased amounts of fibrosis, chronic inflammatory cells, and vascularity, as well as enlarged haversian canals. Thus, although the bone appears denser radiographically, it is more subject to fracture, can bow with weight bearing, especially in the skull, can enlarge as long as the remodeling activity is increased.

The most widely accepted hypothesis for the etiology of PDB is caused by a slow-virus infection of bone cells *(30)*, based on ultrastructural and biochemical evidence. Viral-like inclusions in PDB osteoclasts were first described 24 yr ago *(31)*. Subsequently, using polyclonal and monoclonal antibodies *(32)* against paramyxoviruses, antigens are found in pagetic osteoclasts, suggesting previous infections of involved bone with a measles or respiratory syncitial virus. Antiviral antibody titers to mumps, parainfluenza, and adenovirus have also been detected in PDB *(33)*. In Great Britain, some work suggests that canine distemper virus (CDV) may be an etiologic agent. It has been demonstrated that both in vitro and in vivo infection with CDV produce a dose-dependent increase in the number and size of multinucleated osteoclast-like cells in cultures of canine bone marrow mononuclear cells *(34,35)*. One recent study *(36)* shows increased nucleolar organizer regions (NOR) in osteoclast nuclei of PDB. NOR number is known to correlate with the proliferative activity of the cell population, whether normal or malignant. However, an increase NOR number may not reflect the proliferative activity of osteoclast, because the cells are formed by the fusion of their precursors. Therefore, it is suggested that other mRNA of viral/oncogene origin could be actively transcribed in pagetic patients. This hypothesis is supported by findings that infection of CDV induces mRNA expression of IL-6 and c-*fos* oncogene in canine bone marrow cell cultures, similar to findings in pagetic bone cells *(35)*. Finding measles virus mRNA in other tissues provides further support for the viral infection hypothesis by *in situ* hybridization *(30)*. However, recent studies trying to sequence viral RNA, with the sensitive reverse transcriptase/polymerase chain reaction (RT-PCR) have unsuccessfully detected paramyxoviral RNA *(37,38)*. To date, no virus has been isolated from tissue cultures of pagetic bone cells, but this does not invalidate the theory, because the putative virus is highly defective, and no longer capable of being cultured *(39)*. An animal study *(40)*, using human T-cell leukemia virus-1 (HTLV-1)-infected transgenic mice, has suggested that genetically dependent aberrant host responses to viral proteins may mediate a disease with the same clinical features as PDB.

Scientific interest has turned to focusing on the regulators of osteoclast and osteoblast activity of PDB bone. It has been directly demonstrated increased expression of IL-6 *(41)*, c-*fos* oncogene *(42)*, and TGF *(43)* in Paget's bone by *in situ* hybridization. Roodman et al. *(44)* have also shown increased concentrations of IL-6 in conditioned media from long-term culture of Paget's bone marrow of PDB compared to that from normal bone marrow culture. However, sensitive studies with RT-PCR have found no difference in mRNA expression of IL-6, other cytokines, and growth factor in bone biopsy *(43,45)* and in bone cell culture *(35)* between PDB and normal bone tissue.

Based on published data, it may be hypothesized that development of PDB results from overproduction of cytokines from a slow-viral infection of pagetic bone and individual inheritance abnormalities in inflammatory response, or in genes regulating osteoclast and osteoblast activity. However, further studies must be completed to prove this hypothesis.

CLINICAL MANIFESTATIONS

Patients with PDB present with a wide array of symptoms. Many patients have the diagnosis made incidentally, when an elevated serum alkaline phosphatase level is found on a multiphasic screening panel, or a X-ray is performed that shows an asymptomatic bone lesion. The disease may affect any bone and can be monostotic (one bone) or polyostotic (many bones). Symptoms depend on the number and the site of the bone involved, as well as the activity of the bone remodeling. Indirect evidence suggests that the majority of patients (up to 50–70%) with radiographic evidence of Paget's disease have no symptoms *(46)*.

In patients with symptomatic PDB, the clinic characteristics are mostly composed of local bone pain, sometimes with obvious deformities, and fractures. The disease may also present in a variety of ways, with neurological, cardiovascular, and other miscellaneous signs and symptoms.

The bone pain can be mild to severe, is usually not related to physical activity, and can be variously described as dull aching, burning, or boring in nature. Acute pain may develop as a consequence of a pathologic fracture in an affected bone. Bone pain may also arise from increased vascularity, or from stretching of the periosteum caused by the

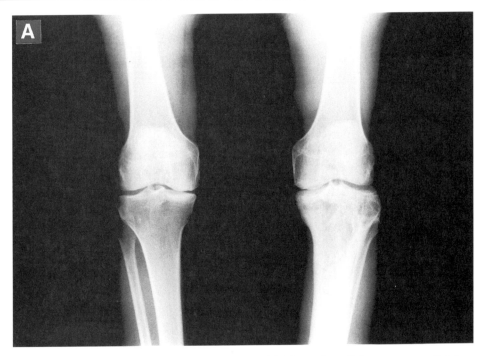

Fig. 1. (A) Standing knee radiographs from a patient with bilateral medial compartment joint space loss from osteoarthritis. The left tibia has PDB. There is thickening of trabeculae, cortical thickening, and areas of lucency.

increased amount of new bone formed in the disorganized bone remodeling (47). Periarticular pain may be the presenting symptom in 50% of symptomatic cases, and is an important diagnostic problem. Secondary osteoarthritis is common in PDB, and affects bone around major joints, such as the hip and knee, as well as those of the spine, with narrowing of the joint spaces and formation of osteophytes (48).

Bowing of weight bearing bone occurs most commonly in the femur and tibia, but also occurs in the humerus and ulna (Figs. 1–3). The bowing seen in the femur and tibia can be associated with stress fractures on the convex surface of the bowed bone. Vertebral bodies with PDB become enlarged and deformed (Fig. 4). Bone deformity alters force transmission through the adjacent joint, causing premature loss of articular cartilage and secondary osteoarthritis, especially in the hip and knee. Degenerative arthritis in joints contiguous to pagetic lesions causes juxta-articular enlargement and altered subchondral bone support. Patients also develop osteoarthritis in unaffected knees as a result of favoring the nonpagetic knee. Protrusio acetabuli occurs in some patients with disease involving the ilium.

Neurological complications reflect the predilection of the disease to affect the axial skeleton. Disease in the skull can cause nonspecific headaches, possibly from increased blood flow. Patients with skull involvement can develop deafness. Pagetic involvement of the temporal bone can cause conductive hearing loss. Involvement of the cochlea results in mixed sensory and conductive deafness. Occasionally, the optic or trigeminal nerves may be involved, resulting in visual loss or tic douloureux (trigeminal neuralgia). Skull deformity may result in enlargement of the vault, with a characteristic appearance particularly of the forehead (frontal bossing) or of the maxilla (leonthasis osseum) (47).

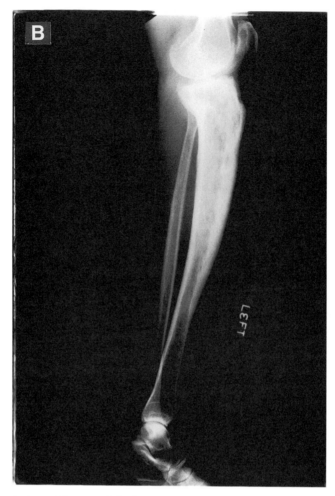

Fig. 1. (B) Lateral view of the same left tibia shows that the proximal two-thirds have evidence of PDB. The tibia also has anterior bowing.

Basilar invagination of the skull can cause symptoms from internal hydrocephalus, with symptom complex of dementia and incontinence, or long tract signs from brainstem compression. Bone enlargement of vertebrae can cause spinal stenosis, resulting in spinal radiculopathy or cauda eolina syndrome *(48)*. Increased blood flow to the highly vascular pagetic bone has been postulated to provoke a "steal syndrome." In this situation, blood is shunted away from the neural elements, exacerbating the neurological symptoms and signs accompanying the stenosis *(49)*. Miscellaneous neurologic complications consist of peripheral neuropathies, carpal/tarsal tunnel syndromes, and hydrocephalic parkinsonism *(50)*.

Pagetic bone fractures more easily, because it is formed more rapidly, without the normal lamellar pattern that normal bone has. In addition to incomplete fissure fractures on convex surfaces of bowed long bones, complete transverse fracture can occur with minimal trauma. These fractures are called chalk stick fractures, because the bone breaks evenly, like a piece of chalk, rather than with jagged fragments, as normal bone does. Such fractures also have a higher rate of nonunion, between 10 and 40%, occurring most commonly in the femur. With involvement of the mandible and maxilla, the

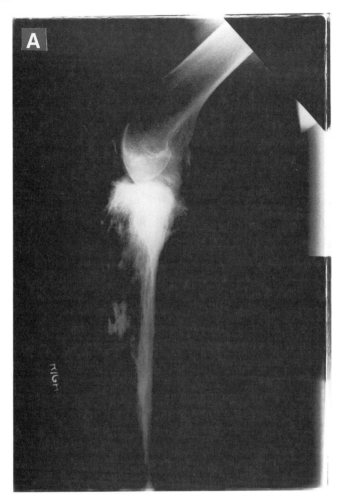

Fig. 2. (A) Lateral radiograph of the right tibia from a patient who had PDB for at least 25 yr that had never been treated. In the proximal two-thirds of the tibia, note the cortical thickening and enlargement.

patients with PDB also have dental complications, including maloccusion, loosening, and hypercementosis *(51)*.

A serious but rare complication of PDB (less than 1.0% of affected patients) is the development of malignant neoplasms *(52)*. Osteosarcomas are the most common type. Chondrosarcomas, fibrosarcomas, giant cell tumors *(53,54)* and tumors of mixed histological characteristic may also develop. These malignant neoplasms are almost always in a preexisting pagetic lesion. Commonest tumor locations are the pelvis, humerus, femur, and skull. They can complicate pathological fractures with acute increasing bone pain and rising level of alkaline phosphatase. Primary giant cell tumors and secondary spread of other cancers to existing pagetic lesions also occurs. When malignant neoplasms occur, they are very aggressive, and, unless the neoplasm can be removed totally (usually limb amputation), the disease is rapidly fatal. At present, there are no data showing that treatment of PDB reduces the occurrence of malignant neoplasms.

With high rates of bone remodeling, some patients with PDB can develop antiresorptive nephrolithiasis *(55)*. Occasionally, when patients with active polyostotic disease

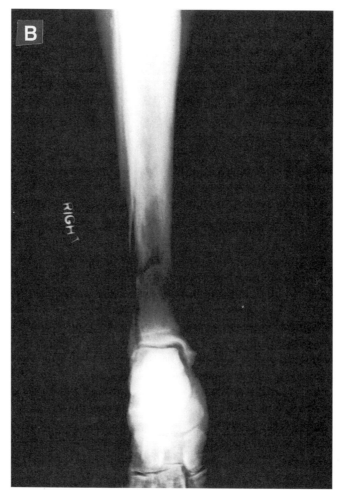

Fig. 2. (B) AP view of tibia at the inferior portion of the tibia. Note the inverted "V" area of lucency, which represents the advancing front of the disease, also known as the "blade of grass" lesion.

must be put in bed, e.g., after a fracture, they can develop hypercalcemia and hypercalcuria. When this occurs, agents must be initiated on an emergency basis to reduce calcium release from bone resorption. Primary hyperthyroidism is usually seen in about 5% of the patients with PDB, but the mechanism of this apparent relationship remains undefined. Hyperuricemia and gout are reported to occur in patients with PDB. It is unclear whether the elevated bone remodeling causes abnormal purine metabolism, or whether gout and PDB are just two common diseases occurring in the same patient.

High-output cardiac failure has been reported to occur in patients with PDB. Generally, patients have more than one third of their skeleton involved with bone turnover lesions *(56)*, but documented occurrences are rare. Other clinic manifestations in the cardiovascular system also occur as medial calcinosis, intimal atherosclerosis, subendocardial calcification, and calcified aortic stenosis. A series of fibrosing or inflammatory disorders are reported to occur with PDB: Dupuytren's contractures, Peyronie's disease, and Hashimoto's thyroiditis *(56–58)*. Whether these inflammatory/fibrotitic disorders are only associated with PDB, or are, in some fashion, caused by the release of cytokines from the areas of increased turnover, will await further study. Angioid streaks

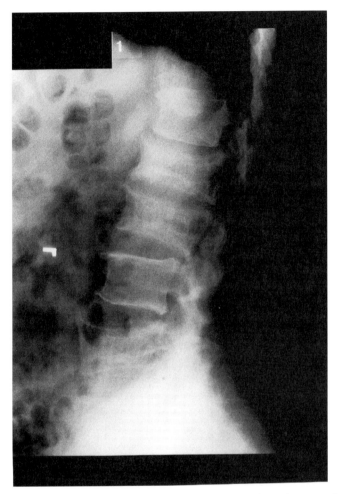

Fig. 3. Lateral lumbar radiograph from a patient with PDB involves the second, third, and fifth lumbar vertebrae. The involved vertebrae are both enlarged and deformed. Note the thickened trabeculae. In the L2 vertebrae, the cortics are thickened, giving it a "picture frame" appearance.

and peripapillary chorioretinal atrophy are associated with PDB, but are more frequently seen with pseudoxanthoma elasticum, and other connective tissue diseases *(59,60)*.

DIAGNOSIS

All patients with PDB should receive a thorough history and physical examination. Because 30–50% of patients have the diagnosis made serendipitously, it may be necessary to reevaluate the patient, seeking symptoms and signs of the disease. All patients with PDB should have a total body bone scan, using a technetium-labeled bisphosphonate. Areas of rapidly remodeling bone will appear as hot spots. This technique is the most sensitive method for localizing the distribution of pagetic areas, and, in addition, probably reveals activity not seen on radiograph. Areas that are hot on bone scan should then have radiographs, to confirm the presence of abnormal remodeling. Radiographs of painful or deformed bones are usually diagnostic, showing the characteristic mixed appearance of areas of lysis from increased osteoclastic resorption with sclerotic areas

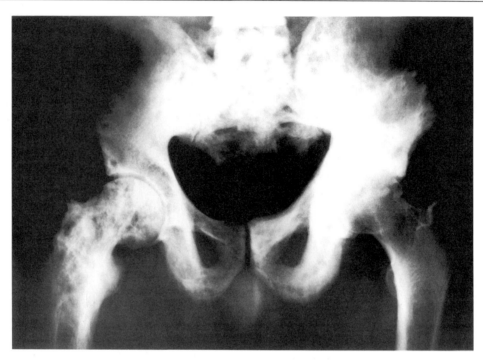

Fig. 4. AP pelvis and proximal femur radiograph from a patient with longstanding PDB. The entire pelvis and sacrum are diseased. The entire right femur shown in the radiograph has PDB. Note the thickened trabeculae increased cortical width, as well as areas of lucency. Also note that the right femoral head is deformed, and the femoral neck now has a coxa vara deformity, in which the angle made by the femoral head and neck with the shaft of the femur is decreased.

from excessive osteoblastic bone formation, as well as cortical thickening. In the early stages of the disease, the changes may be predominantly lytic, with flame-shaped resorption fronts in long bones or osteoporosis circumscripta in the skull. A characteristic appearance that distinguishes PDB from other conditions radiographically is the increased diameter of affected bones, particularly those of the spine or shafts of long bones (61). If spinal stenosis, hydrocephalus, or brainstem compression from basilar skull invagination is suspected, CT or MRI scans may be necessary to confirm these diagnoses.

Measurement of a serum alkaline phosphatase level is the most useful biochemical test for PDB, because it presents the simplest and most sensitive marker of disease activity. This enzyme is located in the plasma membrane of osteoblasts, and levels will be elevated above the normal range in 90% of affected patients. Alkaline phosphatase activity reflects the number and functional state of osteoblasts in patients with the disease (2). The serum level of alkaline phosphatase correlates roughly with the extent of skeletal involvement, as established by radionucleotide bone scans. Serial determinations of alkaline phosphatase provide a useful, simple, and inexpensive biochemical index of skeletal activity. Serum alkaline phosphatase levels do vary from day to day, so that, for a change in levels to represent a change in disease activity or a response to therapy, the level should increase or decrease by 25% to be clinically significant (62). Because 10% of patients with PDB have normal serum alkaline phosphatase levels, it may be helpful to measure bone-specific alkaline phosphatase. This isoenzyme of alkaline phosphatase can be elevated when total alkaline phosphatase levels are normal, and may also be useful

Table 1
Differential Diagnosis of Paget's Disease of Bone

Causes of elevated serum bone alkaline phosphatase level
    Metastatic neoplasm to the skeleton
    Osteomalacia
    Hyperparathyroidism with osteitis fibrosa cystica
    Idiopathic hyperphosphatasia
Causes of skeletal lesions with similar radiographic appearance
    Metastatic neoplasm to the skeleton
    Vertebral hemangioma
    Fibrous dysplasia
    Chronic osteomyelitis
    Metaphyseal dysplasia (Engelmann's disease)
    Familial expansile osteolysis (74)
    Sternocosto clavicular hyperostosis

Modified with permission from ref. 56.

in patients with coexisting liver disease. Measurement of serum osteocalcin level, a vitamin-K-dependent protein made by osteoblasts, has not been useful in diagnosing or following patients with PDB.

Increased bone resorption is the initial abnormality in PDB. Measuring urinary excretion of hydroxyproline, pyridinoline crosslinks, deoxypyridinoline, or n-telopeptide levels can assess bone resorptive activity. The samples can be collected for 2 or 24 h, and a urine creatinine level should always be measured, to assess adequacy of the collection, and to allow for normalization for glomerular filtration rates. All three of these measurements reflect the breakdown rate of bone collagen. Markers of bone resorption change within 7 days after the initiation of therapy for PDB, but it may take 1–2 mo before serum alkaline phosphatase levels show a response to therapy. Once a diagnosis of PDB has been made, and the extent of the bone involvement quantitated, only serum alkaline phosphatase levels need to be followed. In some patients, bone pain can reoccur after successful suppression of disease activity with therapy. When this occurs, and serum alkaline phosphatase levels are normal, measurement of urinary levels of hydroxyproline, pyridinoline crosslinks, or n-telopeptide levels can show an increase in bone resorption activity.

Table 1 lists the diseases that should enter into the differential diagnosis of PDB. These diseases can be categorized as either causing an elevated serum alkaline phosphatase level or causing a radiographic lesion similar to PDB.

In most cases, the diagnosis of PDB is not difficult. An asymptomatic or symptomatic bone lesion with an elevated serum alkaline phosphatase level can be easily resolved by the clinician and a radiologist. Occasionally, the authors have seen an isolated skeletal lesion in the ileum or in a vertebral body that may not have the classical radiographic appearance of PDB and the markers of bone turnover: Serum alkaline phosphatase, urinary hydroxyproline, pyridinoline crosslinks, or n-telopeptide levels are all normal. In these cases, a closed or open bone biopsy is necessary to rule out a neoplasm. Rarely, a patient with PDB of bone may develop a metastasis from another cancer that is in a preexisting pagetic lesion. Recently, one of the authors saw a man whose first recurrence of an adenocarcinoma from his lung primary appeared 2 yr after resection of the primary lesion as a bone metastasis to an area of PDB in his ilium. Finally, fibrous dysplasia can cause diagnostic confusion with PDB because the lesion appears hot on bone scan. An experienced skeletal radiologist or a bone biopsy may be required to clarify this diagnosis.

THERAPY

As with any chronic disease, patient education about PDB is the first and most important aspect of disease management. The Paget Foundation for PDB and Related Disorders, 120 Wall Street, New York, NY 10007, is helpful in providing information to patients and health care professionals.

With current knowledge, not all patients with PDB require treatment. In some cases, the symptoms that cause the patient to seek medical care are caused by active disease and associated complications. Thus, careful consideration of the symptoms and the physical and radiographic findings are necessary to determine whether treatment of PDB is indicated. Medical, surgical, and rehabilitation interventions are available in managing PDB and its complications, but the choice of specific therapy must be individualized for each patient.

Patients with bone pain from associated osteoarthritis should be treated with aspirin, acetaminophen, or nonsteroid anti-inflammatory agents (NSAIDS). Because many patients are elderly, care should be taken to avoid renal and gastrointestinal toxicity from NSAIDS. Some patients with severe joint destruction from PDB who are not candidates for joint replacement may require narcotics to control their pain.

Patients who develop deformities or gait disturbances from their PDB should be evaluated to correct or improve these impairments (63). A cane can be a very important therapeutic device for patients with disease in the pelvis or lower extremities. If the patient has a leg-length deformity, the authors' group tries to correct the deformity with a shoe lift to 50% of the leg-length discrepancy over 3–4 mo. When this has been accomplished, the patients find they ambulate better. Patients with hearing impairments should be referred to an audiologist. When patients have maxillary or mandibular disease, they should be evaluated for malocclusion or other oral complications by a dentist. Once they are stable, patients should be followed semiannually or annually. Alkaline phosphatase should be checked annually, and radiographs performed when symptoms indicate a change in the disease.

The ultimate goal of therapy for PDB is to restore bone remodeling to normal levels, so that all new bone formed is normal. Because the etiology of PDB is unknown, at present all available therapies only control the abnormal remodeling rates and suppress the osteoclast activity, but do not cure the disease.

Two classes of drugs, bisphosphonates and calcitonins, are available to treat PDB (64). Both of these types of drugs control the increased bone remodeling, by inhibiting bone resorption. Any patient who has pain or other symptoms, or an asymptomatic patient with a pagetic lesion that has a risk of complications, should receive antiresorptive therapy. This is means 60–80% of patients with PDB, in the author's experience. Listed in Table 2 are recommendations for the types of patients who should receive therapy. No controlled clinical trials have been performed to support these guidelines. However, such trials may never be performed. The recommendations are generally accepted by experts who treat large numbers of patients.

The development of potent second-generation bisphosphonates has made these agents the mainstay of drugs of choice for the treatment of PDB. This class of drug offers sustained response and greater acceptability. Bisphosphonates are analogs of inorganic

Table 2
Indications for Antiresorptive Therapy in Patients with Paget's Disease

Bone or articular pain
Bone deformity
Bone, articular, or neurologic complications
Asymptomatic disease, but risk of complications because of site
  Base of skull
  Spine
  Long bones of lower extremities
  Ilium, if close to acetabulum
Preparation for orthopedic surgery

Modified with permission from ref. *64.*

pyrophosphate, which binds avidly to the surface of the calcium phosphate mineral phase of bone, and modulates the rate and extent of mineralization. Bisphosphonates have a carbon atom substituted for the oxygen atom in pyrophosphate, and bind to bone hydroxy-appetite, but are resistant to hydrolysis. Different side chains on the central carbon atom confer different activities to bisphosphonates, which bind to bone mineral and are potent inhibitors of osteoclasts. The earliest bisphosphonate, etidronate, inhibited osteoclast activity, but it also impaired bone mineralization. Prolonged use of etidronate was associated with the development of osteomalacia.

Patients with PDB should be treated with bisphosphonates to normalize bone turnover. Treatment is reinitiated when bone turnover increases, or when pain reoccurs. There are now five bisphosphonates approved in the United States for the treatment of PDB: alendronate, tiludronate, pamidronate, risedronate, and etidronate. Alendronate is a recently approved second-generation bisphosphonate. The drug is given in doses of 40 mg daily for 6 mo. More than 60% of patients who receive this drug normalize their serum alkaline phosphatase levels *(65)*. Orally administered alendronate can cause GI disturbances in 17% of patients; in some, esophagitis can be severe enough to cause discontinuation of the drug. Intravenous alendronate is also effective, which results in 65% reduction of pretreatment level of alkaline phosphatase after 3 mo of maximum suppression *(66)*.

Recently, tiludronate, a bisphosphonate more potent than etidronate, but less potent than alendronate or pamidronate, was approved by the FDA *(67)*. It is given as a 400-mg oral dose per day for only 3 mo. This regimen is well tolerated and will normalize alkaline phosphatase levels in 40% of patients *(68)*. Pamidronate is another second-generation bisphosphonate that has been used in Europe for 10 yr. In the United States, it was approved for use by the FDA in 1995 as an iv preparation. It can be administered in doses of 30 or 60 mg intravenously over a 4-h period. Total optimal doses have not been established, but 90 mg can be given over 3 d, with retreatment, if necessary, in 1–6 mo. The advantage of pamidronate is that it can be given intravenously, and thus GI toxicity is avoided. About 20–30% of patients who receive this drug may have an acute-phase response 24–72 h after receiving the medication. This reaction can be controlled with aspirin or acetaminophen, and is self-limited. Recently, the bisphosphonate, risedronate, was approved by the FDA for treatment of PDB. The drug is administered orally in a dose of 30 mg/d for 2 mo *(69)*. It appears to be more effective in controlling alkaline phosphatase levels than etidronate. The final bisphosphonate available for treatment of PDB is etidronate. This is the first bisphosphonate to be used for therapy, and is given for 6 mo at a dose of 5 mg/kg. It is not as potent an inhibitor of osteoclastic bone resorption as alendronate, tiludronate, or pamidronate, and is used less frequently now. It does inhibit resorption, but impairs bone formation with equal potency. Thus, it is only given for 6 mo at a time.

All patients treated with bisphosphonates should receive oral calcium supplements of 1200–1500 mg daily, as well as 800 IU of vitamin D. Also, 20% of patients treated with bisphosphonates may have a transient exacerbation of pain in their pagetic lesions with initiation of therapy. Usually, aspirin or acetaminophen will control this pain, but short-term narcotics may be needed to control this pain, which does resolve.

Calcitonin is a safe and effective treatment for PDB. It acts via activating specific receptors on osteoclasts, which leads to suppression of bone reabsorption, and on pain-relieving pathways of central nervous system. Onset of efficacy is fast, with pain relief within weeks, and with measurable markers of Paget's bone resorption in 3 h. The salmon form is available for use in the United States. The human calcitonin form is no longer manufactured. Calcitonin must be administered subcutaneously, usually daily at first, and after 1–2 mo it is given 3×/wk. Calcitonin can normalize bone turnover indices in mild cases of PDB, but it is clearly not as potent an antiresorptive agent as the bisphosphonates are. Usually, the biochemical response is partial, with about a two-thirds reduction in serum alkaline phosphatase levels. In approx 20% of patients, resistance to chronic salmon calcitonin develops after a successful initial treatment period. Neutralizing antibodies develop to calcitonin, but it is not clear whether these antibodies are responsible for the resistance. Side effects, including nausea, facial flushing, and polyuria, occur in about 20% of patients treated with either salmon or human calcitonin. Recently, nasal salmon calcitonin was approved by the FDA for treatment of postmenopausal osteoporosis. It is not recommended for use in PDB, because only 40% of the drug is absorbed from the nasal mucosa, and thus does not provide a high enough dose of medication. If calcitonin is discontinued, exacerbation of biochemical abnormalities and symptoms usually occurs in 1 yr (70).

Two other drugs have been used to treat PDB: plicamycin and gallium nitrate. Both agents are approved for use in treatment of hypercalcemia of malignancy, and are effective antiresorptive agents. They are not approved by the FDA for use in PDB, and have been supplanted by the more effective second-generation bisphosphonates.

Patients with PDB may need emergency or elective orthopedic surgical procedures, because of complications of their disease. Fractures may require open reduction and internal fixation. Before any operative orthopedic procedure, it is desirable to reduce the remodeling activity, to reduce excessive blood loss. Such a reduction in remodeling activity can be obtained with iv pamidronate or calcitonin, if the surgery is an emergency. Oral bisphosphonates may be used if the procedure is elective. A goal of this form of therapy is to reduce alkaline phosphatase levels by 50% of the baseline level (8). Surgery for spinal stenosis can be effective in relieving symptoms, but most experts suggest a course of bisphosphonates or calcitonin to improve symptoms before undertaking a decompression procedure (2). Total joint replacement, especially for the hip, is a highly effective way to control pain and improve mobility in patients with advanced PDB and degenerative arthritis of the femur or ilium (71). Tibial osteotomy is effective in relieving knee pain in patients who have severe tibial bowing, if the associated osteoarthritis is not too severe (72). Recently, an external fixation device (Ilizarov) has been used in patients with tibial PDB, which allows an osteotomy to be performed, and then gradual changes in external pressure to be used to straighten the bowed tibia, or to allow a nonunion fracture to heal *(73)* (Fig. 4). When any orthopedic procedure is performed, it is important to place the patient on antiresorptive medication after surgery, whenever bone turnover increases, so that prostheses will not loosen with accelerated remodeling, or straightened limbs will not re-bow.

ACKNOWLEDGMENTS

The authors appreciate the help of Sandra D. Giles in preparation of this chapter. Support for this work came from the Veterans Administration Medical Research Service, HD30442 from National Institute of Child Health and Human Development (NICHHD), AG11268 from National Institute of Aging (NIA), and RR-30 from the Division of Research Resources, General Clinical Research Centers Program, National Institute of Health (NIH).

REFERENCES

1. Paget J. On a form of chronic inflammation of bone (osteitis deformans). Trans Med Chir Soc 1977; 60:37–63.
2. Kaplan FS, Singer FR. Paget's disease of bone: pathophysiology diagnosis and management. J Am Acad Orthoped Surg 1995;3:336–344.
3. Siris ES. Management of Paget's disease of bone in the era of new and more potent bisphosdhonates. Endocr Prac 1997;3:264–266.
4. Morales Piga A, Lopez-Abente G, Garcia Vadillo A, Ibanez AE, Gonzales-Lanza M. Features of Paget's disease of bone in a new high-prevalence focus. Med Clin 1990;95:169–174.
5. Kanis JA. Pathophysiology and Treatment of Paget's Disease of Bone. Carolina, London, 1991.
6. Galbraith HJB, Evans E, Lacey J. Paget's disease of bone. A clinical and genetic study. Postgrad Med J 1977;53:33–39.
7. Whyte MP, Daniels EH, Murphy WA. Osteolytic Paget's bone disease in a young man. Am J Med 1985; 78:326–332.
8. Merkow RL, Lane JM. Paget's disease of bone. Orthop Clin N Am 1990;21:171–189.
9. Barker DJP, ed. The epidemiology of Paget's disease. In: Barker DJP, ed. Proceedings of MRC Symposium on Paget's Disease (Scientific Reports No. 5), Medical Research Council, Southhampton, UK, 1983, pp. 1–6.
10. Morales-Piga AA, Rey-Rey JS, Corres-Gonzalez J, et al. Frequency and characteristics of familial aggregation of Paget's disease of bone. J Bone Miner Res 1995;10:663–670.
11. Cundy T. Evidence for a secular change in Paget's disease. Bone 1997;20:69–71.
12. Soafer JA. Evidence for periodicity in incidence of Paget's disease. In: Barker DJP, ed. Proceedings of MRC Symposium on Paget's Disease (Scientific Reports No. 5), Medical Research Council, Southhampton, UK, 1983, pp. 16–21.
13. Siris ES, Ottman R, Flaster E, Kelsey JL. Familial aggregation of Paget's disease of bone. J Bone Miner Res 1991;6:495–500.
14. Fraser WD. Paget's disease of bone. Curr Opin Rheumatol 1997;9:347–354.
15. Barker DJP. The epidemiology of Paget's disease of bone. B Med Bull 1984;40:396–400.
16. Kim GS, et al. Paget bone disease involving young adults in 3 generations of a Korean family. Medicine 1997;76:157–169.
17. Evens RG, Bartter FC. The heredity aspects of Paget's disease. JAMA 1985;205:900–902.
18. Singer FR, Mills BG, Park MS, Takemura S, Terasaki PI. Increased HLA-DRW1 antigen frequency in Paget's disease of bone. Clin Res 1985;33:547A.
19. Godon MT, Carwright EJ, Mercer S, Anderson DC, Sharpe PT. HLA polymorphism in Paget's disease of bone. Semin Arthritis Rheum 1994;23:229.
20. Leach RJ, et al. Evidence of a locus for Paget's disease of bone on human chromosome 18Q. J Bone Mineral Res 1996;11(Suppl 1):S99,S108.
21. Hansen MF, et al. Co-localization on chromosome 18 of a novel osteosarcoma supressor gene with a predisposition for Paget's disease of bone. J Bone Miner Res 1997;12(Suppl 1):S108.
22. Hughes AE, Shearman AM, Weber JL, et al. Genetic linkage of familial expansile osteolysis to chromosome 18q. Hum Mol Genet 1994;3:359–361.

23. Tilyard MW, Gardner RJM, Milligan L, et al. A probable linkage between familial Paget's disease and HLA loci. Aust N Z J Med 1982;12:498–450.
24. Mils BG, Oizumi J, Kudo E, Rude R. Robertsonian translocation in Paget's disease of bone. J Orthop Res 1997;15:477–481.
25. Kaplan FS, Singer FR. Paget's disease of bone: pathophysiology and diagnosis. Instr Course Lect 1993; 42:417–424.
26. Detheridge FM, Guyer PB, Abarker DJP. European distribution of Paget's disease of bone. Br Med J 1982;285:1005–1008.
27. Hamdy RC. Paget's disease of the bone. Clin Geriatr Med 1994;10:719–735.
28. Barker DJP, Chamberlain AT, Guyer AB, et al. Paget's disease of bone: the Lancashire focus. Br Med J 1980;280:1105–1107.
29. Piga AM, Lopez-Abente G, Ibanez AE, et al. Risk factors for Paget's disease: a new hypothesis. Int J Epidemiol 1988;17:198–201.
30. Reddy SV, et al. Detection of measles virus nucleocapsid transcripts in circulating blood cells from patients with Paget's disease. J Bone Miner Res 1997;11:1602–1607.
31. Rebel A, Malkani K, Basle J. Anomalies nucleaires des osteoclasts de la maladie osseuse de Paget. Nouv Presse Med 1974;3:1299–1301.
32. Mills BG, Frausto A, Singer RF, et al. Multinucleated cells formed in vitro from Paget's bone marrow express viral antigens. Bone 1994;15:443–448.
33. Kahn AJ. The viral etiology of Paget's diseases of bone: a perspective. Calc Tissue Int 1990;47: 127–129.
34. Mee AP, May C, Bennett D, Sharpe PT. Generation of multinucleated osteoclast-like cells from canine bone marrow: effects of canine distemper virus. Bone 1995;17:47–55.
35. Mee AP, Hoyland JA, Baird P, Bennett D, Sharpe PT. Canine bone marrow cell cultures infected with canine distemper virus: an in vitro model of Paget's disease. Bone 1995;17(Suppl 4):461s–466s.
36. Chappard D, Retailleau/Gaborit N, Filmon R, et al. Increased nucleolar organizer regions in osteoclast nuclei of Paget's bone disease. Bone 1998;22:45–49.
37. Ralston SH, Digiovine FS, Gallacher SJ, et al. Failure to detect paramyxovirus sequenses in Paget's disease of bone using the polyperase chain reaction. J Bone Miner Res 1991;6:1243–1248.
38. Birch MA, Taylorm W, Fraser WD, et al. Absence of paramyxovirus RNA in cultures of Paget's bone cells and in Paget's bone. J Bone Miner Res 1994;9:11–16.
39. Mills BG, Singer FR. Critical evaluation of viral antigen data in Paget's disease of bone. Clin Orthop 1987;217:16–25.
40. Ruddle NH, Paul N, Horowitz M, et al. HTLV-1 activation of lyphotoxic (TNF-beta) production and high-turnover in bone disease. Calcif Tissue Int 1990;46:A58.
41. Hoyland JA, Freemont AJ, Sharp PT. Interleukin-6, IL-6 receptor, and IL-6 nuclear factor gene expression in Paget's disease. J Bone Miner Res 1994;9:75–80.
42. Hoyland JA, Sharp PT. Upregulation of c-Fos proto-oncogene expression in Paget's osteoclasts. J Bone Miner Res 1994;8:1191–1194.
43. Ralston SH, Hoey SA, Gallacher SJ, et al. Cytokine and growth factor expression in Paget's disease: analysis by reverse transcriptase/polyperase chain reaction. Br J Rheumatol 1994;33:620–625.
44. Roodman GD, Kurihara N, Ohsaki Y, et al. Interleukin-6 a potential autocrine/paracrine factor in Paget's disease of bone. J Clin Invest 1992;89:46–52.
45. Birch AM, Ginty AF, Walsh CA, et al. PCR detection of cytokines in normal human and pagetic osteoblast-like cells. J Bone Miner Res 1993;8:1155–1162.
46. Ooi CG, Fraser WD. Paget's disease of bone. Postgrad Med J 1997;73:69–74.
47. Hosking D, Meunier PJ, Ringe JD, et al. Paget's disease of bone: diagnosis and management. Br Med J 1996;312:491–494.
48. Menwier PJ, Salson C, Mathieu L, et al. Skeletal distribution and biochemical parameters of Paget's disease. Clin Orthop 1987;217:37–44.
49. Hadijipavlou A, Lander P. Paget's disease of the spine. J Bone Joint Surg Am 1991;73:1376–1381.
50. Ikeda K, Kinoshita M, Aiki, K, Tomatsuri A. Hydrocephalic parkinsonism due to Paget's disease of bone: dramatic improvement following ventriculoperitoneal shunt and temporary levodopa/carbidopa therapy. Movement Dis 1997;12:241–242.
51. Smith BJ, Everson JW. Paget's disease of bone with particular reference to dentistry. J Oral Pathol 1981; 10:233–247.
52. Havos AG, Butler A, Bretsky SS. Osteogenic sarcoma associated with Paget's disease of bone: a clinicopathologic study of 65 patients. Cancer 1983;52:1489–1495.

53. Bhambhani M, Lamberty BG, Clements MR, et al. Giant cell tumor in mandible and spine: a rare complication of Paget's disease of bone. Ann Rheum Dis 1992;51:1335–1337.
54. Singer FE, Mills BG. Giant cell tumor arising in Paget's disease of bone. Recurrences after 36 years. Clin Orth Rel Res 1993;293:293–301.
55. Harinck HIJ, Biwoet OLM, Vellenga CJLR, et al. Relation between signs and symptoms in Paget's disease. Q J Med 1986;226:133–151.
56. Crisp AJ. Paget's disease of bone. In: Maddison PJ, et al., eds. Oxford Textbook of Rheumatology. Oxford University, Oxford, 1993, pp. 1025–1031.
57. Morales-Pila M, Rey-Rey JS, Corres-Gonzalee J, et al. Frequency and characteristics of familial aggregation of Paget's disease of bone. J Bone Miner Res 1995;10:663–670.
58. Lyles KW, Gold DT, Newton RA, et al. Peyronies disease is associated with Paget's disease of bone. J Bone Miner Res 1997;12:929–934.
59. Gass JDM, Clarkson JG. Angioid streaks and disciform macular detachment in Paget's disease (osteitis deforrnans). Am J Opthal 1973;75:576–586.
60. Babb TR, Skvoat K. Prevalence of angioid streaks and other ocular complications of Paget's disease of bone. Br J Opthal 1990;74:579–582.
61. Mirra JM, Brien EW, Tehranzaoah J. Paget's disease of bone review with emphasis on radiologic features: part I and part II. Skeletal Radiol 1995;24:163–171 and 173–184.
62. Kanis JA. Pathophysiology and Treatment of Paget's Disease of Bone. Carolina Academic, Durham, NC, 1991, pp. 1–15.
63. Lyles KW, Lammers JE, Shipp KM, et al. Functional and mobility impairments associated with Paget's disease of bone. J Am Geriatr Soc 1995;43:502–506.
64. Delmas BD, Meunier PJ. The management of Paget's disease of bone. N Engl J Med 1997;336:558–566.
65. Siris ES, Weinstein RS, Altman RD, et al. Comparative study of alendronate versus etidronate for the treatment of Paget's disease of bone. J Clin Endocrinol Metab 1996;81:961–967.
66. O'Doherty DP, McCloskey EV, Eyes KS, et al. The effects of intravenous alendronate in Paget's disease of bone. J Bone Miner Res 1995;10:1094–1100.
67. Fleish H. Bisphosphanates in Bone Disease, 3rd ed. Parthenon, New York, 1997, pp. 69–83.
68. Siris ES. Management of Paget's disease of bone in the era of new and more potent bisphosphonates. Endocr Prac 1997;3:264–266.
69. Hosking DJ, Eusebro RA, Chingz AA. Paget's disease of bone: reduction of disease activity with oral risedronate. Bone 1998;22:51–55.
70. Bockman RS, Weinerman SA. Medical treatment for Paget's disease of bone. Instr. Course Lect 1993; 42:425–433.
71. Ludkowski P, Wilson-MacDonald J. Total arthroplasty in Paget's disease of the hip: a clinical review and review of the literature. Clin Orthop 1990;255:160–167.
72. Meyers MH, Singer FR. Osteotomy for tibia virus in Paget's disease under cover of calcitonin. J Bone Joint Surg Am 1978;60:810–814.
73. Lovette EL, Lammens T, Rabry G. The ilizarov external fixator for treatment of deformities in Paget's disease. Clin Orthop Related Res 1996;323:298–303.
74. Hughes AD, Shearman AM, Weber JL, et al. Genetic linkage of familial expansile osteolysis to chromosome 18q. Hum Mol Genet 1995;3:359–361.

9

Testosterone

John E. Morley, MB, BCH

CONTENTS

INTRODUCTION

"The seventh age drifts into the lean and slippered pantaloon,
His youthful hose well saved, a world too wide
For his shrunk shrank and his manly voice
Turning again towards childish treble pipes
And whistles in his song"

William Shakespeare—*As You Like It*

From: *Contemporary Endocrinology: Endocrinology of Aging*
Edited by: J. E. Morley and L. van den Berg © Humana Press Inc., Totowa, NJ

This quotation from Shakespeare beautifully describes the signs and symptoms of male hypogonadism. Despite the clear similarities between the effects seen in young men with low testosterone levels and the major changes reported in older males, there has been a reluctance to pursue hormonal replacement therapy in the male. Why is this the case? Although there are clearly many contributory reasons, it seems that the major reason was, until recently, the complete male dominance of the medical profession. Males have had little problem perceiving females, who, as the "other" sex, went through a hormonal change that diminished them as reproductively useful individuals. On the other hand, the very essence of maleness is their virility. The concept that males, too, may have a waning of their sex hormones with age reaches into the deepest taboos of the male psyche. Their macho image was seriously threatened by the hints of this male "imperfection." It is for this reason that, in the area of sex hormones, we know far more about their effects in females than in males. This stands in stark contrast to most other areas of medicine, in which women have been essentially ignored until recently.

As outlined in this chapter, it is clear that males go through a menopause or climacteric similar to that undergone by women, although more insidious in onset. Gail Sheehy has characterized this occurrence in her book *New Passages* as a viropause, stressing that the major observable effect in the male is a decline in virility. This chapter will first examine the evidence that testosterone declines with age, and the controversy surrounding these findings; then it reviews the historical studies of the nineteenth century and the first half of this century, which attempted to produce rejuvenating effects with testicular extracts. Focus then shifts to the established effects of testosterone injection in older males, and the dark side of testosterone administration. Finally, a few words are ventured about emerging studies on the potential role of testosterone in menopausal women.

DOES TESTOSTERONE DECLINE WITH AGE?

The study sponsored by the National Institute of Aging, known as the Baltimore Longitudinal Study, nearly obscured forever the fact that testosterone declines with age [1]. This study has been carefully following healthy men through the aging process and examining a variety of physiological processes. They published a cross-sectional study purporting to demonstrate that, in healthy males, there was no change in testosterone with aging. They claimed that studies such as those from Australia [2] and the carefully carried-out studies by Vermeulen [3], which showed a decline in testosterone with aging, were because these investigators included in their studies persons who had diseases. They argued that the work done by Distiller and the author [4–6], which showed that sickness produced hypogonadism, invalidated all studies except those done by them in their healthy, carefully screened population. Vermeulen's studies were further invalidated by the fact that he had carried them out in Belgian monks, whose presumed lack of sexual experience and proclivity for alcohol made them a bad model for normal men [7].

Fortunately for science, techniques improved, and it was realized that the majority of testosterone in the circulation is strongly bound to a protein, sex-hormone-binding globulin, and, as such, is not available to the tissues. Measurements of free testosterone and bioavailable testosterone were demonstrated to better approximate the trace concentrations of testosterone seen by the cells on which it acts.

Utilizing this information, Korenman and the author [8] demonstrated that bioavailable testosterone levels decline even more markedly with age than testosterone levels in a group of healthy males on no medications attending a health fair in Los Angeles. More than half of the males over 50 yr of age had bioavailable testosterone levels lower than any values seen in young males 20–40 yr of age. Similar data in smaller groups was obtained by Bremner et al. *(9)* and Nankin and Calkins *(10)*. Subsequently, Kaiser and the author repeated these findings in a group of healthy, medically screened males from the Midwest *(11)*. Both studies also found a decline in total testosterone levels with aging, as had the Boston Normative Aging Study *(12)*. Gray et al. *(13)* undertook a review of the effects of aging on testosterone, and utilized a statistical technique called meta-analysis, which found that testosterone did indeed decline with age, and that this decline was independent of associated disease processes.

How did the investigators running the Baltimore Longitudinal Study of Aging get it all wrong? The answer is that, although they were more gerontologist than they were endocrinologist. All endocrinologists know that there is a circadian rhythm to testosterone secretion, with levels being higher in the morning and lower in the afternoon. The blood samples obtained from the Baltimore Longitudinal Study were drawn in the afternoon. Kaiser *(14)* and the author have shown, as has Bremner et al. *(9)*, that, when specimens are obtained throughout the day, older persons lack this dramatic circadian rhythm. As testosterone levels decrease in young males in the afternoon, they tend to overlap those values seen in older persons. On the other hand, bioavailable and free testosterone levels do not overlap between young and old men, even in the afternoon, when both groups are healthy.

Many researchers in the aging field are suspicious of cross-sectional studies such as those described above, because they may represent a cohort effect. The argument goes as follows: Different groups of persons live through different life experiences; for example, older persons living today went through the Great Depression and World War II, experiences that middle-aged and younger persons have not had. Could the differences between different age groups result from these experiences, rather than from true aging differences? Most young-old today seem to be less functionally impaired than those who lived 50 yr ago. To get around this conundrum, most epidemiologists like to see longitudinal studies that follow the same group (cohort) over a period of time, before they will agree that a change is truly age-related.

For this reason, in collaboration with Garry from Albuquerque, and with Vellas from Toulouse, France, the author studied the changes in testosterone levels over a 15-yr period in a healthy group of seniors living in New Mexico *(15)*. We found that these older males, aged 61 yr old and above, showed a decline in their testosterone levels of approx 100 ng/dL per decade, or slightly more than 10% of their starting values—proof positive that testosterone declines with aging.

Another reason why it has taken so long for the decline in the male hormone with age to be recognized is that the mechanism for the decline is different from that seen in women. In women, the ovaries fail, resulting in an increase in the pituitary hormone, luteinizing hormone (LH), as it attempts to drive the failing ovary to produce sex steroids. In rats, menopause in both males and females occurs because of a failure of the hypothalamus to produce sufficient gonadotrophin-releasing hormone (GnRH) to drive pituitary release of LH, and subsequently the gonadal hormones. In human males, the fall in testosterone, at least at middle age, is predominantly caused by a failure of the hypothalamic–pituitary unit *(16)*.

There appear to be multiple reasons for the failure of LH release from the pituitary in response to falling testosterone levels in the aging male. Korenman and the author *(8)* found a decreased sensitivity of the pituitary gland to GnRH, a finding previously reported by investigators at Johns Hopkins *(17)*. There is some evidence that, with aging, testosterone may more potently inhibit LH release from the pituitary. Veldhuis *(18)* has performed elegant studies demonstrating an alteration in the secretion of GnRH from the hypothalamus, based on mathematical modeling of alterations in LH secretary bursts in the circulation.

Hershman, Carlson, and the author *(19)* showed that the secretions of LH in humans was inhibited by β-endorphin, the body's own morphine. These findings created an industry for other scientists studying the mechanisms by which opioids (peptide hormones that act like morphine) modulate hormones. The authors used the blocker of opiate action, naloxone, to show that β-endorphin inhibited LH.

Billington and the author found that a long-acting naloxone-like drug, nalmefene, increased LH and testosterone levels in middle-aged males with low testosterone levels and inappropriately normal LH levels *(20)*. This suggested that the reason for the failure of the hypothalamus to adequately drive the release of LH and testosterone was excessive endorphin tone. Vermeulen et al. showed that, over the age of 70 yr, the opioid tone is no longer elevated, and in a longitudinal study, found that, at that age, LH levels started to rise *(21)*. The ability of the testes to produce testosterone also declines with age *(22)*, and the number of testosterone-producing Leydig cells also declines with age *(23)*. It seems that very old men eventually develop hormonal failure similar to that seen with menopausal women.

It is well recognized that even 90-yr-old males can still father children, but this does not mean that there is no deterioration in sperm production with aging. Sperm decreases in both quantity and quality with aging *(24)*, but, as has often been pointed out, it takes only one successful swimmer to impregnate an egg. Both the semineferous tubules and the Sertoli cells, which are responsible for sperm production, deteriorate with aging. This is demonstrated by the finding that, unlike LH, follicle-stimulating hormone (FSH), another pituitary hormone, increases with age. Secretion of FSH is normally inhibited by a hormone produced by the Sertoli cells, called inhibin. Levels of inhibin fall with age *(25)*. Thus, a second component of the male viropause is the decline in reproductive capacity, but this is not nearly as dramatic as occurs in women at the menopause.

Male hormonal alterations that occur with age are summarized in Table 1.

TESTICULAR EXTRACTS AND THE REJUVENATION CRAZE

A series of fascinating studies were conducted by Charles Edouard Brown-Sequard when his strength and energy failed him in old age. Brown-Sequard, a famous French physiologist, is best known for his precise description of the neurological changes that accompany hemisection of the spinal cord. Brown-Sequard has been also considered the "father of endocrinology."

In 1875, at Nahant near Boston, he tested his hypothesis that "the weakness of older men is partly due to decreasing function of the testicles." In these experiments, he grafted young Guinea pig testes into six old dogs. He only had success in old animals, which led him to "decide to perform upon myself studies to be, in every respect, more decisive than those on the experimental animals" *(26)*.

Table 1
Anatomical and Hormonal Changes Associated with Male Aging

Anatomy
  Decreased testicular size and weight
  Decreased number of Leydig cells
  Intra-Leydig-cell vacuolizations and lipofusin
  Atherosclerotic vessels
  Patchy seminiferous tubule degeneration
  Peritubular fibrosis
  Impairment of sperm maturation
  Altered sperm morphology
  Thickened basement membrane
  Decreased Sertoli cell number
Hormones
  Decreased testosterone
  Increased sex-hormone-binding globulin
  Decreased free and bioavailable testosterone
  Mild decrease in dihydrotestosterone
  Decreased androstenedione
  Decreased dehydroepiandrosterone and its sulfate
  Minimal changes in estradiol and estrone
  Decreased luteinizing hormone response to gonadotrophin-releasing hormone
  Luteinizing hormone remains in normal range
  Decreased inhibin and increased follicle stimulating hormone

At the time of his experiments in 1888, Brown-Sequard (27) was 72 yr of age, and had noted "my general vigor, which had been considerable, has greatly and gradually diminished during the past 10 to 12 years." In particular, he found that he could not work in the evening, after returning from work at 6 PM. (It should be noted that he started work at 3 to 4 AM). For these reasons, he injected himself with sc injections of a water extract of crushed dog or guinea pig testes. Testosterone in the testes is joined to fatty acids, and therefore were expected to be water soluble. He first injected the mixture about 20× into a very old dog, to assure that the liquid was innocuousness. He noted that the injections caused extreme pain for 12 h and was still painful 10 d later.

Within 2 d of the first injection, he regained the strength he had had a number of years previously. He was less fatigued. He could work after dinner and could "now without difficulty, even without thinking of it, ascend and descend stairs almost on the run something I had always done until the age of 60." Using a dynamometer, he found an increase in his grip strength of 6 to 7 kg. He had an increase in the "length of the path of the urine jet in reaching the toilet bowl." He also noted that intellectual work became much easier. Brown-Sequard noted that Dr. Hack Tuke had written a book on the "Illustration of the influence of the mind upon the body," and acknowledged that the majority of changes that he observed could have been brought about solely by "suggestion in the human organism." Today, this concept is well recognized as the placebo effect.

Within a year of these first reports, numerous physicians had treated patients with testicular extracts. Vanot in Paris reported on three males, aged 51, 56, and 68 yr, who had improved appetite, strength, defecation, and "sexual power." Three American physicians, H. P. Loomis and W. A. Hammond of New York and Brainerd of Cleveland, all utilized sheep testicular fluid, and reported improvement in functioning.

Based on his own experiments and those of others, Brown-Sequard wrote the following: "If the degenerations, of the senile alterations are diseases a day will come when it will be possible to cure them. The question is certainly not whether the injections rejuvenate the question is to know if one can approximate the strength of a younger person, and to me THAT APPEARS CERTAIN."

EARLY TWENTIETH CENTURY:
SEX GLANDS AS FOUNTAIN OF YOUTH

The concepts of Brown-Sequard were carried forward into this century by Serge Voronoff *(28)*, a Russian who emigrated to France when he was 18 yr old. After training in medicine, he spent some years as the physician to the court of Abbas II, the Khedive of Egypt. During this time, he noted that the castrated eunuchs who guarded the king's harem appeared to age more rapidly than males who had not been castrated. This led him to conclude that testicular hormones protected against the aging process.

In 1919, Voronoff was appointed to the faculty at the prestigious College de France. He began his research by transplanting the testes of young rams into senile rams, and claimed to have rejuvenated the older rams. These successful experiments led him in 1920 to have sufficient enthusiasm to transplant chimpanzee testes into two men who had become hypogonadal secondary to tubercular destruction of the testes. This failure did not distress him, and he continued these experiments. Soon, he was claiming superb results, and reported that monkey-gland transplants could put back human aging by twenty to thirty years. He was highly successful at public relations, and developed a villa clinic on the Italian Riviera, where he transplanted monkey-glands, obtained from thousands of chimpanzees from the African jungles, into the aging rich of Europe. His charges reached as high as $5,000 a transplant, making him an rich man. Voronoff's only regret was that he could not find a similarly successful treatment for women: "In the meantime I can only offer this consolation: the mortality statistics of every land prove that women live much longer than men. Hence they already have an advantage of us and consequently may still wait a few more years before the experiments in course of developments bring them the remedy which is to intensify and prolong their existence."

The most scientifically successful disciple of Voronoff was an Australian physician, Henry Leighton Jones *(29)*, who had undertaken his medical and dental training in Kentucky and Pennsylvania, and in Scotland. Jones completed a successful career not only as a physician, but also as a pharmacist and dentist, and retired from the general practice of medicine in 1928 at 60 yr of age. Having read about the work of Voronoff, he went to Paris to learn Voronoff's technique for himself. He clearly had a close personal interest, because, in 1929, Jones had Voronoff do a monkey testicular graft on him. During this time, while assisting Voronoff, he became enamored of Voronoff's secretary from England, Nora Elizabeth Barrett. He and his new bride then returned to his house on Lake Macquarie in Australia. He contacted his friend, the Sultan of Johore, to provide him with a supply of rhesus monkeys, and, in 1931, started doing transplant surgery in a small hospital in Monsset. Jones did approx 30 testicular grafts on males between 26 and 74 years of age. In two cases, these were repeat grafts done 5 yr after the first successful transplant.

Jones reportedly had a much lower rejection rate than Voronoff. The reason appears to be that he stopped using baboons and chimpanzees, and used rhesus monkeys instead.

Their tissue type is closer to humans, and he would check that the monkey's and the human's blood type were compatible before attempting the transplant. He, in fact, was taking the first crude steps toward tissue typing for transplant recipients, which today allows surgeons to successfully transplant hearts, kidneys, and livers. Unlike Voronoff, Jones did not seek notoriety or become rich from his work.

Many other physicians throughout the world popularized the Voronoff monkey-gland technique, which had its hey day in the twenties and thirties. Testicular extracts were used to treat a wide variety of ailment besides aging, including asthma, epilepsy, diabetes, impotence, influenza, tuberculosis, hysteria, and a variety of other disorders. Those physicians who popularized testicular extract implants were known as the "Erector" doctors. According to one of the leading endocrinologists following World War II, Gregory Pincus *(30)*, testes transplants were "obnoxiously publicized in the late nineteenth and twentieth centuries." In his opinion, the development of endocrinology was slightly derailed by "the exploitation of the idea of rejuvenation by hormones."

The possibility of testosterone having any real rejuvenating effect was further obscured by a parallel theory concerning the role of sperm in the aging process *(31)*. The sperm were first clearly identified as "motile animacules" by the pioneering Dutch microscopist, Anton von Leeuwenhoek, in 1672. In 1891, von Poehl thought that the active ingredient of sperm was a substance named "spermin." Spermin was widely used for the treatment of hypogonadism. The concept that it was sperm rather than testosterone that was the active testicular ingredient responsible for rejuvenation was taken up by Eugene Steinach. In 1912, Steinach was appointed director of the Biological Institute of the Viennese Academy of Sciences (the Vienna Vivarium). He was a consummate experimentalist, and in his early experiments demonstrated that castration in young animals produced many features similar to those seen in older animals. These included appetite and weight loss, changes in hair, fatigue, and an unsteady gait. Steinach theorized that, if one could prevent sperm escaping the testes, this would reverse the aging process. He tied the vas deferens (the tubes that carry sperm from the testes to the penile urethra), and reported increased activity and regression in senile rats.

Steinach convinced Robert Lichtenstein, an urologic surgeon, to carry out this operation on a human in 1918. The first person who was rejuvenated by this procedure was a 43-yr-old coachman. Ligations of the vas deferens reversed the premature senility seen in this young man. Lichtenstein then decided that this "Steinach" operation was such a success that he went on to do 400 more operations: From the 1920s into the 1930s, numerous surgeons joined the frenzy to make money from the Steinach rejuvenation craze. Its credibility was enhanced when luminaries, such as Sigmund Freud, the father of modern psychiatry, and William Butler Yeats, romantic poet, both underwent the operation as they began to feel the effects of aging.

Clearly, this mixture of science and quackery in the first part of the century took its toll, and retarded the development of the understanding of the role of testosterone in the aging process. Only in the past 20 yr have respectable scientists been prepared to again attempt to tilt at these gonadal windmills.

THE ULTIMATE APHRODISIAC

Raoul Schiavi, a psychologist working in New York, has done pioneering studies in older men, demonstrating that the fall in testosterone with age is closely correlated with sexual enthusiasm or libido *(32)*. He found that lower levels of bioavailable testosterone were associated with a decreased frequency of sexual thoughts, frequency of desire for sex, easiness of becoming aroused, degree of coital erections, and frequency of sleep erections.

Earlier, Julian Davidson *(33)*, a psychologist at Stanford University, had shown that testosterone injections increased the enthusiasm for sex in young hypogonadal men. John Money *(34)* in England had similar findings, suggesting the importance of testosterone in the maintenance of libido. Libido is the enthusiasm for sexual behavior, and is different from potency, which refers to the ability to have penile erections.

Recently, one of the author's fellows, Ramzi Hajjar *(35)*, has examined the outcome of patients in Kaiser's impotence clinic, who had low bioavailable testosterone levels and either elected to receive testosterone injections or declined the treatment. By 2 yr of follow-up, over 80% of those receiving testosterone had increased libido, but, in those not receiving testosterone shots, the majority had had a decline in their libido. In addition, males receiving testosterone tend to feel much more enthusiastic about life. So much so that many of them opt to regularly be venesected (donate blood) to keep their circulating levels of red blood cells at a low enough level to continue to receive their testosterone.

STRENGTH

In general, males are stronger than females, and it is the male hormone testosterone that is the major determinant of this difference. Animal studies have suggested that testosterone primarly effects the fore (upper) limbs. With Baumgartner et al. in the New Mexico Process Study, the author has found that one of the major factors that predicts the amount of muscle tissue in older males is the free testosterone level. This study found that, along with testosterone, the other predictors of muscle bulk in older men were physical activity and a measure of growth hormone secretion (unpublished observations).

To study whether testosterone could, in fact, enhance strength in older males, the author et al. has conducted two studies *(36,37)*. In the first study, testosterone injections were administered (200 mg) every 2 wk for 3 mo to males over 70 yr of age who had been part of the Systolic Hypertension in the Elderly (SHEP) trial, and compared the results to a control group of males from the same study. The outstanding result of this study was an improvement in grip strength in the dominant hand of the men receiving injections *(36)*.

This led to a second study, undertaken by Sih *(37)*, which recruited larger numbers of males over 50 yr of age who had low bioavailable testosterone levels. They received 200 mg testosterone cypionate injections or a placebo injection every 2 wk for 1 yr. Again, the major finding of this study was that testosterone increased both right and left arm muscle strength, and this effect was maintained for the full 12 mo of the study.

Randall Urban et al. *(28)* examined the effect of testosterone injections for 4 wk on men with a mean age of 67 yr. They found an increase in leg muscle strength, and an increase in the ability of the muscle after testosterone treatment to make new protein. They also found an increase in insulin-like growth factor I in the muscle, suggesting that local production of this growth-promoting substance may play a role in the increase in muscle protein synthesis.

There is a report in the literature of a single patient who had severe muscle weakness in association with testosterone deficiency *(39)*. Testosterone replacement therapy in this man resulted in marked improvement in muscle strength.

Grip strength is an excellent proxy for functional status. For this reason, studies by the author et al. strongly suggest that testosterone therapy may prove an appropriate approach to improve function in the frail elderly.

DOES HIGH-DOSE TESTOSTERONE INCREASE STRENGTH IN YOUNG MEN?

Athletes have long taken testosterone-like compounds (so-called anabolic steroids) to increase strength. So pervasive is this drug use or abuse that testosterone has been declared a habit-forming drug in the United States. Its possible effectiveness was highlighted when the Canadian, Ben Johnson, lost his world record in the 100 m when anabolic steroids were detected in his urine. Numerous studies have suggested that testosterone improves strength in young weight lifters, and a number of weight lifters have been found to be sterile (unable to produce sperm), a side effect of ingestion of large amounts of male hormone *(40)*.

Recently, Shalender Bhasin et al. *(41)*, at the Charles R. Drew University of Medicine and Science in Los Angeles, carefully examined the effects of high doses of testosterone (600 mg/wk for 10 wk) in 43 healthy young men. Bhasin also examined the interaction of testosterone with exercise, to see if its effects were supra-additive: In males who received only testosterone without exercise, there was no increase in muscle bulk nor in upper or lower strength. When exercise was combined with testosterone, there was a tendency to see even greater improvements in muscle strength. Despite these high doses of testosterone, no changes in mood or behavior could be detected by these men or their spouses.

The study by Bhasin et al. *(41)* has clearly demonstrated that high doses of testosterone can increase strength in normal young men. This raises the ethical question of whether or not testosterone should be used by young competitive athletes. Given that, under excessive training conditions, testosterone may decline to hypogonadal levels, it could be argued that testosterone replacement may be appropriate. Others would argue that the use of performance-enhancing agents in competitive sports is inappropriate. Whether long-term use of inappropriately high doses of testosterone have severe adverse effects is not yet known. It would seem, however, that, as man continues to reach for greater sporting achievements, at least low-dose testosterone replacement in those athletes with depressed testosterone levels will become the Olympic state-of-the-art.

MEMORY

James Flood and the author *(42)* found that testosterone, injected into the head of mice, enhances the ability of the mice to learn a simple task. Flood and Morley had been studying a spontaneous mutant mouse, the senescence-accelerated mouse P8 (SAMP8) *(43)*. This mouse develops problems with learning and memory at a young age (about 8 mo), and lives about half of its life-span with memory problems. Flood and Morley have found that the memory problems of this mice are caused by an excessive production of a protein, β-amyloid protein. This protein is also overproduced in persons with Alzheimer's disease, the most devastating disease of cognitive dysfunction effecting older persons. The SAM P8 mouse also has a deficit in the functioning of acetylcholine in the brain. These and other findings have led us to postulate that SAMP8 mice are an animal model for Alzheimer's disease. Further studies by this group have shown that testosterone levels fall precipitously in SAMP8 mice, so that the levels of testosterone seen in most 8-mo-old mice are in the hypogonadal range. When the author et al. found this, the testosterone in these animals was replaced, using a slow-release testosterone system. After replacement of testosterone, the older mice could learn and remember as easily as 4-mo-old mice. This suggests that, in males, loss of the male hormone may allow excessive production of the β-amyloid protein, and predispose to the development of an Alzheimer's-like syndrome. As pointed out in Chapter 11, women appear to be less predisposed to developing Alzheimer's disease when they take estrogen following the menopause. Thus, there is increasing evidence that the decrease in sex hormones with age may predispose to age-related cognitive deficits, and perhaps to Alzheimer's disease.

In studies of healthy males across the life-span, the author et al. have found that, as testosterone and its bioavailable form fall with aging, there is a similar fall in a number of standard tests of memory function *(44)*. The tight correlation between testosterone and memory function over the life-span further suggests, but does not prove, that testosterone is involved in age-related cognitive decline that everyone experiences with aging.

Janowsky et al. *(45)* have undertaken a well-designed study in older males to examine the effect of testosterone administration on memory. They found that testosterone improved the ability of older males to match two different pairs of blocks to one another. This is a test of visuospatial memory, an area in which males are particularly proficient. Powell *(46)*, a psychologist at Harvard, has demonstrated that the most rapid decline in cognition with aging is in the visuospatial domain. This decline in visuospatial decline explains why there are few baseball, basketball, or football players over the age of 40. Although there are still a minimum of studies on the effects of testosterone on cognition, the hope that, at a minimum, testosterone replacement will decrease the age-related decline in visuospatial memory seems to be not an unreasonable one.

It should not be expected that testosterone will positively effect all types of cognition. Sherwin *(47)* has shown that, of the seven major kinds of memory she has studied, females perform better on four and males on three.

HEART DISEASE

Females live, on average, 5 yr longer than males, but they are also more likely to have functional impairment at any given age than are the male survivors. The factor(s) that are lethal in males may also be responsible for their increased physical function. Much of this increased mortality in males appears to be caused by a higher rate of ischemic (athero-slerotic) heart disease.

In a study that examined heart disease in countries with very high and very low rates, it was found that males invariably were more likely to die from heart disease. This has been presumed to be, in part, because of the effects of testosterone on lipids. Following puberty, males have a rapid rise in the bad low-density lipoprotein (LDL) cholesterol, and have lower levels of the good high-density lipoprotein (HDL) cholesterol, than do females. When testosterone levels are lowered artificially (as occurs when a male is castrated), or in young males with testosterone deficiency, lipid levels tend to approximate the healthier findings seen in premenopausal females.

Although it is generally believed that testosterone increases cholesterol levels, the majority of studies suggest that this belief is based on questionable data utilizing chemically altered forms of testosterone. In young males, five studies have found no effect of testosterone on LDL cholesterol. The three interventional studies in older males found either a decrease in LDL or no effect on LDL and HDL *(36,37,48)*.

Epidemiological studies that have examined the relationship of testosterone to lipids have tended to find that, the higher the testosterone, the higher the HDL cholesterol *(49,50)*. In a study of the retirement community living in Rancho Bernado, outside San Diego, CA, Barrett-Connor et al. *(51)* have found that, the higher the testosterone, the lower the cholesterol, the blood pressure, and the prevalence of obesity. This would suggest that testosterone may be protective against heart disease. Low testosterone levels have also been associated with more abdominal (visceral) fat, which is an independent risk factor for heart disease *(52,53)*.

There have been more than 30 epidemiological, cross-sectional studies examining the relationship of testosterone to heart disease. According to Barrett-Connor, two-thirds of these studies found low testosterone levels as a predictor of heart disease *(54)*. In three prospective studies, in which testosterone levels were obtained before the men had heart attacks or angina, no association could be found between testosterone and subsequent heart disease *(55–57)*.

In retrospective analyses of the sexual dysfunction clinic established by Korenman *(58)* at UCLA and the Sepulveda Veterans Administration Medical Center, and the St. Louis University Sexual Dysfunction Clinic run by Kaiser *(35)*, no association with angina or heart attacks (myocardial infarction) could be seen in those men with low bioavailable testosterone levels who opted for testosterone treatment, compared to those who did not receive testosterone. Finally, a few studies have compared testosterone levels to the degree of atheroma seen in coronary angiograms (a technique in which a radio-opaque dye is injected into the heart vessels). These studies suggested that low testosterone levels were highly associated with a greater abundance of atheroma in the vessels of the heart *(59)*.

Overwhelmingly, these studies seem to suggest that, at least in middle-aged and older males, low testosterone is more likely to be associated with atherosclerotic heart disease than is a high testosterone level. Clearly, the generally held belief of endocrinologists, that testosterone is bad for the heart, does not appear to be acceptable. As succinctly put by Barrett-Connor: "Being male is good for men, / Being female is good for females."

BONE

It is generally believed that testosterone is as important for maintaining bone mass in men as estrogen is in women. There is, however, minimal data to support this viewpoint. The evidence most often quoted about this is questionable. A study done in Eastern Europe on a group of men who were castrated for sexual offenses *(60)*. In this study, in which bone density was followed for a number of years following castration, there was a rapid decrease in bone tissue in these eunuchs.

A study in males with Klinefelter's syndrome found that bone mineral deficiency was only prevented when testosterone therapy was started before 20 yr of age, with later testosterone therapy having no effect on the bone *(61)*. The syndrome is a genetic defect in which a male has an extra female (X) chromosome. Thus, these males have an XXY chromosome pattern, rather than the normal XY pattern. Their testes fail to develop normally, and they have very low testosterone levels and high LH levels.

A number of epidemiological studies have suggested that, in males, bone density drops along with age *(62,63)*. However, the tight correlation of testosterone with age has not allowed a clear-cut association to be made between the age-associated fall in testosterone and the decrease in bone mineral density. Two studies in older males with hip fractures have been able to successfully demonstrate that males who fracture their hips are more likely to have lower testosterone levels than those of the same age who do not have hip fractures *(64,65)*.

Neither of the author's testosterone treatment studies of older men have demonstrated a change in the blood measurements of enzymes that are normally associated with increased bone manufacture *(36,37)*.

Overall, it would appear that testosterone is extremely important for early bone growth, and for bone to reach its maximal size in the early years following puberty. However, in older males, testosterone appears to play a minimal role in bone strength in males who have had normal declines in testosterone with age.

PROSTATE

Medical wisdom dictates that testosterone will cause prostate growth, and that high testosterone levels will increase the chances of a male developing prostate cancer. The basis for this belief appears to be some early studies, which showed that, when testosterone at physiological doses was mixed with prostate tumor cell lines in a test tube, the growth of the tumor was enhanced. However, pharmacological doses of testosterone tended to slow prostate growth. The other roots of the belief that testosterone enhances prostatic growth and prostate cancer is the simple observation that men have testosterone and old men get these conditions. However, we now know that older men have lower testosterone levels than young men. It would appear that this may be another example of conventional medical mythology. Let us explore what is really known about testosterone and the prostate.

Most of the effects of testosterone on the prostate appear to be mediated by the conversion of testosterone to dihydrotestosterone (DHT) in the prostate by the enzyme, 5α-reductase. Some, but not all, parts of the prostate, appear to be effected by DHT. The fact that it is DHT that is the active agent in modulating prostate growth has been utilized in the treatment of benign prostatic hyperplasia (BPH) with finasteride (Proscar, Merck and Co., Inc., Rahway, NJ). Proscar has been shown to decrease prostate size by about 25%, and to improve the strength of the urine stream *(66)*. More recent studies have been less enthusiastic about the effects of Proscar than the original company-sponsored studies. Lisa Tenover at Emory University is in the process of conducting a National Institute of Aging-sponsored study, attempting to see whether, when estosterone is administered with finasteride, there is an inhibition of prostatic growth (unpublished observations).

The evidence that testosterone increases prostatic growth is minimal. Levels of prostatic-specific antigen (PSA) circulating in the blood have been thought to be a measure of the activity of androgen-dependent prostatic tissue. In the past few years, a number of epidemiological studies have failed to demonstrate a relationship between testosterone and circulating PSA levels *(67,68)*. Further, a number of studies, including two studies by the author et al., have failed to find a significant increase in PSA during testosterone treatment *(36,37)*. The author's experience, with Korenman *(58)*, and Kaiser *(35)*, has failed to find any increase in BPH in the patients treated, compared to those with low testosterone levels who did not opt to be treated.

Similarly, the author et al. have not seen an increase in prostatic cancer in older patients treated with testosterone. Some years ago, Moon and the author measured testosterone levels in patients with prostatic cancer. Contrary to expectations, the levels of testosterone found were much lower than those in males with BPH. Subsequently, a number of studies finding low testosterone levels in males with prostatic cancer have been published *(69,70)*. It would appear that prostatic cancer is responsible for producing these low levels.

The Baltimore Longitudinal Study of Aging followed testosterone levels in males for 7–25 yr before the diagnosis of prostate cancer was made. In this study, no differences were found in testosterone levels for the males who developed prostate cancer, compared to those who did not, for up to 10–15 yr before diagnosis *(71)*.

Much of the belief that testosterone effects prostatic cancer is based on the findings in the Veterans Affairs co-operative study, that castration provided symptomatic relief (but not extension of the survival time) in males with prostate cancer *(72)*. Today, many men receive injections of analogs of GnRH to reduce their circulating testosterone levels.

In 1981, Fowler and Whitmore *(73)* retrospectively reviewed their experience in 67 patients with adenocarcinoma of the prostate that had spread to other tissues, who were administered exogenous testosterone. Unfavorable responses were seen in 45 patients and favorable ones in seven patients. This study seems to suggest that testosterone is potentially dangerous in persons who have prostate cancer that has metastasized to other tissues.

These studies suggest that testosterone therapy is unlikely to cause major changes in the prostate in older males. However, prudence dictates that males receiving testosterone therapy should have a minimum of a digital rectal examination and a PSA every 6 mo while receiving testosterone therapy. There appears to be no need for these males to have a prostatic ultrasound (a somewhat unpleasant procedure), unless the physician detects a problem during the rectal examination.

BALDING

Hair and its growth patterns often differentiate males from females, and males are more likely to lose hair than females *(74)*. Hair loss classically occurs on the top of the head, with hair receding above the temples. Hair at the level of the ears and below is much less likely to be lost. In contrast, the male tends to maintain facial hair growth as he is losing scalp hair. Some hair, such as the eyelashes and the lower part of the scalp hair, does not depend on male hormones (androgens) for its growth. Testosterone inhibits the growth of scalp hair by being converted to another androgenic hormone, DHT. In the case of the beard, testosterone promotes hair growth, and is not converted to DHT.

Will testosterone therapy accelerate balding? There is at present no answer to this question. Clearly genes play a major role in balding, and testosterone can at worst accelerate this phenomenon when the appropriate genetic milieu exists. No studies have examined the effect of testosterone replacement therapy on hair loss. However, Proscar (finasteride), a drug that converts testosterone to DHT, has been shown in preliminary studies to improve hair growth in balding men *(75)*.

DEPRESSION

Persons who are severely depressed have been found to have low testosterone levels. Corticotropin-releasing hormone (CRF), the hormone in the hypothalamus that coordinates the body's responses to stress, is elevated in persons with depression. CRF has been shown to inhibit the release of LH from the pituitary *(76)*. As LH drives the testes to produce testosterone, this provides a mechanism by which depression may reduce testosterone levels.

Low testosterone levels are associated with fatigue, and many men, when taking testosterone, have a general feeling of well being. These findings have led to the suggestion that testosterone may be useful for enhancing happiness in men with depression. In reality, it seems unlikely that testosterone will become a major antidepressant. The present drugs available for treating depression appear to be much more powerful than testosterone. However, as already alluded to, it seems clear that testosterone can certainly enhance the enthusiasm for life in many aged and older men.

THE DARK SIDE OF TESTOSTERONE

The major side effect of testosterone appears to be its ability to increase the amount of red blood cells in the circulation. With aging, the hematocrit, a measure of the number of red blood cells in the body, declines in males, but not in females. When males are administered testosterone, there is invariably an increase in the hematocrit. In some cases, this may be good: Testosterone has been used in the past to treat the anemia (very low hematocrit) seen in patients with renal disease. However, in a number of males, the hematocrit level increases so much that the blood can sludge and result in the person developing a stroke. This is not just a theoretical occurrence. The author has seen strokes occur in persons on testosterone whose hematocrit was too high.

Because of this effect on hematocrit, it is essential that persons who receive testosterone injections have a complete blood count measured every 3 mo. If the hematocrit is above 55, it is essential that testosterone injections are stopped until the hematocrit falls below this level. As already mentioned, some men opt to have blood withdrawn from their veins to lower the hematocrit, and allow them to continue to receive testosterone injections. Some have pointed out that any drugs that may occasion the use of such an archaic therapy should be avoided.

Men who smoke, or who have lung disease (chronic obstructive pulmonary disease, emphysema, bronchitis), are particularly prone to develop an elevated hematocrit. Another group of males who may have soaring hematocrits with testosterone injections are those with sleep apnea. Sleep apnea is a condition in which the person has periods when he stops breathing while asleep. This leads to a drop in the blood oxygen level. Breathing is reinitiated when the oxygen level falls so low as to make the brain feel as though it is starved for oxygen. Many would consider the use of testosterone to be absolutely contraindicated in males with sleep apnea *(77)*. The author has treated some men with this condition with testosterone, but with extreme caution. Treatment starts at half the usual dose, and for the first few months the hematocrit is monitored at monthly intervals. In a year-long study of testosterone treatment in middle-aged and older males, the most common reason for males to stop taking testosterone was an elevated hematocrit *(37)*.

A second unpleasant effect of testosterone is that it can cause an unpleasant tingling in the breasts, and even growth of one or both breasts (gynecomastia). This occurs because, when testosterone is administered to testosterone-deficient men, it is first converted into fat by a process known as aromatization to the female hormone, estrogen. When men with low male hormone levels experience a testosterone surge it is associated with breast growth, as is well recognized in pubertal boys. Many young boys at the time of puberty experience a modicum of growth of breast tissue, which can make them the butt of many hurtful jokes in the locker room. It is absolutely essential to warn males concerning this potential feminizing effect of testosterone. In most cases, breast growth is minor, and resolves with continued testosterone administration.

Another side effect of testosterone is water retention. In most men, this has little effect, with perhaps the male noticing a small amount of ankle swelling at the end of the day. However, in males with severe heart failure, testosterone can make the heart failure worse, and even precipitate pulmonary edema (a condition in which the lungs become waterlogged, and it becomes extremely difficult to breathe). Because of the water retention, testosterone can also cause high blood pressure to worsen.

AGGRESSION

"For it is the semen, when possessed of vitality which makes us to be men, hot, well-braced in limbs, well-voiced, spirited, strong to think and act."

Aretaeus of Cappadocia, 150 AD

The first great Renaissance man, Leonardo da Vinci, carried out a number of experiments in which he demonstrated that castration was associated with a decrease in aggression in animals *(78)*. Most parents of teenage boys have little doubt that testosterone causes aggression and bizarre behavior, as the young man learns to deal with his testosterone surge.

Overall, males are more likely to take part in aggressive activities (American football, boxing), and to be involved in violent crimes, than are females. Some of this may be caused by socialization, but there is little doubt that testosterone plays a role in this clear difference between the sexes, but it has been much more difficult to demonstrate that variations in testosterone levels in individual males is associated with more or less violent behavior. Violent male criminals do not have higher testosterone levels than their less violent counterparts.

Although it is unlikely that wholesale testosterone replacement will result in 80-yr-olds forming gangs to roam the streets and beat up other seniors, it is possible that testosterone will enhance lesser levels of aggressive behavior. In some instances, a small increase in aggression may be considered useful, such as in a middle-aged executive who is not able to keep up with his younger colleagues.

PATCH, TABLET, OR INJECTION?

In the United States, the only form of testosterone available is methyltestosterone, which can be particularly damaging to the liver. For this reason, the use of oral forms of testosterone is not recommended for men living in the United States.

In Canada, Europe, and the rest of the world, there is an oral form of testosterone, testosterone undecanoate, which is much less likely to cause liver damage. Unlike methyltestosterone, which is absorbed from the gut directly into the blood stream, and bathes the liver in high amounts of testosterone, testosterone undecanoate is absorbed into the lymphatic system, allowing it to be diluted throughout the body before it is seen by the liver. A few studies have suggested that the absorption of testosterone undeconate varies from day to day. Testosterone undecanoate has been used for many years around the world, with minimal side effects *(79)*.

There are three forms of testosterone patches available at the moment, with a third under development by Alza. The first of these transdermal delivery systems to become available in the United States was Testoderm *(80)* from Alza. This patch is placed on the shaved scrotum. The scrotum is utilized because the skin in this area is thinner and more permeable than that in the rest of the body, allowing better absorption of testosterone. This scrotal skin patch results in normal levels of testosterone, but slightly elevated levels of DHT. The increased levels of DHT are caused by increased levels of the enzyme 5α-reductase, that converts testosterone to DHT in scrotal skin. There is no information available on whether the increased levels of DHT are potentially harmful over a long period of time. Because testosterone is well absorbed from the scrotum, testoderm does not include skin permeation enhancers, and is associated with a very low occurrence of skin irritation at the site of application. Occasionally, a male who has had long-standing hypogonadism may have a very small scrotal surface area, which will prevent him from applying the patch. Testoderm patches contain 4 or 6 mg of testosterone that is absorbed over 24 h. They cost $71.76/d, compared to less than $4 per dose for the injectable forms of testosterone, which need to be used only every 2 wk.

The second testosterone patch is called Androderm *(81)*, and is manufactured by Thera Tech in Salt Lake City for Smith Kline Beecham. A single 24-h dose (two 2.5 mg testosterone patches) costs more than testoderm: $97.50. The putative advantage of Androderm is that it can result in direct absorption of testosterone across nonscrotal skin. Two Androderm patches need to be applied each day to the skin on the back, abdomen, thighs, or upper arms. Besides testosterone, the reservoir in the Androderm patches contains alcohol, glycerine, glycerol monooleate, and methyl laureate, gelled with an acrylic acid copolymer to enhance absorption of the testosterone through the skin. These additional permeation enhancers appear to be responsible for the much greater level of skin irritation seen in patients using the Androderm patches *(82)*. Virtually every patient using the system develops mild-to-moderate redness at the site of application at some time during the treatment. Over one-third of patients develop itching at the site of the patch. Blisters at the application site occur in more than 1 in 10 persons using the system. Chronic skin irritation is present in about 5% of patients, necessitating discontinuation of therapy. Milder irritation has been treated with local over-the-counter hydrocortisone cream or antihistamines. A handful of patients have had severe local allergic reactions within the first 8 wk of using Androderm *(82)*. In most cases, this appears to be caused by skin sensitization to alcohol. There are no published controlled clinical trials of the nonscrotal androgen patch. Studies by Meikle et al. *(83)*, and his colleagues without adequate controls, have suggested an improvement in libido and sexual function. They have also reported less fatigue and hair growth in young males who had inadequate hair growth (nonvirilized) previously.

Arver and Meikle *(83)* reported that they had treated 82 men for more than 4 yr with Androderm. In the summary to their presentation, they claimed this was "a convenient and patient friendly modality for treatment of male hypogonadism" *(83)*. This system is expensive and clearly causes an unacceptable level of side effects, and has no proven efficacy in a controlled trial. The patch cannot be applied over bony areas such as the shoulders and the hips; sites of applications should be rotated, with a 7-d period between applications to the same site, and the patch should not be applied to oily or damaged skin.

Two forms of injectable testosterone are available in the United States: testosterone enanthate and cypionate. In dose-finding studies by Peter Snyder *(86)*, the ideal dose seems to be 200 mg every 2 wk or 300 mg every 3 wk. Most clinicians use the 200 mg every 2 wk dosing schedule. The injection may hurt slightly, but otherwise there are minimal side effects. As already pointed out, the injectable forms are incredibly cheap, costing less than $4 every 2 wk. I have taught many patients to self-inject at home, taking away the inconvenience of doctor's office visits every 2 wk. Clearly, unless you are incredibly needle-shy, testosterone injections are the way to go.

For those who do not want to take regular testosterone shots, there is an alternative: testosterone pellet implants. These have been shown to produce physiological levels of testosterone for 4–5 mo. These pellets of testosterone are implanted in the subcutaneous tissue and slowly release testosterone into the circulation. There are minimal experimental publications on this form of therapy, though a few physicians who have used this form of therapy on their patients successfully over extended periods of time.

TESTOSTERONE AND DISEASE

In 1979, Shlomo Melmed and the author (85) pointed out that many diseases caused a decrease in testosterone. Despite this, few studies of the effect of testosterone have been undertaken in young and middle-aged men with disease. Testosterone has clearly been demonstrated to increase the hemoglobin levels in patients with renal failure, and it was widely used for this purpose prior to the discovery of the hormone, erythropoetin, which is more effective at increasing hemoglobin levels and treating anemia.

Testosterone levels can decrease to low levels males with AIDS (86). Testosterone treatment is widely used by patients with AIDS, but there are minimal studies available on its effectiveness (87). In one study, Rabkin et al. treated 72 men with AIDS for at least 8 wk (88). Sexual interest and function improved in 85%, and mood improved in two-thirds of the subjects who had problems at baseline. There was no improvement in immune (T-cell) function in those receiving testosterone.

Male patients with rheumatoid arthritis often have hypogonadism. In an European study, seven men received oral testosterone undeconate daily for 6 mo (89). These men showed a reduction in the number of joints affected by arthritis, and also required less pain medication for their arthritis. They had a decrease in the circulating immunoglobulin (IgM) rheumatoid factor in the blood, which is a measurement of the degree of activity of their rheumatoid arthritis. These are particularly exciting results, if they can be confirmed in better controlled studies.

Finally, Reid et al. (90) studied 15 men with asthma who were receiving steroid treatment. Steroids are well recognized to cause bone loss (osteoporosis). The asthmatics' average age was 61 yr. All men received testosterone injections for 12 mo and had a period in which they were not treated for 12 mo. Testosterone increased bone mass and prevented the loss of lean mass in the asthmatics during the treatment period. Testosterone, or, in females, an anabolic steroid, should be considered for addition to steroids in persons undergoing long-term treatment with this type of drug.

TESTOSTERONE IN WOMEN

Some women at the time of the menopause complain that, despite estrogen replacement therapy, they do not feel quite right. Sherwin and Gelfand (91) have suggested that, in these women, the addition of testosterone preparations provides some decrease in nonspecific symptoms.

Following the menopause, the production of testosterone is decreased to approximately one-quarter of the amount made before the menopause. This decrease is non-testosterone caused by a decrease in other androgens, such as androstenedione, which are converted into testosterone by peripheral tissues.

Burger et al. *(92)* have undertaken a number of studies suggesting some improvement in a women's libido at the menopause when she receives testosterone. He has also completed a study that showed an improvement in bone strength and a decrease in body fat in women receiving testosterone in combination with estrogen.

Two forms of oral estrogen–androgen combinations are available in the United States: Estratest manufactured by Solvay (Marietta, GA) and Premarin with methyltestosterone, manufactured by Wyeth-Ayerst. Both of these preparations contain methyltestosterone, and can be taken orally. Estratest contains between 1.25 and 2.5 mg of methyltestosterone, compared to the higher doses of 5–10 mg in the Premarin with methyltestosterone preparations. As pointed out in the subheading on male hormone replacement, methyltestosterone may damage the liver, and lead to the person becoming jaundiced. Methyltestosterone has been associated with the formation of blood blisters in the liver, with bleeding into the abdominal cavity. This condition is known as peliosis hepaticus, and can be fatal. Methyltestosterone has also been associated with the formation of liver tumors, including cancer. Another side effect of methyltestosterone is swelling of the ankles. However, the doses being used in women are much lower than those used in men.

Should menopausal women use testosterone? Kaiser (personal communication), gives an unequivocal "No." She feels the risks of liver disease are too great to offset the benefits. Perhaps, in this case, Kaiser is being a little too radical. There clearly are potential uses for testosterone in a small group of women at the time of menopause. These are women who have symptoms that do not respond to estrogen replacement therapy alone. Like Kaiser, the author wishes that the available preparations did not contain methyltestosterone.

ANDROGEN DEFICIENCY IN AGING MALES (ADAM)

The author et al. have developed a screening questionnaire for androgen deficiency in aging males (Table 2). This questionnaire was validated in 310 Canadian physicians. It has high sensitivity and acceptable specificity.

SHOULD I FUEL MY ENGINES WITH TESTOSTERONE?

Although there is not yet sufficient data to give an absolute answer to whether males over the age of 50 yr should consider taking testosterone, sufficient evidence exists to provide some guidance to the aging male. The presentation by Tenover at the 1998 Endocrine Society Meeting further supports this viewpoint.

The author is 50 and would not consider taking testosterone unless symptoms developed that could be reversed by testosterone. What are these symptoms? A marked decrease in enthusiasm for sex would be the first symptom. Before considering testosterone, one should take a week or so of vacation, because hard work and stress are more common causes of decreased libido than is a low testosterone. In addition, if one found a marked decrease in strength or ability to aggressively pursue physical or mental tasks, this could be caused by low testosterone.

Table 2
St. Louis University Androgen Deficiency in Aging Males Questionniare

1. Do you have a decrease in libido (sex drive)?
2. Do you have a lack of energy?
3. Do you have a decrease in strength and/or endurance?
4. Have you lost height?
5. Have you noticed a decreased "enjoyment of life"?
6. Are you sad and/or grumpy?
7. Are your erections less strong?
8. Have you noted a recent deterioration in your ability to play sports?
9. Are you falling asleep after dinner?
10. Has there been a recent deterioration in your work performance?

Positive answers to questions 1 or 7 or any three other questions suggests testosterone deficiency.

With any of these symptoms, one could measure bioavailable testosterone, which the author prefers to a free testosterone level, but that would be an acceptable second best. Measuring a straight testosterone level is a waste of time, and may give misleading information. If bioavailable testosterone level was below the normal range for young males, then one could start taking testosterone injections (200 mg every 2 wk). Changes in libido could be carefully monitored by keeping a diary, strength could be measured using a handheld dynamometer, and the time it takes to walk 6 yd. If these improved, injections would continue. Like Brown-Sequard, as long as one felt better, he could care less whether this was a real or a placebo effect. To monitor for side effects, hematocrit (hemoglobin) would be measured at 3 mo, and then every 6 mo thereafter (3 mo, if it was greater than 50). One would have a digital rectal examination and liver function enzymes measured every 6 mo. The one question to which the author has no answer is how long this should continue this: The pragmatic answer is that one should continue testosterone until the hassles of treatment were greater than its perceived benefits.

It is clear that the time has come for some men over the age of 50 to take testosterone. Just who this should be and for how long is not certain. Testosterone is a controlled substance (treated like marijuana and cocaine), and, for this reason, many physicians may be loath to provide this treatment. However, it is clear that testosterone used appropriately is much less dangerous than tobacco or alcohol (both of which are freely available), and probably as therapeutically effective and less likely to produce side effects than digoxin, a drug obtained from the foxglove, and used to treat heart failure.

REFERENCES

1. Harman SM, Tsitouras PD. Reproductive hormones in aging men. I. Measurement of sex steroids, basal luteinizing hormone, and Leydig cell response to human chorionic gonadotropin. J Clin Endocrinol Metab 1980;51:35–40.
2. Baker HW, Burger HG, deKretser DM, Hudson B, O'Connor S, Wang C, et al. Changes in the pituitary-testicular system with age. Clin Endocrinol 1976;5:349–372.
3. Vermeulen A. Clinical review 24: androgens in the aging male. J Clin Endocrinol Metab 1991;73:221–224.
4. Sagel J, Distiller LA, Morley JE, Isaacs H, Kay G, Van Der Walt A. Myotonia dystrophica: studies on gonadal function using luteinizing hormone-releasing hormone (LRH). J Clin Endocrinol Metab 1975; 40:1110–1113.
5. Distiller LA, Morley JE, Sagel J, Pokroy M, Rabkin R. Pituitary-gonadal function in chronic renal failure: the effect of luteinizing hormone-releasing hormone and the influence of dialysis. Metabolism 1975;24:711–720.

6. Distiller LA, Sagel J, Morley JE, Oxenham E. Assessment of pituitary gonadotropin reserve using luteinizing hormone-releasing hormone (LRH) in states of altered thyroid function. J Clin Endocrinol Metab 1975;40:512–515.
7. Deslypere JP, Vermeulen A. Leydig cell function in normal men: effect of age, life-style, residence, diet, and activity. J Clin Endocrinol Metab 1984;59:955–962.
8. Korenman SG, Morley JE, Mooradian AD, Davis SS, Kaiser FE, Silver AJ, Viosca SP, Garza D. Secondary hypogonadism in older men: its relation to impotence. J Clin Endocrinol Metab 1990;71: 963–969.
9. Tenover JS, Dahl KD, Vale WW, Rivier JE, Bremner WJ. Hormonal responses to a potent gonadotropin hormone-releasing hormone antagonist in normal elderly men. J Clin Endocrinol Metab 1990;71:881–888.
10. Nankin HR, Calkins JH. Decreased bioavailable testosterone in aging normal and impotent men. J Clin Endocrinol Metab 1986;63:1418–1420.
11. Morley JE, Kaiser F, Raum WJ, Perry HM 3rd, Flood JF, Jensen J, Silver AJ, Roberts E. Potentially predictive and manipulable blood serum correlates of aging in the healthy human male: progressive decreases in bioavailable testosterone, dehydroepiandrosterone sulfate, and the ratio of insulin-like growth factor 1 to growth hormone. Proc Natl Acad Sci USA 1997;94:7537–7542.
12. Gray A, Feldman HA, McKinlay JB, Longcope C. Age, disease, and changing sex hormone levels in middle-aged men: results of the Massachusetts Male Aging Study. J Clin Endocrinol Metab 1991;73: 1016–1025.
13. Gray A, Berlin JA, McKinlay JB, Longcope C. An examination of research design effects on the association of testosterone and male aging: results of a meta-analysis. J Clin Epidemiol 1991;44:671–684.
14. Kaiser FE, Morley JE. Gonadotropins, testosterone, and the aging male. Neurobiol Aging 1994;15: 559–563.
15. Morley JE, Kaiser FE, Perry HM 3rd, Patrick P, Morley PM, Stauber PM, et al. Longitudinal changes in testosterone, luteinizing hormone, and follicle-stimulating hormone in healthy older men. Metabolism 1997;46:410–413.
16. Veldhuis JD, Iranmanesh A, Weltman A. Elements in the pathophysiology of diminished growth hormone (GH) secretion in aging humans. Endocrine 1997;7:41–48.
17. Blackman MR, Tsitouras PD, Harman SM. Reproductive hormones in aging men. III: Basal and LHRH-stimulated serum concentrations of the common alpha-subunit of the glycoprotein hormones. J Gerontol 1987;42:476–481.
18. Veldhuis JD. Altered pulsatile and coordinate secretion of pituitary hormones in aging: evidence of feedback disruption. Aging 1997;9:19–20.
19. Morley JE, Baranetsky NG, Wingert TD, Carlson HE, Hershman JM, Melmed S, et al. Endocrine effects of naloxone-induced opiate receptor blockade. J Clin Endocrinol Metab 1980;50:251–257.
20. Billington CJ, Shafer RB, Morley JE. Effects of opioid blockade with nalmefene in older impotent men. Life Sci 1990;47:799–805.
21. Vermeulen A, Deslypere JP, DeMeirleir K. A new look to the andropause: altered function of the gonadotrophs. J Steroid Biochem 1989;32:163–165.
22. Vermeulen A. Androgen secretion after age 50 in both sexes. Hormone Res 1983;18:37–42.
23. Paniagua R, Nistal M, Saez FJ, Fraile B. Ultrastructure of the aging human testis. J Electron Microsc Technique 1991;19:241–260.
24. Neaves WB, Johnson L, Petty CS. Seminiferous tubules and daily sperm production in older adult men with varied numbers of Leydig cells. Biol Reprod 1987;36:301–308.
25. Tenover JS, McLachlan RI, Dahl KD, Burger HG, de Kretser DM, Bremner WJ. Decreased serum inhibin levels in normal elderly men: evidence for a decline in Sertoli cell function with aging. J Clin Endocrinol Metab 1988;67:455–459.
26. Brown-Sequard CE. Effects in man of subcutaneous injections of freshly prepared liquid from guinea pig and dog testes. CR Seances Soc Biol Ser 9 1889;1:415–419.
27. Brown-Sequard CE. The physiological and therapeutic of animal testicular extract based on several experiments in man. Physiol Norm Pathol 1889;115:739–746.
28. Carruthers M. Maximizing Manhood. Harper Collins:Hammersmith, London, 1997.
29. Hamilton D. The Monkey Gland Affair. Chatto and Windus, New York, 1986.
30. Jensen EV. Remembrance: Gregory Pincus—catalyst for early receptor studies. Endocrinology 1992; 131:1581–1582.
31. Hoberman JM, Yesalis CE. The history of synthetic testosterone. Sci Am 1995;272:76–81.

32. Schiavi RC, Schreiner-Engel P, White D, Mandeli J. The relationship between pituitary-gonadal function and sexual behavior in healthy aging men. Psychosom Med 1991;53:363–374.

33. Davidson JM, Chen JJ, Crapo L, Gray GD, Greenlead WJ, Catania JA. Hormonal changes and sexual function in aging men. J Clin Endocrinol Metab 1983;57:71–77.

34. Money J. The therapeutic use of androgen-depleting hormone. Int Psychiatry Clin 1971;8:165–174.

35. Hajjar RR, Kaiser FE, Morley JE. Outcomes of long-term testosterone replacement in older hypogonadal males: a retrospective analysis. J Clin Endocrinol Metab 1997;82:3793–3796.

36. Morley JE, Perry HM 3rd, Kaiser FE, Kraenzle D, Jensen J, Houston K, Mattammal M, Perry HM Jr. Effects of testosterone replacement therapy in old hypogonadal males: a preliminary study. J Am Geriatr Soc 1993;41:149–152.

37. Sih R, Morley JE, Kaiser FE, Perry HM 3rd, Patrick P, Ross C. Testosterone replacement in older hypogonadal men: a 12-month randomized controlled trial. J Clin Endocrinol Metab 1997;82:1661–1667.

38. Urban RJ, Bodenburg YH, Gilkison C, Foxworth J, Coggan AR, Wolfe RR, Ferrando A. Testosterone administration to elderly men increases skeletal muscle strength and protein synthesis. Am J Physiol 1995;269:E820–E826.

39. Orrell RW, Woodrow DF, Barrett MC, Press M, Dick DJ, Rowe RC, Lane RJ. Testosterone deficiency myopathy. J Royal Soc Med 1995;88:454–456.

40. Elashoff JD, Jacknow AD, Shain SG, Braunstein GD. Effects of anabolic-androgenic steroids on muscular strength. Ann Intern Med 1991;115:387–393.

41. Bhasin S, Storer TW, Berman N, Callegari C, Clevenger B, Phillips J, et al. The effects of supraphysiologic doses of testosterone on muscle size and strength in normal men. N Engl J Med 1996;335:1–7.

42. Flood JF, Morley JE. Learning and memory in the SAMP8 mouse. Neurosci Biobehav Rev 1998;22: 1–20.

43. Flood JF, Farr SA, Kaiser FE, La Regina M, Morley JE. Age-related decrease of plasma testosterone in SAMP8 mice: replacement improves age-related impairment of learning and memory. Physiol Behav 1995;57:669–673.

44. Morley JE, Kaiser F, Raum WJ, Perry HM 3rd, Flood JF, et al. Potentially predictive and manipulable blood serum correlates of aging in the healthy human male: progressive decreases in bioavailable testosterone, dehydroepiandrosterone sulfate, and the ratio of insulin-like growth factor 1 to growth hormone. Proc Natl Acad Sci USA 1997;94:7537–7542.

45. Janowsky JS, Oviatt SK, Orwoll ES. Testosterone influences spatial cognition in older men. Behav Neurosci 1994;108:325–332.

46. Powell DH. Profiles in Cognitive Aging. Harvard University Press, Cambridge, MA, 1994.

47. Sherwin BB. Sex hormones and psychological functioning in postmenopausal women. Exp Gerontol 1994;29:423–430.

48. Tenover JS. Effects of testosterone supplementation in the aging male. J Clin Endocrinol Metab 1992; 75:1092–1098.

49. Nanjee MN, Rajput-Williams J, Samuel L, Wootton R, Miller NE. Relationships of plasma lipoprotein concentrations to unbound, albumin-bound and sex hormone-binding globulin-bound fractions of gonadal steroids in men. Eur J Clin Invest 1989;19:241–245.

50. Deutscher S, Bates MW, Caines MJ, LaPorte RE, Puntereri A, Taylor FH. Determinants of lipid and lipoprotein level in elderly men. Atherosclerosis 1986;60:221–229.

51. Khaw KT, Barrett-Connor E. Endogenous sex hormones, high density lipoprotein cholesterol, and other lipoprotein fractions in men. Arterioscler Thromb 1991;11:489–494.

52. Risssanen J, Hudson R, Ross R. Visceral adiposity, androgens, and plasma lipids in obese men. Metabolism 1994;43:1318–1323.

53. Khaw KT, Barrett-Connor E. Lower endogenous androgens predict central adiposity in men. Ann Epidemiol 1992;2:675–682.

54. Barrett-Connor EL. Testosterone and risk factors for cardiovascular disease in men. Diabete Metab 1995;21:156–161.

55. Wu S, Weng X. Therapeutic effect of andriol on serum lipids and apolipoproteins in elderly male coronary heart disease patients. Chin Med Sci J 1992;7:137–141.

56. Zhao SP, Li XP. The association of low plasma testosterone level with coronary artery disease in Chinese men. Int J Cardiol 1998;63:161–164.

57. Phillips GB, Pinkernell BH, Jing TY. The association of hypotestosteronemia with coronary artery disease in men. Arterioscler Thromb 1994;14:701–706.

58. Hartnell J, Korenman SG, Viosca SP. Results of testosterone enanthate therapy in older men. Proceedings of the 72nd Annual Meeting of the Endocrine Society, 1990, p. 428.

59. Barth JD, Jansen H, Hugenholtz PG, Birkenhager JC. Post-heparin lipases, lipids and related hormones in men undergoing coronary arteriography to assess atherosclerosis. Atherosclerosis 1983;48:235–241.

60. Stephan JJ, Lachman M. Castrated men with bone loss: effect of calcitonin treatment on biochemical indices of bone remodeling. J Clin Endocrinol Metab 1989;69:523–527.

61. Foresta C, Ruzza G, Mioni R, Meneghello A, Baccichetti C. Testosterone and bone loss in Klinefelter syndrome. Horm Metab Res 1983;15:56–57.

62. Ongphiphadhanakul B, Rajatanavin R, Chailurkit L, Piaseu N, Teerarungsikul K, Sirisriro R, Komindr S, Puavilai G. Serum testosterone and its relation to bone mineral density and body composition in normal males. Clin Endocrinol 1995;43:727–733.

63. Wishart JM, Need AG, Horowitz M, Morris HA, Nordin BE. Effect of age on bone density and bone turnover in men. Clin Endocrinol 1995;42:141–146.

64. Jackson JA, Riggs MW, Spiekerman AM. Testosterone deficiency as a risk factor for hip fractures in men: a case-control study. Am J Med Sci 1992;304:4–8.

65. Stanley HL, Schmitt BP, Poses RM, Deiss WP. Does hypogonadism contribute to the occurrence of a minimal trauma hip fracture in elderly men? J Am Geriatr Soc 1991;39:766–771.

66. McConnell JD, Bruskewitz R, Walsh P, Andriole G, Lieber M, Holtgrewe HL, et al. The effect of finasteride on the risk of acute urinary retention and the need for surgical treatment among men with benign prostatic hyperplasia. Finasteride Long-Term Efficacy and Safety Study Group. N Engl J Med 1998;338:557–563.

67. Vatten LJ, Ursin G, Ross RK, Stanczyk FZ, Lobo RA, Harvei S, Jellum E. Androgens in serum and the risk of prostate cancer: a nested case-control study from the Janus serum bank in Norway. Cancer Epidemiol Biomarkers Prev 1997;6:967–969.

68. Ribeiro M, Ruff P, Falkson G. Low serum testosterone and a younger age predict for a poor outcome in metastatic prostate cancer. Am J Clin Oncol 1997;20:605–608.

69. Monda JM, Myers RP, Bostwick DG, Oesterling JE. The correlation between serum prostate-specific antigen and prostate cancer is not influenced by the serum testosterone concentration. Urology 1995; 46:62–64.

70. Mermall H, Sothern RB, Kanabrocki EL, Quadri SF, Bremner FW, Nemchausky BA, Scheving LE. Temporal (circadian) and functional relationship between prostate-specific antigen and testosterone in healthy men. Urology 1995;46:45–53.

71. Carter HB, Pearson JD, Metter EJ, Chan DW, Andres R, Fozard JL, Rosner W, Walsh PC. Longitudinal evaluation of serum androgen levels in men with and without prostate cancer. Prostate 1995;27:25–31.

72. Group (VACURG) Veterans Administration Cooperative Urology (VACUR). Treatment and survival of patients with cancer of the prostate. Surg Gynecol Obstet 1967;124:1011–1027.

73. Fowler JE Jr, Whitmore WF Jr. The response of metastatic adenocarcinoma of the prostate to exogenous testosterone. J Urol 1981;126:372–375.

74. Thornton MJ, Messenger AG, Elliott K, Randall VA. Effect of androgens on the growth of cultured human dermal papilla cells derived from beard and scalp hair follicles. J Invest Dermatol 1991;97:345–358.

75. Dallob AL, Sadick NS, Unger W, Lipert S, Geissler LA, Gregoire SL, et al. The effect of finasteride, a 5 alpha-reductase inhibitor, on scalp skin testosterone and dihydrotestosterone concentrations in patients with male pattern baldness. J Clin Endocrinol Metab 1994;79:703–706.

76. Tsukamura H, Nagatani S, Cagampang FR, Kawakami S, Maeda K. Corticotropin-releasing hormone mediates suppression of pulsatile luteinizing hormone secretion induced by activation of alpha-adrenergic receptors in the paraventricular nucleus in female rats. Endocrinology 1994;134:1460–1466.

77. Sandblom RE, Matsumoto AM, Schoene RB, Lee KA, Giblin EC, Bremner WJ, Pierson DJ. Obstructive sleep apnea syndrome induced by testosterone administration. N Engl J Med 1983;308:508–510.

78. Morley JE, Krahn DD. Endocrinology for the psychiatrist. In: Nemeroff CB, Loosen PT, eds. Handbook of Clinical Psychoneuroendocrinology. Guilford, New York, 1987, pp. 3–41.

79. Gooren LJ. A ten-year safety study of the oral androgen testosterone undecanoate. J Androl 1994;15: 212–215.

80. Place VA, Nichols KC. Transdermal delivery of testosterone with Testoderm to provide a normal circadian patern of testosterone. Ann NY Acad Sci 1991;618:441–449.

81. Arver S, Dobs AS, Meikle AW, Caramelli KE, Rajaram L, Sanders SW, Mazer NA. Long-term efficacy and safety of a permeation-enhanced testosterone transdermal system in hypogonadal men. Clin Endocrinol 1997;47:727–737.

82. Jordan WP Jr. Allergy and topical irritation associated with transdermal testosterone administration: a comparison of scrotal and nonscrotal transdermal systems. Am J Contact Derm 1997;8:108–113.
83. Arver S, Dobs AS, Meikle AW, Allen RP, Sanders SW, Mazer NA. Improvement of sexual function in testosterone deficient men treated for 1 year with permeation enhanced testosterone transdermal system. J Urol 1996;155:1604–1608.
84. Snyder PJ, Lawrence DA. Treatment of male hypogonadism with testosterone enanthate. J Clin Endocrinol Metab 1980;51:1335–1339.
85. Morley JE, Melmed S. Gonadal dysfunction in systemic disorders. Metabolism 1979;28:1051–1073.
86. Holzman D. Testosterone wasting and AIDS. Mol Med Today 1996;2:93.
87. Grinspoon S, Corcoran C, Askari H, Schoenfeld D, Wolf L, Burrows B, et al. Effects of androgen administration in men with the aids wasting syndrome: a randomized, double-blind, placebo-controlled trial. Ann Intern Med 1998;129:18–23.
88. Rabkin JG, Rabkin R, Wagner GJ. Testosterone treatment of clinical hypogonadism in patients with HIV/AIDS. Int J STD AIDS 1997;8:537–545.
89. Hall GM, Larbre JP, Spector TD, Perry LA, DaSilva JA. A randomized trial of testosterone therapy in males with rheumatoid arthritis. Br J Rheumatol 1996;35:568–573.
90. Reid IR, Wattie DJ, Evans MC, Stapleton JP. Testosterone therapy in glucocorticoid-treated men. Arch Intern Med 1996;156:1173–1177.
91. Sherwin BB, Gelfand MM. Differential symptom response to parenteral estrogen and/or androgen administration in the surgical menopause. Am J Obstet Gynecol 1985;151:153–160.
92. Davis SR, Burger HG. Use of androgens in postmenopausal women. Curr Opin Obstet Gynecol 1997; 9:177–180.

10   Gynecomastia

Harold E. Carlson, MD

CONTENTS

INTRODUCTION
PATHOGENESIS
GYNECOMASTIA ACROSS THE LIFE-SPAN
SPECIFIC CONDITIONS ASSOCIATED WITH GYNECOMASTIA
TREATMENT
REFERENCES

INTRODUCTION

Enlargement of the male breasts, termed gynecomastia, is a common problem. In adult men, the prevalence of gynecomastia increases with age, and it may result in both psychosocial and, less often, physical discomfort. Male breast enlargement may occur as a side effect of many medications; occasionally, gynecomastia is a clue to the presence of disease elsewhere in the body. This chapter will review the pathogenesis of gynecomastia, its investigation as a clinical problem, and current approaches to treatment.

PATHOGENESIS

Histologically, gynecomastia is characterized by proliferation of mammary ductules, embedded in a connective tissue stroma: true glandular acini are rarely seen. In gynecomastia of recent onset, the ductules are relatively prominent, and the stroma is loose and edematous; with time, the ductules become less conspicuous, and the stroma becomes more fibrous and hyalinized *(1)*. As in the female breast, it is likely that there is a local, paracrine interaction between the ductular and stromal tissue, with the products of one influencing the proliferative activity of the other *(2)*.

There is abundant evidence that estrogens stimulate the proliferation of mammary ductular tissue in men; there is also evidence, albeit less extensive, that androgens inhibit the proliferation of ductular cells. Thus, the concept has evolved that gynecomastia may, in most cases, be a reflection of an imbalance of these two opposing influences. An increase in estrogenic stimulation, a decrease in androgenic inhibition, or a combination of these two factors may lead to male breast enlargement. Although one traditionally thinks of circulating sex steroid concentrations as determining tissue effects, much recent investigation has suggested that local production or destruction of steroid hormones may

From: *Contemporary Endocrinology: Endocrinology of Aging*
Edited by: J. E. Morley and L. van den Berg © Humana Press Inc., Totowa, NJ

be as important as delivery from the systemic circulation *(2)*; recent studies *(3)* of female breast cancer support the concept that locally produced estrogens may contribute significantly to the hormonal milieu in the breast. Although mostly unexplored, it is possible that many diseases and drugs associated with gynecomastia may alter the *in situ* hormonal balance without significantly perturbing serum estrogens or androgens; such alterations would result in an apparent change in the sensitivity of the breast to circulating sex steroids.

Peptide growth factors may also play a role in the genesis of gynecomastia. Prolactin appears to be a minor factor; prolactin receptors have rarely been demonstrated in gynecomastia tissue *(4)*. The prolactin receptor is generally limited in its mammary expression to glandular acini, rather than ductules or stroma, and prolactin action on the breast is more concerned with lactation than with ductular proliferation. Nevertheless, prolactin may occasionally play a role in the genesis of gynecomastia by causing hypogonadism, with a resultant imbalance in the circulating estrogen:androgen ratio. Other peptide growth factors, such as insulin-like growth factors, transforming growth factors-α and -β, and epidermal growth factor may be more important, perhaps as mediators of steroid hormone effects, but they have been virtually ignored in investigation to date.

There has also been little investigation of the role of genetic factors in gynecomastia. The best-known association is with Klinefelter's syndrome, in which the presence of an extra X chromosome leads to characteristic somatic abnormalities and moderately severe primary hypogonadism; it is not clear how the additional X chromosome damages the testis, or if certain genes on the second X chromosome are actively expressed, and important pathogenically. A second category involves deficiencies in androgen receptor function caused by mutations or deletions in the androgen receptor gene. These abnormalities often result in gynecomastia, presumably as a result of a decrease in androgen-mediated inhibition of breast growth; testicular feminization and its variants are prime examples of this mechanism *(5)*. Finally, a few instances have been described of gynecomastia caused by familial abnormalities in steroid metabolizing enzymes, which lead either to estrogen overproduction or failure of androgen synthesis *(6,7)*.

GYNECOMASTIA ACROSS THE LIFE-SPAN

Gynecomastia occurs physiologically in the newborn period, and again during puberty; in both of these situations, there appears to be a temporary increase in the circulating estrogen:androgen ratio. Pubertal gynecomastia is found in about 60–70% of normal boys; it generally regresses after 1–2 yr, so that, at age 20, about 20% of men have palpable breast tissue. Thereafter, there is a slow, gradual increase in the prevalence of palpable breast tissue, with about 30–40% of middle-aged men and 50–60% of older men demonstrating this finding *(8–10)*. There appears to be a positive correlation with adiposity, and also with systemic illness; about 70% of hospitalized men in their seventh decade were found to have palpable gynecomastia *(10)*. Adipose tissue is a source of estrogen, because the aromatase enzyme that converts androgens to estrogens is located there, and obese men probably produce more estrogen than thin men, both systemically and locally, in mammary adipose tissue. The role of illness is less clear; systemic illness may decrease testicular function, and may also activate aromatase, via inflammatory cytokines *(11)*. Elderly men also frequently have hypogonadism, often secondary, with low serum testosterone and modest elevations in sex-steroid-binding globulin, which lowers free testosterone further *(12)*.

It is important and useful to draw a distinction between this background gynecomastia, which is so prevalent in normal men, and the occurrence of new-onset gynecomastia, which is more likely to be caused by disease or drugs. In addition to the patient's report of a change in the breasts, the presence of breast pain or tenderness is often an indication that the breast enlargement is of recent onset. In such cases, a more detailed investigation is in order.

SPECIFIC CONDITIONS ASSOCIATED WITH GYNECOMASTIA

Hypogonadism

Primary hypogonadism is commonly associated with gynecomastia. Several mechanisms account for the alteration in the estrogen:androgen ratio. First, testicular disease limits androgen production, lowering both total and free serum testosterone. Second, increased serum luteinizing hormone (LH) results in a disproportionate stimulation of Leydig cell aromatase (13), raising testicular estradiol production, and further increasing the estrogen:androgen ratio. In addition, estrogens continue to be produced in hypogonadal patients from peripheral aromatization of adrenal-derived estrogen precursors, such as androstenedione. Patients with secondary (central) hypogonadism may also develop gynecomastia, primarily attributed to androgen deficiency; estrogen production from adrenal-derived precursors also continues in adipose tissue and other sites. Finally, hypogonadal men may have an increased adipose tissue mass; it is not known if this plays an important role in overall estrogen production.

As previously mentioned, Klinefelter's syndrome has a particularly high incidence of gynecomastia (65%); it is possible that the presence of the second X chromosome plays a unique role in determining this incidence. The incidence of male breast cancer is increased 16-fold in Klinefelter's syndrome (14,15), the only cause of gynecomastia in which this is the case; for this reason, it is reasonable for men with Klinefelter's syndrome to perform regular breast self-examination, and for their physicians to be alert to the increased risk of breast cancer.

Estrogen-Producing Tumors

Leydig cell tumors of the testis are rare neoplasms; about 90% are benign. These tumors tend to be small, and are very efficient producers of estrogen. The direct overproduction of estradiol raises serum estrogen levels; the estrogen excess tends to suppress LH release from the pituitary, leading to a decrease in serum testosterone. Estrogen also stimulates the production of sex-steroid-binding globulin (SSBG), the carrier protein for both testosterone and estradiol; because testosterone is more tightly bound than estradiol, free testosterone levels are lowered whenever SSBG rises, further raising the ratio of free estradiol to free testosterone. In this way, SSBG is said to act as an estrogen amplifier. Although some Leydig cell tumors are too small to be palpated, they may be detected by testicular sonography or thermography. Leydig cell tumors are treated surgically. Although most Leydig cell tumors occur in young and middle-aged men, about 10% occur after age 60 yr (16,17).

Estrogen-producing adrenal tumors are generally malignant; they are also among the rarest of adrenal neoplasms. Adrenal carcinomas tend to be relatively inefficient producers of steroid hormones, and are often quite large when discovered; indeed, about 50% of patients with estrogen-producing adrenal carcinomas have a palpable abdominal mass at the time of presentation *(18)*. Essentially all feminizing adrenal carcinomas can be visualized on CT scans of the abdomen. Many of these tumors also produce other hormonal products, and serum DHEA-sulfate or urinary 17-ketosteroids may be useful as tumor markers *(18,19)*. In some instances, gynecomastia may result when adrenal tumors produce estrogen precursors (e.g., androstenedione), which are aromatized in peripheral tissues to active estrogens. The estrogen excess suppresses pituitary LH secretion, which lower serum testosterone, and further alters the estrogen:androgen balance. The treatment of feminizing adrenal tumors is surgical, although the prognosis is poor. Most feminizing adrenal tumors occur in men between the ages of 20 and 50 yr.

A variety of other tumors may also produce estrogen; these are generally those that also produce human chorionic gonadotropin (hCG) and are considered in the next section.

Tumors Producing hCG

The placental hormone, hCG, is similar to LH in its structure and action on the testis. Thus, elevated serum levels of hCG disproportionately stimulate estradiol secretion from normal testicular Leydig cells, with a resultant rise in serum estradiol; estradiol also stimulates hepatic production of SSBG, and results in a decrease in free serum testosterone. In addition, hCG-secreting tumors, like normal placenta, often have the capacity to take up estrogen precursors from the circulation, and aromatize them into active estrogens *(20)*. Many testicular cancers produce hCG, often from chorionic elements in the tumor. A wide variety of other carcinomas are also associated with ectopic hCG production; lung, liver, and gastric tumors are among the more common. Measurement of serum hCG by an immunoassay directed against the specific β-subunit of hCG should be used for detection; normal men have undetectable serum hCG in commercially available assays (i.e., <5 mIU/mL).

Liver Disease

Gynecomastia has commonly been thought to be associated with liver disease, particularly with alcoholic cirrhosis, although this association has also been questioned *(21,22)*. Nevertheless, a variety of abnormalities are present in patients with liver disease that would be expected to lead to an increased prevalence of gynecomastia. Patients with cirrhosis are frequently hypogonadal, often caused by a combination of testicular damage from ethanol and central defects in gonadotropin secretion *(23)*; thus, serum testosterone levels are lowered. SSBG levels are often elevated, further lowering free testosterone concentrations. Serum estrogen levels are increased, primarily because of increased extrahepatic aromatization *(24)*. Finally, some alcoholic beverages may contain plant-derived phytoestrogens, with estrogen-agonist actions on the breast *(25)*. Standard liver function tests will reveal evidence of hepatic dysfunction in men with gynecomastia caused by liver disease.

Thyrotoxicosis

In men with thyrotoxicosis, serum concentrations of SSBG are often remarkably increased, probably as a direct effect of thyroid hormone excess; this results in a marked increase in total serum testosterone and total serum estradiol concentrations. As previously mentioned, SSBG acts as an estrogen amplifier by binding testosterone more tightly than estradiol, so that free testosterone levels are normal, but free estradiol levels are high *(26)*. There is also some evidence for excessive estrogen production in thyrotoxicosis, apparently from peripheral sites *(27)*. About 10–40% of men with thyrotoxicosis have been reported to have gynecomastia; the breast enlargement resolved as euthyroidism was restored *(28)*.

Refeeding

During and after World War II, it was noted that inmates liberated from prison camps commonly developed gynecomastia within a few weeks of resuming an adequate diet; the tender breast enlargement persisted for 1–2 yr, and then spontaneously regressed *(29)*. Similar occurrences have been noted in more recent studies of refugee populations around the world *(30)*. Although the pathogenesis of refeeding gynecomastia is not entirely clear, it has been proposed that testicular function is shut down during periods of starvation; when gonadal function resumes following refeeding, there may be a temporary imbalance of estrogen vs androgen production, akin to normal puberty. Complicating this interpretation is the frequent co-occurrence of chronic medical illnesses in malnourished populations; because testicular function is frequently depressed in chronic illness *per se (31)*, concurrent treatment of the illness may have as much effect on testicular function as the reversal of malnutrition. Additionally, specific nutrients may have effects on gonadal function; for example, high-protein diets have been reported to depress serum testosterone in normal men *(32)*.

Dialysis

A small number of men beginning dialysis therapy develop transient gynecomastia *(33)*. The cause is not known; although there are major perturbations of gonadal function in renal failure, there do not seem to be any further alterations caused by dialysis *(34)*. Dialysis-associated gynecomastia is generally a self-limited process, lasting 1–2 yr or less; it may be a variant of refeeding, since the initiation of dialysis often leads to a reversal of the uremic state, a liberalization of dietary intake, and weight gain.

Medications

Drugs are a relatively frequent cause of gynecomastia. A wide variety of agents may cause breast enlargement, acting through several mechanisms. Estrogens (e.g., given for palliation of prostate carcinoma) directly stimulate the breast; hCG stimulates estradiol production by normal Leydig cells. Digitoxin has estrogen-agonist-like effects, binding to the estrogen receptor *(35)*. Testosterone preparations may occasionally produce gynecomastia, perhaps by conversion to estrogens in the breast or other peripheral tissues; the observation that nonaromatizable androgens, such as methyltestosterone, may also produce gynecomastia suggests that additional mechanisms may be involved, as well *(36,37)*.

Drugs that lower serum testosterone concentrations can cause gynecomastia. Analogs of gonadotropin-releasing hormone, which lower pituitary LH secretion, are given to induce a hypogonadal state in men with prostate carcinoma; serum estrogen concentrations may be maintained by aromatization of adrenal-derived precursors, leading to an elevation in the estrogen:androgen ratio. Cytotoxic chemotherapy frequently damages testicular Leydig cells, impairing testosterone production, and resulting in a rise in serum LH; this elevation of LH stimulates excessive estradiol production by remaining Leydig cells. Chemotherapy-induced hypogonadism and gynecomastia are often transient *(38)*. Spironolactone, ketoconazole, and, perhaps, metronidazole can interfere with testosterone biosynthesis, lowering serum testosterone concentrations *(39–41)*. Spironolactone also acts as an androgen receptor antagonist, blocking the action of testosterone on the breast, as do cimetidine, flutamide, and cannabis *(42–45)*.

Many drugs that act on the central nervous system have been reported to cause gynecomastia, including methyldopa, amphetamines, reserpine, diethylpropion, tricyclic antidepressants, diazepam, and phenytoin. The mechanisms of action are unknown; although methyldopa and reserpine may raise serum prolactin modestly, the magnitude of this increase is probably not sufficient to produce hypogonadism.

Recently, calcium channel blockers have been reported to produce gynecomastia and, occasionally, mild hyperprolactinemia *(46)*; the mechanism of breast enlargement is unclear. Theophylline, amiodarone, and D-penicillamine have also been reported to occasionally cause gynecomastia. Recombinant human growth hormone, which is being used more frequently as replacement therapy in elderly individuals with functional growth hormone deficiency, may occasionally cause gynecomastia *(47)*.

Male Breast Cancer

Male breast cancer accounts for only 0.2% of all malignancies in men; breast cancer is about 150× less frequent in men than in women. Despite its rarity, many patients with gynecomastia (and frequently their physicians as well) are concerned that the breast enlargement may be caused by breast cancer. As in women, the characteristics of a breast mass that suggest malignancy include unusual hardness, irregularity, fixation or ulceration, an eccentric (rather than subareolar) location, and axillary adenopathy. In the absence of one or more of these features, breast biopsy is generally not needed. Mammography may occasionally provide evidence supporting suspicions of malignancy, but is generally not required in most cases of gynecomastia. Breast biopsy should, however, be performed whenever suspicious findings are encountered on examination; biopsy may be performed using either a fine-needle aspiration technique or excision *(48)*. In general, gynecomastia does not seem to predispose men to the development of breast cancer, with the exception of Klinefelter's syndrome, in which the risk of breast cancer is 16× that of the general male population.

INVESTIGATION OF THE PATIENT WITH GYNECOMASTIA

Because a large proportion of normal men have asymptomatic palpable breast tissue, it is evident that such men should not undergo an expensive, prolonged evaluation in a search for underlying disease. In these men, the physician should perform a careful examination of the breasts to determine if there is any clinical finding suggestive of breast cancer. If not, no further evaluation is needed in an otherwise healthy man.

However, in men with newly developed, progressive, or tender gynecomastia, a more thorough evaluation should be performed, because, in these patients, it is more likely that a specific cause will be identified. A careful history should be taken, focusing on the use of medications or hormonal preparations, symptoms of hypogonadism, hyperthyroidism, liver disease, chronic illness, and weight gain. Physical examination should be directed at uncovering testicular abnormalities or masses, hypogonadism, thyrotoxicosis, features of liver disease, abdominal masses, or lymphadenopathy.

Laboratory testing should, in general, be guided by the findings on history and physical examination. A screening examination may be performed in patients with no localizing findings, and could consist of measurements of serum thyroid-stimulating hormone, liver enzymes and serum albumin, serum hCG, testosterone, estradiol, LH, follicle stimulating hormone, and prolactin.

TREATMENT

Several conditions (puberty, refeeding, dialysis) that cause gynecomastia are self-limited, and the breast enlargement will spontaneously regress. Reassurance is usually the only treatment needed in such instances. Hypogonadism and gynecomastia induced by cancer chemotherapy are also often transient. Treatment of an underlying medical condition will frequently alleviate the associated gynecomastia (e.g., hyperthyroidism, removal of a tumor), as will withdrawal of an offending drug.

Patients with hypogonadism may benefit from administration of testosterone; this raises serum testosterone and also suppresses LH-mediated estradiol secretion from the testes.

Medical treatment with antiestrogens has been reasonably successful. Although clomiphene has occasionally been used, most published reports have utilized tamoxifen; doses of 10–20 mg/d have been given for periods up to 6 mo, with good results *(49)*. Danazol, a weak androgen that suppresses gonadotropin secretion and lowers estradiol production by the testes, has also been used *(50)*, as has testolactone, a peripheral aromatase inhibitor *(51)*.

In men with prostate cancer, prophylactic irradiation of the breast prior to starting estrogen therapy has been quite successful in preventing the development of painful gynecomastia *(52)*.

Surgery may be indicated for patients with persistent, large, or painful breasts that cause physical or psychological disability. Suction lipectomy has been used successfully in many cases, when there is not extremely dense breast tissue *(53)*.

REFERENCES

1. Nicolis GL, Modlinger RS, Gabrilove JL. A study of histopathology of human gynecomastia. J Clin Endocrinol Metab,1971;32:173–178.
2. Sasano H, Kimura M, Shizawa S, Kimura N, Nagura H. Aromatase and steroid receptors in gynecomastia and male breast carcinoma: an immunohistochemical study. J Clin Endocrinol Metab 1996;81:3063–3067.
3. Santner SJ, Pauley RJ, Tait L, Kaseta J, Santen RJ. Aromatase activity and expression in breast cancer and benign breast tissue stromal cells. J Clin Endocrinol Metab 1997;82:200–208.
4. DiCarlo R, Muccioli G, Bellussi G, Lando D, Mussa A. Presence and characterization of prolactin receptors in human benign breast tumours. Eur J Cancer Clin Oncol 1984;20:635–638.
5. Griffin JE, Leshin M, Wilson JD. Androgen resistance syndromes. Am J Physiol 1982;243:E81–E87.
6. Castro-Magana M, Angulo M, Uy J. Male hypogonadism with gynecomastia caused by late-onset deficiency of testicular 17-ketosteroid reductase. N Engl J Med 1993;328:1297–1301.
7. Stratakis CA, Vottero A, Brodie A, Kirschner LS, DeAtkine D, Lu Q, et al. Aromatase excess syndrome is associated with feminization of both sexes and autosomal dominant transmission of aberrant P450 aromatase gene transcription. J Clin Endocrinol Metab 1998;83:1348–1357.
8. Nuttall FQ. Gynecomastia as a physical finding in normal men. J Clin Endocrinol Metab 1979;48:338–340.
9. Carlson HE. Gynecomastia. N Engl J Med 1980;303:795–799.
10. Niewoehner CB, Nuttall FQ. Gynecomastia in a hospitalized male population. Am J Med 1984;77: 633–638.
11. Reed MJ, Purohit A. Breast cancer and the role of cytokines in regulating estrogen synthesis: an emerging hypothesis. Endocr Rev 1997;18:701–715.
12. Korenman SG, Morley JE, Mooradian AD, Davis SS, Kaiser FE, Silver AJ, Viosca SP, Garza D. Secondary hypogonadism in older men: its relation to impotence. J Clin Endocrinol Metab 1990;71: 963–969.
13. Forest MG, Lecoq A, Saez JM. Kinetics of human chorionic gonadotropin-induced steroidogenic response of the human testis. II. Plasma 17α-hydroxyprogesterone, Δ⁴-androstenedione, estrone, and

17β-estradiol: evidence for the action of human chorionic gonadotropin on intermediate enzymes implicated in steroid biosynthesis. J Clin Endocrinol Metab 1979;49:284–291.

14. Scheike O, Visfeldt J, Petersen B. Male breast cancer. 3. Breast carcinoma in association with the Klinefelter syndrome. Acta Pathol Microbiol Scand 1973;81:352–358.

15. Sasco AJ, Lowenfels AB, Pasker-deJong P. Epidemiology of male breast cancer: a meta-analysis of published case-control studies and discussion of selected aetiological factors. Int J Cancer 1993;53: 538–549.

16. Gabrilove JL, Nicolis GL, Mitty HA, Sohval AR. Feminizing interstitial cell tumor of the testis: personal observations and a review of the literature. Cancer 1975;35:1184–1202.

17. Bercovici J-P, Nahoul K, Tater D, Charles J-F, Scholler R. Hormonal profile of Leydig cell tumors with gynecomastia J Clin Endocrinol Metab 1984;59:625–630.

18. Gabrilove JL, Sharma DC, Wotiz HH, Dorman RI. Feminizing adrenocortical tumors in the male: a review of 52 cases including a case report. Medicine 1965;44:37–79.

19. Boyar RM, Nogeire C, Fukushima D, Hellman L, Fishman J. Studies of the diurnal pattern of plasma corticosteroids and gonadotropins in two cases of feminizing adrenal carcinoma: measurements of estrogen and corticosteroid production. J Clin Endocrinol Metab 1977;44:39–45.

20. Kirschner MA, Cohen FB, Jespersen D. Estrogen production and its origin in men with gonadotropin-producing neoplasms. J Clin Endocrinol Metab 1974;39:112–118.

21. Baker HWG, Burger HG, DeKretser DM, Dolmanis A, Hudson B, O'Connor S, et al. A study of the endocrine manifestations of hepatic cirrhosis. Q J Med 1976;45:145–178.

22. Cavanaugh J, Niewoehner CB, Nuttall FQ. Gynecomastia and cirrhosis of the liver. Arch Intern Med 1990;150:563–565.

23. Van Thiel DH. Ethanol: its adverse effects upon the hypothalamic-pituitary-gonadal axis. J Lab Clin Med 1983;101:21–33.

24. Kley HK, Niederau C, Stremmel W, Lax R, Strohmeyer G, Kruskemper HL. Conversion of androgens to estrogens in idiopathic hemochromatosis: comparison with alcoholic liver cirrhosis. J Clin Endocrinol Metab 1985;61:1–6.

25. Gavaler JS, Rosenblum ER, Van Thiel DH, Eagon PK, Pohl CR, Campbell IM, Gavaler J. Biologically active phytoestrogens are present in bourbon. Alcohol Clin Exp Res 1987;11:399–406.

26. Chopra IJ, Tulchinsky D. Status of estrogen-androgen balance in hyperthyroid men with Graves' disease. J Clin Endocrinol Metab 1974;38:269–277.

27. Southren AL, Olive J, Gordon GG, Vittek J, Brener J, Rafii F. The conversion of androgens to estrogens in hyperthyroidism. J Clin Endocrinol Metab 1974;38:207–214.

28. Ashkar FS, Smoak WM, Gilson AJ, Miller R. Gynecomastia and mastoplasia in Graves' disease. Metabolism 1970;19:946–951.

29. Klatskin G, Satter WT, Humm FD. Gynecomastia due to malnutrition. I. Clinical studies. Am J Med Sci 1947;213:19–30.

30. Linn S, Almagor G, Lamm S. Gynecomastia among Ethiopian Jews. Pub Hlth Rep 1986;101:237.

31. Semple CG, Gray CE, Beastall GH. Male hypogonadism—a non-specific consequence of illness. Q J Med 1987;64:601–607.

32. Anderson KE, Rosner W, Khan MS, New MI, Pang S, Wissel PS, Kappas A. Diet-hormone interactions: protein/carbohydrate ratio alters reciprocally the plasma levels of testosterone and cortisol and their respective binding globulins in man. Life Sci 1987;40:1761–1768.

33. Schmitt GW, Shehadeh I, Sawin CT. Transient gynecomastia in chronic renal failure during chronic intermittent hemodialysis. Ann Intern Med 1968;69:73–79.

34. Morley JE. Melmed S. Gonadal dysfunction in systemic disorders. Metabolism 1979;28:1051–1073.

35. Rifka SM, Pita JC, Loriaux DL. Mechanism of interaction of digitalis with estradiol binding sites in rat uteri. Endocrinology 1976;99:1091–1096.

36. Swerdloff RS, Palacios A, McClure RD, Campfield LA, Brosman, SS. Male contraception: clinical assessment of chronic administration of testosterone enanthate. Int J Androl 2(Suppl):731–747.

37. McCullagh EP, Rossmiller HR. Methyl testosterone. I. Androgenic effects and the production of gynecomastia and oligospermia. J Clin Endocrinol Metab 1941;1:496–502.

38. Saeter G, Fossa SD, Norman N. Gynaecomastia folllowing cytotoxic therapy for testicular cancer. Br J Urol 1987;59:348–352.

39. Rose LI, Underwood RH, Newmark SR, Kisch ES, Williams GH. Pathophysiology of spironolactone-induced gynecomastia. Ann Intern Med 1977;87:398–403.

40. Pont A, Goldman ES, Sugar AM, Siiteri PK, Stevens DA. Ketoconazole-induced increase in estradiol-testosterone ratio. Probable explanation for gynecomastia. Arch Intern Med 1985;145:1429–1431.
41. Fagan TC, Johnson DG, Grosso DS. Metronidazole-induced gynecomastia. JAMA 1985;254:3217.
42. Loriaux DL, Menard R, Taylor A, Pita JC, Santen R. Spironolactone and endocrine dysfunction. Ann Intern Med 1976;85:630–636.
43. Winters SJ, Lee J, Troen P. Competition of the histamine H2 antagonist cimetidine for androgen binding sites in man. J Androl 1980;1:111–114.
44. Boccon-Gibod L, Fournier G, Bottet P, Marechal JM, Guiter J. Rischman P, et al. Flutamide versus orchiectomy in the treatment of metastatic prostate carcinoma. Eur Urol 1997;32:391–396.
45. Purohit V, Ahluwahlia BS, Vigersky RA. Marihuana inhibits dihydrotestosterone binding to the androgen receptor. Endocrinology 1980;107:848–850.
46. Tanner LA, Bosco LA. Gynecomastia associated with calcium channel blocker therapy. Arch Intern Med 1988;148:379–380.
47. Cohn L, Feller AG, Draper MW, Rudman IW, Rudman D. Carpal tunnel syndrome and gynaecomastia during growth hormone treatment of elderly men with low circulating IGF-I concentrations. Clin Endocrinol (Oxford) 1993;39:417–425.
48. Lilleng R, Paksoy N, Vural G, Langmark F, Hagmar B. Assessment of fine-needle aspiration cytology and histopathology for diagnosing male breast masses. Acta Cytol 1995;39:877–881.
49. McDermott MT, Hofeldt FD, Kidd GS. Tamoxifen therapy for painful idiopathic gynecomastia. South Med J 1990;83:1283–1285.
50. Buckle R. Danazol in the treatment of gynecomastia. Drugs 1980;19:356–361.
51. Zachmann M, Eiholzer U, Muritano M, Werder EA, Manella B. Treatment of pubertal gynecomastia with testolactone. Acta Endocrinol 1986;113(Suppl 279):218–226.
52. Fass D, Steinfeld A, Brown J, Tessler A. Radiotherapeutic prophylaxis of estrogen-induced gynecomastia: a study of late sequelae. Int J Radiat Oncol Biol Phys 1986;12:407–408.
53. Rosenberg GJ. Gynecomastia: suction lipectomy as a contemporary solution. Plast Reconst Surg 1987;80:379–385.

11

Menopause

Morris Notelovitz, MD, PHD,

INTRODUCTION

The menopause has become a twentieth-century phenomenon simply because women are living longer. This is a global reality, and has led to an ever-increasing societal health issue: care of elderly women. Most women can now expect to live 25–30 yr beyond their menopause *(1)*. Thus, female longevity is no longer a major issue, but the quality of this expanded life-span, certainly is. The solution to the burgeoning cost of menopause-related conditions rests with the understanding of the pathophysiology of the changes associated with the menopause, and the recognition of the following salient points:

1. By definition, the menopause is the last natural menstrual period, and therefore lasts 1 wk. It is a diagnosis that can only be made retrospectively, and is usually postdated after at least 1 yr of amenorrhea.
2. The menopause is preceded and followed by at least 15 yr of physical and other changes directly associated with the downregulation of ovarian steroid genesis. This 30-yr time-span—the climacteric—represents the period during which clinically obvious symptoms and physical changes occur (often far removed from the reproductive tract), and which is still incorrectly referred to as "the menopause."
3. Many postmenopausal concerns, such as cardiovascular disease (CVD) and osteoporosis, are confounded by variables such as the individual's genetic constitution; early adolescent and premenopausal nutrition, exercise, lifestyle, and societal behavior; and the effect of chronological aging *per se.*

With the advent of modern technology, it is possible to identify and quantify some of these variables, and to separate issues that are clearly hormonal from those that are not.

From: *Contemporary Endocrinology: Endocrinology of Aging*
Edited by: J. E. Morley and L. van den Berg © Humana Press Inc., Totowa, NJ

It is also feasible to define women who are experiencing their menopausal transition normally from those who have evidence of latent or overt (but silent) disease. Thus, it is now practical and relevant to differentiate the management of healthy menopausal women from those who need treatment for specific reasons.

The menopausal experience is individualized and varied. Socioeconomic and cultural factors not infrequently color the attitude, and hence the behavior, of menopausal women. The physiology of the menopause, however, is generic to all women, but in reality there is (or should be) no generic treatment. Individualization is the key to optimal climacteric health care.

CLIMACTERIC HORMONAL PHYSIOLOGY

The classical symptoms and signs of the climacteric and menopause are caused by changes in the synthesis and secretion of estrogen, progesterone, and androgens. The pattern of this change is similar in all women, but there are considerable inter- and intra-individual differences. The clinical response to a similar degree of estrogen deprivation also varies between women. The modern approach to hormonal therapy is predicated on a better appreciation of these hormonal variables. Thus, lower-dose hormone prescription, based on an individual's specific needs and adjusted to their response and requirements over time, is replacing the standardized one-dose-suits-all approach.

The predominant estrogen in premenopausal women is estradiol. The mean serum levels vary during the menstrual cycle: early follicular phase (first week), 40–80 pg/dL; mid-to-late follicular phase (second week), 80–300 pg/dL; early-to-late luteal period (third week), 100–150 pg/dL; and the late luteal phase (fourth week), 40 pg/dL. The average value over a 28-d cycle is 100 pg/dL. Estrone is derived primarily from the metabolism of estradiol, and from the peripheral aromatization of the androgen, androstenedione, in adipose tissue. Serum levels of estrone, including the menstrual cycle, vary from 40 to 170 pg/dL. The estradiol:estrone ratio is usually greater than one *(2)*.

With progressive atresia of the ovarian follicles, the estradiol values fall to below 20 pg/dL, and the predominant estrogen is estrone, with a resultant estradiol:estrone ratio of less than 1. Postmenopausal estrone is derived primarily from the peripheral aromatization of androstenedione and testosterone to estrone, and averages about 30 pg/dL. Progesterone is not measurable postmenopausally. Thus, postmenopausal women have an absolute lack of progesterone, and have variable degrees of estrogen deficiency, with estrone as the predominant estrogen *(2)*.

As follicular function declines, plasma levels of follicle stimulating hormone (FSH) and luteinizing hormone (LH) increase, with values of the former exceeding 40 mIU/L. The plasma level of plasma FSH is further influenced by the two ovarian peptides, inhibin and activin, and their various subunits. On average, serum FSH levels in postmenopausal women are 10–15× higher than early follicular levels in young women. Plasma LH levels increase threefold (probably because inhibin has little control over LH secretions).

Premenopausal women synthesize the androgens, androstenedione and testosterone, from both the ovaries and the adrenal glands. The ovaries also synthesize and secrete small amounts of dehydroepiandrosterone (DHEA). The adrenal gland is the primary source for both DHEA and its sulphate derivative (DHEAS). About 50% of the plasma testosterone premenopausally is derived from the conversion of androstenedione in peripheral tissues; 50% of testosterone postmenopausally comes from the ovary. Plasma levels of testosterone remain constant throughout the menstrual cycle, at about 50 ng/dL *(3)*.

The biologic function of both estrogen and testosterone is dependent on an individual's tissue sensitivity and binding affinity for sex steroids, and the physical state of the steroids in plasma. Additionally, the availability of 5α-reductase activity is needed to convert testosterone to the biologically active androgen, DHEA. Plasma binding of both estrogen and testosterone is dependent on attachment primarily to sex-hormone-binding globulin (SHBG), and, to a lesser extent, albumin, and, in the case of estrogen, a specific liver-derived estrogen-binding globulin. Only about 1% of estradiol and testosterone is biologically active or free, a value that will vary with SHBG synthesis and binding. Exogenous oral estrogen and thyroid therapy, for example, increases SHBG levels; conditions characterized by insulin resistance or hyperinsulinism (obesity, noninsulin-dependent diabetes, and polycystic ovarian syndrome) are associated with low SHBG (2).

A recent major discovery, which may explain why women respond differently to estrogen deprivation and estrogen-replacement therapy, is the identification of at least two estrogen receptors (Ers): α and β (5). There is a variable distribution of ERα and ERβ in different tissues and organs. Within individuals, there may also be a heterogeneity of receptor type that is specific to that person. The ERα tends to predominate in tissues such as the breast and endometrium, and the ERβ in the brain, and possibly the vascular tree, and bone. A new generation of synthetic target tissue-specific drugs have now become available—selective estrogen receptor modulators (SERMS)—which have both estrogen agonist (ERβ) and estrogen antagonist (ERα) activity.

DEFINING THE CLIMACTERIC SYNDROME

It is clinically expedient to subdivide the 30-yr climacteric (age 35–65 yr) into three decades of varying clinical presentation and health care need: the early climacteric (from age 35 to 45 yr), the perimenopause (age 46–55 yr), and the late climacteric (from age 56 to 65 yr). In addition, management of the active elderly (age 66–75 yr) frequently involves treatment similar and pertinent to women in their late climacteric.

Technology makes it possible to identify and quantify deviations from normal, irrespective of a woman's chronologic or menopausal age. With this evidence-based approach, treatment can now be selectively and individually prescribed. The traditional "pelvic and Pap" adult women's annual examination needs to be expanded to a much broader general examination, to include additional tests such as mammograms, lipid profiles, bone density tests (including selective measurement of bone markers), and, occasionally, hormone profiles. The scope of this chapter precludes detailed discussion of this aspect.

Given the physiologic nature of the climacteric and menopause, the majority of climacteric women will be found to be normal, and can be managed conservatively with exercise, nutrition, and counseling. Although there are some practitioners who regard the menopause as an endocrinopathy, HT should be restricted to women with a valid indication. If HT is contraindicated, nonhormonal therapy, such as SERMs, or drugs to treat specific confounding medical problems, such as hypertension or hypercholesterolemia, should be prescribed.

ESTROGEN THERAPY

Indications

The type of estrogen preparation(s) prescribed varies with both the phase of the climacteric and indications for HT.

EARLY CLIMACTERIC

The author strongly advocates an in-depth evaluation at age 35–40 yr, including mammograms, lipid profiling, and bone density testing. Apart from identifying latent disease or significant risk factors, this approach serves as an important education experience for the patient, and places into perspective the value of general management principles involving nutrition, exercise, and lifestyle, together with other strategies needed for the prevention of CVD, osteoporosis, and even Alzheimer's disease.

The most prevalent medical problem of women in the early climacteric is dysfunctional uterine bleeding. This condition, plus the need for contraception, can be conveniently and effectively met with low-dose oral contraception. The latter is perfectly safe in women over age 40 (if they do not smoke), and, in addition, have significant other noncontraceptive benefits: reduced prevalence of later ovarian and endometrial cancer, less benign cystic breast disease, and a lowered risk of ectopic pregnancy and pelvic inflammatory disease (6). Oral contraceptives (OCs) do not increase the risk of breast cancer. Two less-well-recognized advantages of low-dose OC use include management of climacteric symptoms (including hot flashes) indistinguishable from those associated with the menopause, and the management of premenopausal osteopenia (7). Recent studies have confirmed that women on low-dose OCs do have greater bone mineral density (BMD) than untreated age-matched peers.

Clinically useful caveats when prescribing OCs for climacteric women include:

1. Preference for OC formulation that includes low-dose ethinyl estradiol in all 28 tablets, because climacteric women develop their symptoms during their estrogen-free placebo week of therapy.
2. For improvement in osteopenia, the OCs should contain at least 1 mg norethindrone (NE) (or equivalent) (7).
3. When converting a woman from OC use to HT (when indicated), the patient's FSH should be assayed on the day prior to initiation of a new cycle of treatment. A value in excess of 20 mIU/mL is indicative of ovarian follicular downregulation and impending failure. This approach is only applicable to traditional OC formulations. Women taking continuous low-dose ethinyl estradiol OCs need to stop their OCs for at least 1 (or preferably 2) mo, before testing their FSH. Alternative barrier contraception will be required during this period.

PERIMENOPAUSE

Assessing Risk Factors. By concentrating on the treatment of a predominant presenting symptom, more significant and potentially more harmful conditions may be overlooked. Irrespective of the patient's complaints, appropriate examination and tests should be performed in all perimenopausal women as part of their annual examination. Risk factors (or evidence of) CVD, osteoporosis, Alzheimer's disease, and cancer (colon, breast, endometrium, and ovary) should be evaluated.

Vasomotor Symptoms. A frequently held misconception is that typical menopausal symptoms—hot flashes, insomnia, mood swings, irritability, and so on—in menstruating women are not caused by estrogen deficiency. In reality, a significant percentage (if not the majority) of menopausal women experience vasomotor instability prior to developing amenorrhea and/or other target tissue evidence of estrogen deprivation, such as atrophic vaginitis and urogenital symptoms. When estrogen levels fall below an individual's minimal brain estrogen threshold, irrespective of their age or menstrual function, symptoms triggered by the brain's vasomotor center will occur *(8)*. In menstruating women, this typically occurs during the late luteal phase and during menstruation, when estradiol values drop. The symptoms usually respond to appropriate estradiol supplementation, but can be exacerbated if too much estrogen is given. In most women, relatively low values of estradiol will control central nervous system (CNS) symptoms. In one study, symptomatic women using low-dose transdermal estrogen (25 µg estradiol patch) achieved total estradiol values of between 40 and 50 pg/dL, and decreased the frequency of hot flashes by 84% *(9)*.

Menstrual migraine is yet another common estrogen threshold-related problem. A relative drop in plasma estradiol perimenstrually stimulates intracerebral vasoconstriction, followed by extracerebral vasodilation and a typical vascular headache. The vascular tone can frequently be stabilized, and the initiating cerebral vascular spasm prevented, by maintaining constant estradiol values. This is best, and most physiologically, achieved with transdermal estradiol administered during the second half of the menstrual cycle, including menstruation, thus augmenting endogenous luteal-phase estradiol production. Low doses of estrogen are usually required. It is not necessary to add a progestin or progesterone, as long as regular withdrawal bleeding still occurs.

Atrophic Vaginitis. Urogenital disorders are the most prevalent consequence of the menopause, and, according to some experts, involve 50% of all perimenopausal women *(10)*. The urogenital response to HT is mediated by estrogen and progesterone receptors situated in the vagina, urethra, bladder trigone, and related pelvic floor and ligaments.

Patients are often reluctant to volunteer that they have significant vaginal or bladder problems. Also, whereas the clinical features of advanced atrophic vaginitis are usually self-evident, the physical appearance of mild-to-moderate changes in the vaginal epithelium are subtle, and the diagnosis of atrophic vaginitis can be easily missed.

In addition to direct questioning and examination, the vaginal pH should be tested. Secretion should be taken from the lateral vaginal wall at the junction of the upper one-third and lower two-thirds of the vagina. A lack of estrogen is reflected in an increase in the vaginal pH. In premenopausal women, estrogen facilitates vaginal colonization with lactobacilli, which produce lactic acid from vaginal glycogen, thus maintaining a low vaginal pH. After menopause, the vaginal pH increases as lactobacilli disappear from the vaginal flora. Estrogen replacement, locally applied or by oral administration, improves vaginal wall glycogenization and vaginal blood flow, resulting in the restoration of a normal vaginal bacterial flora, and a concomitant lowering of the vaginal pH.

The gold standard for diagnosing atrophic vaginitis is still cytohormonal analysis of the vaginal epithelium. Several ratios are used karyopyknotic index, maturation values, and the maturation index, all of which are expressed as a numeric value. From the patient's point of view, this number is meaningless, and, in addition, the result is usually made available sometime after the examination. Bedside testing of the vaginal pH yields a result that the patient can actually visualize at the time of her examination. Demonstration of an improved pH on subsequent exams encourages treatment compliance. Persistence of an elevated pH is indicative of inadequate dosing, incorrect usage of treatment, or noncompliance.

The route of administration, and possibly the type and dose of estrogen used, influences the clinical outcome. In one report *(11)*, 40% of women on oral HT had persistent complaints of vaginal dryness, and, in another investigation *(12)*, 55% of women with documented urethral syndrome/trigonitis (also an estrogen-sensitive disorder) were on oral therapy. This idiosyncracy may relate to the route of estrogen therapy and the distribution/affinity of ERα and ERβ in the lower genital tract of responsive vs non-responsive subjects. In this context, local therapy seems to work better for the management of urogenital atrophy. However, depending on the product used, and its dose, estrogen is avidly absorbed through the vaginal epithelium, and could function as a systemic drug. In all probability, vaginally administered estrogens have both local and systemic effects, mostly directly on the local target tissue. The ideal is to choose those preparations that have a minimal systemic absorption.

A number of options are available for local estrogen therapy. These include estrogen-based vaginal creams containing either conjugated equine estrogen, micronized estradiol or diethylstilbestrol, vaginal estriol pessaries, estradiol vaginal rings, and a specially formulated slow-release 17β-estradiol matrix vaginal tablet. Using a cellulose ether polymer, the tablets, when placed deep in the vagina (via a disposable applicator), dissolve and adhere to the vaginal mucosa. The latter preparation is currently in clinical trial in the United States.

Bladder Dysfunction. Estrogen increases the resistance to urinary tract injection (UTI) by lowering the pH, decreasing the carriage of *Escherichia coli* bacteria, and increasing the vaginal colonization of lactobacilli. For example, topically applied vaginal estradiol cream has been shown to significantly reduce the incidence of UTI from 5.9 to 0.5 episodes per patient year, compared with women given a placebo. This was accompanied by return of lactobacilli in the vaginal cultures of the treated women, a decrease in *E. coli* colonization, and a significant decrease in vaginal pH *(13)*.

Women with urinary incontinence do have a significant improvement in bladder control when treated with estrogen. This is especially true for women with genuine stress incontinence. Patients with low urethral pressures increase the pressure significantly after treatment with estrogen, as evidenced by an increase in the maximal urethral closure pressure *(14)*.

LATE CLIMACTERIC

Numerous observational studies have linked estrogen therapy with the prevention of CVD, osteoporosis, and even Alzheimer's disease. Yet, most of these diseases arise well before the menopause. Atherogenesis is known to commence in early adolescence, and an individual's peak bone mass is determined by bone mineral accrual between puberty and early adulthood. Given the obvious protection of endogenous ovarian function during the formative and early reproductive years, it is still the impact of lifestyle, nutrition, and physical activity that eventually determines the pathogenesis of these diseases *(15)*. Postmenopausal HT should therefore play a secondary role when planning the long-term health care needs of premenopausal women, but deserves primary consideration in women who are already postmenopausal, or who are at high risk for CVD and/or osteoporosis.

Cardiovascular Disease. The pathogenesis of CVD involves two separate but interrelated processes: atherothrombosis and vascular smooth muscle hypertrophy and hyperreactivity. Estrogen therapy has a protective effect by influencing both aspects *(16)*. A recent review *(17)*, citing over 30 observational studies, concluded that postmenopausal women on estrogen therapy reduced their risk of CVD by 50%. The overall effect of estrogen therapy is dose-dependent, and, to some extent, varies with the route of estrogen administration.

Atherothrombosis. An atheromatous plaque results from interrelated abnormalities in lipid and carbohydrate metabolism, and hemostasis. Levels of total plasma low density lipoprotein (LDL) cholesterol are lowered with estrogen therapy, and those of high-density lipoprotein (HDL) cholesterol are increased. The latter effect is greater with oral than with parenteral estrogen. Estrogen also reduces LDL oxidation. Although the clinical relevance awaits further study, traditional doses of oral estrogen therapy frequently increases the level of triglycerides by as much as 20%, and may be associated with an increase in levels of potentially atherogenic small-molecule LDL particle size *(18)*. Elevated level of triglycerides are associated with hyperinsulinemia and an increase in procoagulation factors. Low-dose natural oral estrogen (for example, esterified estrogen, 0.3 mg) *(19)* and transdermal estradiol therapy maintain or reduce levels of plasma triglycerides and fasting plasma insulin, and increase hepatic insulin clearance *(20)*. Low-dose natural oral estrogen therapy and transdermal estrogen have not been found to have a clinically relevant adverse effect on hemostasis *(21)*.

The main cardioprotective effect of estrogen is mediated by influence on the arterial endothelium and smooth muscle. Thus, estrogen therapy enhances the synthesis of vasodilatory factors such as nitric oxide *(22)* and prostacyclin *(23)*, and also inhibits the synthesis of the vasoconstrictor, endothelin-I *(23)*. In addition, estrogen acts as a calcium channel blocker of vascular smooth muscle cells, and decreases the activity of angiotensin-converting enzyme by 20% *(24)*. The net result is a decrease in the vascular resistance and an increase in blood flow, together with a concomitant lowering of blood pressure, a clinical end point demonstrated with both oral and transdermal estrogen therapy. There are occasional exceptions to this response. Less than 5% of women on oral estrogen therapy have an idiosyncratic reaction, with a resulting increase in blood pressure. This may be caused by stimulation of the renin–angiotensin system. Patients are less likely to be affected when taking nonoral estrogens.

Monitoring the clinical cardioprotective efficacy of estrogen therapy is problematic. The biological parameters usually measured are for the recognition of risk factors related to the clinical end point (myocardial infarction), but are not necessarily reflective of endothelial health and function. Plasma estradiol may serve as a valuable surrogate measure. Animal studies indicate that a plasma estradiol level of 60–100 pg/dL is consistent with vascular endothelial health and appropriate coronary artery vasodilatory activity *(25)*.

Osteoporosis. Postmenopausal osteoporosis is clearly linked to estrogen deprivation. Estrogen has a direct effect on bone cells inhibiting osteoclast activity and stimulating osteoblasts, and so indirectly modulating osteoclast recruitment. Estrogens also stimulate osteoblasts to synthesize progesterone receptors, and to secrete bone matrix collagen. Estrogen also has an indirect influence on calcium homeostasis and regulation by actions affecting calcium absorption from the intestine, renal excretion, and the control of certain hormones, such as parathyroid hormone, calcitonin, and activated vitamin D. This subject has been extensively reviewed *(7)*. Estrogen therapy is associated with an increase in bone density, and is effective in women with osteopenia and no vertebral fractures (prevention), as well as for older women with established osteoporotic-related fractures (treatment).

All estrogens effectively inhibit bone loss, as long as an adequate dose is prescribed and the estrogen is biologically active. The dose of estrogen will also be governed according to the need to maintain or increase bone mass. For example, in a recent 2-yr study, 50 µg transdermal estradiol maintained the lumbar bone density of a group of menopausal women; those treated with 100 µg estradiol had a 3.7% mean increase in their lumbar BMD *(26)*. Women in the placebo group lost 6.5% of their spinal bone density. Respective mean plasma estradiol levels were 62 pg/dL, 108 pg/dL, and 13 pg/dL *(26)*.

Not all women respond to the same dose of estrogen. Approximately 10–15% of women taking 0.625 mg of conjugated equine estrogen or 1 mg of micronized 17β- estradiol continue to lose bone mass *(27)*. This may result from individual variations in the dose needed, the absorption of estrogen, or to the enhanced metabolism and/or binding of estrogen as it traverses the enterohepatic pathway. Transdermal estradiol and equivalent doses of oral estrogen increase bone density to a similar degree *(28)*.

Estrogen therapy reduces the risk of hip fracture by 50–60% *(29)*, and vertebral deformation by as much as 90% *(30)*. Key issues are continuance with estrogen therapy, because bone density is lost once estrogen therapy is stopped, and tailoring the dose of estrogen to the individual's need. The minimal serum level of estradiol needed to prevent post-menopausal bone loss has been estimated at 60–90 pg/dL, although more recent studies have shown that much lower doses of either natural or transdermal estrogen can effectively prevent bone loss *(31)*. In one dose-ranging study, 0.3 mg/d of esterified estrogen administered for 2 yr increased the BMD of the lumbar spine by 1.9%, compared to a 2.9% loss in placebo-treated controls—a difference of 4.8% *(19)*. In addition, the unopposed, esterified, estrogen-treated patients had the same incidence of endometrial hyperplasia as the placebo group subjects (1.7%), and, as a group *(32)*, showed modest but significant lowering of cholesterol and LDL cholesterol, without a compensatory increase in plasma triglycerides *(19)*.

Given the variable response to estrogen therapy eluded to above, bone density testing with dual-energy X-ray absorptiometry technology, and the selective use of bone markers, such as urinary collagen crosslink excretion and urinary calcium/creatinine ratio, is essential, because the results allow practitioners to decide on the dose of estrogen therapy needed, and, with continued monitoring, to ensure that the patient is taking her treatment, and that the treatment prescribed is efficacious *(7)*.

The Brain, Cognition, and Alzheimer's Disease. Estrogen has a direct effect on many functions of the brain via nuclear receptors in the pituitary gland, hypothalamus, and cerebral cortex, as well as in areas affecting emotion (limbic system) and memory (hippocampus). Estrogen influences the biochemistry of cerebral neurotransmission by modulation of serotonin biochemistry, synthesis, and release. Estrogen also induces choline acetyltransferase, an enzyme needed to synthesize acetylcholine. Estrogen stimulates a number of nerve- and brain-derived growth factors, resulting in a greater number of dendrites and synapses between nerve cells. Estrogen may prevent the deposition of amyloid in the senile plaques and neurofibrillary tangles characteristic of Alzheimer's disease, by suppressing plasma levels of apolipoprotein E *(33)*. Estrogen also increases the cerebral and cerebellar blood flow, and restores the normal vasodilatory response to acetylcholine in women with cerebral arteriosclerotic disease *(34)*. Verbal memory is improved when mean plasma estradiol levels of 136 pmol/L (±45 pg/dL) are achieved *(35)*. Cerebral and cerebellar blood flow, on the other hand, is increased in women with mean plasma estradiol levels of 150 pg/dL.

Although some researchers believe that long-term estrogen therapy may decrease Alzheimer's disease by almost 50%, there is still sufficient conflicting information to preclude a general consensus. Given the increasing longevity of postmenopausal women, and the increased prevalence of Alzheimer's disease with advancing age (3% in women age 65–74 yr; 18.7% among those age 75–84 yr, and 47.2% in individuals over 85 yr of age) *(36)*, the need to clarify the role of estrogen therapy in Alzheimer disease prevention/ treatment is self-evident.

Table 1
Estimated Serum Estradiol and Estrone Levels
and Biological Potency After Oral Estrogen Therapy

	CEE	ME	EV
Dose: (mg)	0.625	1	1
Estradiol (pg/mL)	30–50	30–50	50
Estrone (pg/mL)	153	150–300	160
Potency			
FSH	1.4	1.3	
CBG	2.5	1.9	
SHBG	3.2	1.0	
A	3.5	0.7	

CEE, conjugated equine estrogen; ME, micronized estradiol; EV, estradiol valerate; CBG, cortisol binding globulin; A, serum angiotensinogen. Adapted with permission from ref. 2.

Clinical experience confirms that estrogen therapy, in estrogen-deficient women, has a profound positive influence on depression and cognition, resulting in enhanced mood and a feeling of well-being. This effect is usually dose-dependent, and, in the author's experience, more apparent in women taking nonoral estrogen.

Colon Cancer. Colon cancer is the third commonest cancer in women. It has been hypothesized that bile acids are co-carcinogenic or promotional agents in the colon (37). Steroid receptors have been found in colon tumors, and have been associated with defective ER gene function (38). Progestins and estrogen reduce the production of secondary bile acids, and their use has been found in many studies (but not all) to be associated with a reduced risk for colon cancer. In a recent study (37), postmenopausal hormone use was associated with a significant reduction in colon cancer incidence: 30% in ever-users and 46% in recent users. The protective effect was noted both in women on estrogen therapy alone and in women on combination HT. The protective effect of HT is lost 5–10 yr after cessation of treatment (39).

Prescribing Estrogen Therapy

The term "estrogen replacement therapy" is a misnomer, except when applied to the treatment of premature or surgically menopausal women, because it is normal for a naturally menopausal woman to be estrogen-deficient, and abnormal for them to be estrogen replete. However, although the use of estrogen therapy is pharmacologic (and not physiologic), the benefit of estrogen therapy usually outweighs the risk for the majority of women (40).

PHARMACOLOGY

All oral estradiol- and estrone-based estrogens result in higher estrone levels than estradiol, because estradiol is metabolized by the intestinal mucosa during the first passage, to estrone (2). Table 1 summarizes the approximate serum estradiol and estrone levels after the administration of commonly used oral estrogen preparations (2). Although the serum estrogen levels may be similar, the bioequivalence and potency is not necessarily the same. For example, conjugated equine estrogen, which is extracted from the urine of pregnant mares, contains so-called B-ring estrogens that are not native to humans (equilin sulfate [25%]; 17α-dihydroequilin sulfate [15%], and traces of many other equilin derivatives and metabolites), with a resultant greater potency in stimulating binding proteins, such as cortisol-binding globulin and thyroid-binding globulin (2). Estradiol binds to a variable degree to both albumin and SHBG (30–40%), leaving only 1–1.5% estradiol unbound, and therefore physiologically active (2). For some women (fortunately a minority), the daily bolus of oral estradiol results in peaks and valleys of estrogen. This results in those women who are sensitive to fluctuations in estradiol levels becoming symptomatic. Also, some women appear to bind estradiol excessively, rendering the therapy biologically ineffective or inadequate. This situation is readily diagnosed by assaying plasma estradiol and FSH levels 12 h after oral dosing. Women with estradiol binding have adequate estradiol values (consistent with the dose of estrogen prescribed), but, in addition, have elevated FSH levels (above 40–50 mIU/mL).

Maximum absorption and, therefore, blood levels are achieved 4–6 h after oral ingestion of estrogen. Vasomotor symptoms and sleep disturbances are maximal in the early hours of the morning (4 AM); consequently, optimal symptomatic control is achieved by patients taking their estrogens before going to sleep.

Estradiol is the predominant estrogen when administered transdermally. For example, utilizing a 7-d patch, average levels of estradiol peak at around 100–50 pg/dL, 12–48 h after the application of a 100- and 50-μg patch, respectively (41). The 7-d patch results in fewer fluctuations in serum estradiol levels, compared with a twice-weekly applied patch. However, some patients become symptomatic on d 5–7 of the 7-d patch, and respond better to twice-weekly dosing estrogen patches.

CLINICAL APPLICATION

Given the above, it is possible to replicate the premenopausal milieu using the transdermal approach (estrogen replacement therapy) or elect to maintain, but enhance, the natural postmenopausal milieu with oral estrogen (estrogen replenishment therapy). The decision about the route of administration and dose will depend on the patient's underlying medical condition and her preference (Fig. 1). For example, women with low HDL cholesterol levels should be treated with oral estrogen, and those with high triglycerides should be managed with transdermal or low dose natural (esterified) oral estradiol. Other relative indications for transdermal estrogen include nonresponse to oral estrogen, oral estrogen-induced hypertension, high risk for cholelithiasis, smoking, and perioperative estrogen therapy (20).

Either natural oral estrogen (for example, micronized estradiol) or transdermal estrogen is preferable for women requiring close monitoring and titration of the plasma estradiol levels. For example, maintaining a biologically active plasma estradiol level, between 40 and 80 pg/dL, may be one of the more reliable means of ensuring estrogen-induced cardiovascular protection. With the use of complex estrogens, it is not possible to measure the additional estrogen subfractions, many of which are known to be fairly potent estrogens. The various estrogen preparations available in the United States is listed in Table 2.

To improve the benefits and reduce the risk of estrogen therapy, the following prescribing practices are recommended:

1. Individualize treatment by comprehensive patient examination and selective testing.
2. Use the lowest effective dose of estrogen (hormones) to accomplish the goal of therapy. Recent research has shown that ultra-low doses of estrogen can frequently meet the patient's needs, for example, the control of vasomotor symptoms (9,19), improvement in the lipid profiles, and preventing bone loss (19).

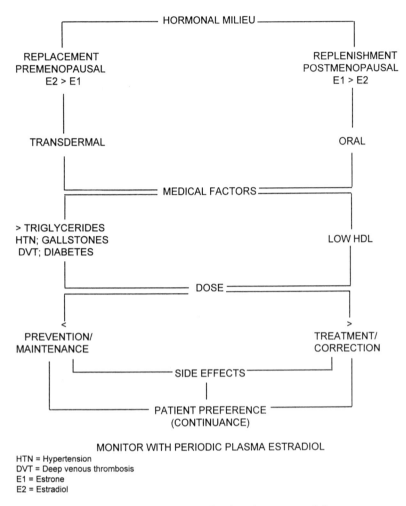

HTN = Hypertension
DVT = Deep venous thrombosis
E1 = Estrone
E2 = Estradiol

Fig. 1. Estrogen therapy selecting the route and dose.

3. Monitor the patient's response to therapy and adjust the treatment accordingly: initially, 3 mo after starting therapy, and thereafter annually.
4. Choose the route and the type of estrogen therapy that will optimize compliance. HT is only effective as long as the patient takes it.
5. Consider the use of natural estrogens to mimic the hormonal milieu of the peri- and postmenopausal woman.
6. Educate the patient. Only an educated consumer can make informed decisions. This leads to improved patient acceptance and continuance with HT *(42)*.

PRESCRIBING PROGESTINS

There is only one indication for adding progestins to estrogen therapy: the prevention of endometrial hyperplasia and endometrial cancer. Thus, with occasional exceptions, hysterectomized women should not be given progestins.

Apart from natural progesterone, there are two synthetic progestins that are commonly used in practice: drugs structurally related to progesterone (for example, medroxyprogesterone acetate [MPA]), and those that are developed from the testosterone molecule

Table 2
Postmenopausal Hormonal Preparations

Brand name	Type of hormone	Available dosages (mg)	Manufacturer
Oral estrogens			
Estrace	Micronized estradiol	0.5, 1.0, 2.0	Bristol-Myers Squibb
Estratab	Esterified estrogens	0.3, 0.625, 2.5	Solvay Pharmaceuticals
Menest	Esterified estrogens	0.3, 0.625, 1.25, 2.5	SmithKline Beecham
Ogen	Estropipate	0.625, 1.25, 2.5	Pharmacia Upjohn
Ortho-Est	Estropipate	0.625, 1.25	Ortho
Premarin	Conjugated equine estrogens	0.3, 0.625, 0.9, 1.25, 2.5	Wyeth Ayerst Labs
Parenteral estrogens (injections, pellets, patches)			
Alora	Transdermal	1.5, 2.3 and 3.0	Procter & Gamble
Climara	Transdermal estradiol	0.05, 0.1	Berlex
Estraderm	Transdermal estradiol	0.05, 0.1	CibaGeneva
FemPatch	Transdermal	10.3	Parke-Davis
Vivelle	Transdermal estradiol	0.0375, 0.05, 0.075, 0.1	CibaGeneva
Vaginal estrogen			
Estrace	Micronized estradiol	1.0	Bristol-Myers Squibb
Ogen vaginal cream	Estropipate	1.5	Pharmacia Upjohn
Ortho Dienestrol	Dienestrol	0.1%	Ortho-McNeil
Premarin vaginal cream	Conjugate equine estrogens	0.625	Wyeth-Ayerst
Estring	Estradiol	2-mg reservoir	Pharmacia Upjohn
Progestogens			
Amen	Medroxyprogesterone acetate	10	Carnrick
Aygestin	Norethindrone acetate	5	ESI-Lederle
Cycrin	Medroxyprogesterone acetate	2.5, 5, 10	ESI-Lederle
Megace	Megestrol acetate	20, 40, 160	Bristol-Myers Squibb
Micronor	Norethindrone	0.35	Ortho
Nor-QD	Norethindrone	0.35	Searle
Ovrette	Norgestrel	0.075	Wyeth-Ayerst Labs
Progesterones			
–	Micronized oral progesterone	100	Solvay
–	Progesterone vaginal suppositories	25, 50	–
Oral androgens			
Android	Methyltestosterone	10	ICN
Halotensin	Fluoxymesterone	5	Pharmacia Upjohn
Testred	Methyltestosterone	10	ICN
Injectable androgens			
Deca-Durabolin	Nandrolone decanoate	50, 100 mg/mL	Organon
Delatestryl	Testosterone enanthate	10 mg/mL	BTG Pharmaceuticals
Depo-testosterone	Testosterone cyponate	50 mg/mL	Pharmacia Upjohn
Durabolin	Nandrolone phenpropionate	25–50 mg/mL weekly	Organon
Estrogen/androgen or progestogen combinations			
Estratest tablets	Esterified estrogens	1.25	Solvay Pharmaceuticals
	Methyltestosterone	2.5	
Estratest H.S.	Esterified estrogens	0.625	Solvay Pharmaceuticals
	Methyltestosterone	2.5	
Prempro	Conjugated estrogens	0.625	Wyeth-Ayerst Labs
	Medroxyprogesterone acetate	2.5	
Premphase	Conjugated estrogens	0.625	Wyeth-Ayerst Labs
	Medroxyprogesterone acetate	2.5	

(for example, norethindrone [NE], and norethindrone acetate [NETA]). Other progestins are available, but most hormone regimens include either MPA or NE *(43)*.

NE has a slightly greater binding affinity for the endometrium and myometrium than MPA, and this may account for its better menstrual hemostatic properties *(43)*. In the author's experience, NE in doses equivalent to MPA, used in clinical practice, is less likely to result in side effects such as depression and mood dysfunction.

Relatively little is known about the pharmacokinetic properties of both MPA and NE, certainly in the doses now recommended for HT. Approximately 90% of MPA is bound to albumin; 95% of NE is bound to SHBG and albumin. There is large inter- and intra-patient variability regarding to the absorption of both of these progestins *(43)*.

Progestins may dilute the coronary artery vasodilating effect of estrogen therapy, induce an increased peripheral resistance to insulin, and reduce the lipid-lowering effect of estrogen-alone therapy *(44)*. However, the clinical impact of these side effects is minimal, and most epidemiological studies have confirmed that estrogen therapy and combination HT afford similar cardiovascular protection *(44–46)*. Two important applied clinical caveats: It is advisable to use the lowest dose of progestin, and to vary the amount prescribed, with the dose of estrogen therapy needed for a given indication and patient. Also, natural micronized progesterone is now available, and is the recommended preparation in women at risk for CVD, and in women who are intolerant of synthetic progestins. Thus, the author prefers a flexible approach to combination HT.

Three progestin regimens may be considered:

1. For patients who request/require amenorrhea, estrogen and progestins are taken daily and continuously *(47,48)*.
2. Patients with significant risk factors for CVD, or with persistent breakthrough bleeding on a continuous combined regimen, are prescribed progestins, in a slightly higher dose, for the first 10–12 d of each month. The patient will experience a withdrawal bleed in the middle of each month *(49,50)*.
3. Progestins (in a dose similar to that prescribed for monthly cycling) can be prescribed every 3 mo for 2 wk per cycle *(51)*.

Hormone-induced endometrial cancer is rare, and, in some studies, the risk of endometrial cancer in women on combination HT is less frequent than spontaneously developing endometrial cancer in untreated postmenopausal women *(52)*. Despite this reassurance, regular clinical surveillance, with selective vaginal probe ultrasound and endometrial sampling, is advocated.

PRESCRIBING ANDROGENS

It is normal for postmenopausal women to have reduced, but significant, amounts of circulating androgens. An exception to this are surgically menopausal women.

Androgens, when added to estrogen therapy, enhance the symptomatic relief of hot flashes, improve libido, and increase patients' general feeling of well-being. Androgens also selectively ameliorate certain estrogen-induced side effects, such as headaches and mastalgia *(53)*.

Combined estrogen–androgen therapy is also very effective in treating women with osteopenia/osteoporosis *(53)*. This is especially true in women with little or no improvement in BMD on adequate doses of estrogen therapy. In both pharmacokinetic and clinical studies *(53,54)*, testosterone has been shown to stimulate osteoblasts and, therefore, new bone formation. This response can be conveniently monitored by measuring plasma bone-specific alkaline phosphatase and urinary collagen crosslink excretion. Apart from its anabolic effect on muscle and bone, testosterone decreases SHBG, and may increase plasma levels of free estradiol.

Two forms of testosterone are available in clinical practice: natural testosterone; synthetic testosterone (methyltestosterone). Either form should always be used in conjunction with estrogen. Natural testosterone is poorly absorbed from the gastrointestinal tract, and is currently available by injection or pellets (as a sc implant). Testosterone patches are in development. Methyltestosterone is available as a sublingual (oral) tablet, and in conjunction with esterified estrogen.

Methyltestosterone, added to estrogen, may depress HDL cholesterol levels, and patients need to have this factor monitored at 6-mo intervals *(53)*. However, the same androgen–estrogen combination lowers triglycerides, cholesterol, and LDL cholesterol *(53)*, and does not impair estrogen-induced vasodilation of the coronary artery *(55)*. Natural testosterone does not lower HDL cholesterol. Apart from the systemic benefit of testosterone, locally applied testosterone cream is effective for treating atrophic vulvar dystropy, and for enhancing clitoral sensitivity in anorgasmic women.

In the doses recommended for clinical use, side effects are relatively uncommon, but may include oily skin, acne, hirsuties, and deepening of the voice. The latter change may become permanent *(53)*. Testosterone does not inhibit the endometrium, so additional progesterone is needed to prevent endometrial hyperplasia. To reduce the additional androgenic effect of synthetic progestins, natural progesterone is preferred when prescribing estrogen–androgen HT.

RISKS OF HORMONE THERAPY

There are two potentially significant risks associated with estrogen therapy: breast and endometrial cancer. In addition, there are some women who may respond in an idiosyncratic fashion by developing hypertension. Thrombosis and thrombophlebitis are rarely encountered, but some studies have demonstrated a modest relationship between estrogen therapy and documented thrombosis, the risk increasing from 1/10,000 in untreated to 3/10,000 events in women on various doses of estrogen therapy *(56)*. Some women are intolerant to HT, and present with problems such as mastalgia, nausea, headache, and, when taking certain progestins, depression. A more important concern in women on combination HT is breakthrough bleeding, and sometimes even scheduled withdrawal bleeding. These nuisance issues are more concerned with therapy compliance than with true risk *(42)*.

Breast Cancer

The fear of breast cancer is so strong that many patients refuse HT or take HT for a limited period. Breast cancer is a disease of aging. About one in eight American women will have a lifetime probability of developing breast cancer. The risk of developing breast cancer from birth to 39 yr is 1 in 217; at 40–50 yr, the risk is 1 in 26, increasing to 1 in 15 from 60–79 yr *(57)*. With the greater use of screening mammography, breast cancer is now diagnosed earlier, and the 5-yr survival for localized breast cancer has risen to 93% *(58)*.

Breast cancer is susceptible to hormonal manipulation, but estrogen probably serves as a promoter rather than an initiator of breast cancer. The use of progesterone (and progestins) is more controversial, because mitotic activity of breast tissue (unlike the situation in the endometrium) peaks during the progesterone-dominant luteal phase. The impact of this accepted physiologic event on the pathogenesis of breast cancer remains unclear, especially concerning the use of synthetic progestins.

There are over 40 observational studies examining the relationship between HT and breast cancer, and no consensus opinion *(58)*. This is surprising, given over 50-yr experience with estrogen therapy and its use by millions of women. An in-depth review of the subject concludes that doses of estrogen known to be effective in preventing osteoporosis and CVD (for example, conjugated equine estrogen 0.625 mg/d; estradiol 1 mg/d) are not associated with a meaningful increased risk of breast cancer *(58)*. Adding a progestin does not appear to increase the risk *(59)*, and there is some data *(59)* to suggest that the risk may even be lower, although the information in this regard is still too limited.

Patients ask for and deserve answers regarding their risk for HT-associated breast cancer. The results of five meta-analyses suggest that the duration of therapy (and the dose of estrogen therapy) may be the determining factor. Thus, after 15 yr of conjugated equine estrogen use, the risk of breast cancer may increase by 30% *(58)*. The risk is further increased in women with a family history of breast cancer. Current use of estrogen therapy may also be relevant. The increase in relative risk, however, overstates the case, compared to the absolute increase in breast cancer cases. Two studies illustrate the point: The most recent report from the Nurses Health Study *(60)* concluded that the relative risk for current use of estrogen therapy for 10 or more years was 1.46: a 46% increase. Put another way, the risk for a woman age 60 yr not on HT developing breast cancer over the next 5 yr is approx 1.8%; this will increase to 3% in women on estrogen therapy. A reanalysis of 51 published studies *(61)* concluded that, whereas 45 cases of breast cancer would occur in 1000 untreated women over a 20-yr period from 50–70 yr of age, 47/1000 would occur in women taking HT for 5 yr, and 51/ 1000 if HT was continued for 10 yr. This slight increase in risk has to be balanced with a 50% decrease in risk for CVD. A final reassuring point: Most studies evaluating the mortality rates of women taking estrogen therapy at the time of the diagnosis of their breast cancer, note an improvement in survival. This may be the result of both earlier diagnosis and better-differentiated tumors, and is consistent with a 19% reduction in death from breast cancer reported in the *Leisure World* follow-up study *(62)*.

Endometrial Cancer

The relationship between unopposed estrogen therapy and endometrial cancer is well established. Retrospective epidemiological case-control studies conclude that estrogen-alone users have a 1.7–20-fold increased relative risk for developing adenocarcinoma of the endometrium *(52)*.

The type of cancer produced is usually an early-stage tumor, and is thus readily amenable to cure. In one center, the 5-yr survival rate was 96.7% *(63)*. This is primarily the result of early detection and the presence of well-differentiated tumors. Further experience has determined that estrogen therapy-related endometrial cancer usually develops progressively from simple through complex hyperplasia, without and with cellular atypia, to adenocarcinoma. The risk of simple endometrial hyperplasia progressing to cancer is less than 5%; this increases to 25% in women diagnosed with complex hyperplasia without atypia, and to 50% in patients with atypical complex hyperplasia *(64)*. The estrogen therapy-induced cancer has to be differentiated from a more aggressive nonhormone-dependent endometrial cancer, which may occur spontaneously, or in conjunction with estrogen therapy.

The cyclic addition of progestins reverses the risk of endometrial hyperplasia. It soon became apparent that the duration of progestin use was what determined the successful reversal or prevention of endometrial hyperplasia. The type of progestin prescribed is less important than the relative potency of the progestin and its duration of use *(65)*. Thus, natural micronized progesterone, medroxyprogesterone acetate, and NE acetate have all been shown to effectively protect the endometrium, and need to be prescribed as noted previously. The dose of progestin originally advocated was intended to induce a secretory endometrium. It was subsequently shown that doses of progestin (sufficient to result in a proliferative endometrium) was equally effective in preventing endometrial hyperplasia and progression to cancer.

The type and dose of estrogen may also be important. Patients taking unopposed 0.3 mg of esterified estrogen for 2 yr showed no increase in hyperplasia, compared to placebo-treated controls *(32)*. Longer exposure (8 yr) to unopposed 0.3 mg of conjugated estrogen was linked to an increased risk of endometrial cancer *(66)*. Although the studies were of different lengths, it is possible that the pharmacologic composition of estrogen may affect clinical outcomes. The clinical message: Equal-dose estrogens do not necessarily have the same target-tissue biological effect, thus necessitating adjustment of progestin dosing.

SELECTIVE ESTROGEN RECEPTOR MODULATORS

SERMs are a series of compounds that have estrogen agonist and antagonist activity. Raloxifene is the first of this class of drug that has been FDA-approved for the prevention of bone loss. Other compounds still in clinical trials include droloxifene, levomeloxifene, and idoxifene.

Recent research *(68)* has demonstrated that raloxifene fits into the ER domain cavity, but has a side chain that projects outside the cavity, thus disabling the activation factor (AF-2) domain of the receptor needed to initiate gene transcription in tissues, such as the breast and endometrium (rich in ERα). In these tissues, raloxifene acts as an estrogen antagonist. Raloxifene does not disable the activation function (AF-1) domain, with consequent estrogen-like activity in tissues such as bone, and possibly the cardiovascular system and brain *(68)*.

In a recent phase III clinical trial *(69)*, 60 mg raloxifene given daily was found to have no stimulating effect on the endometrium, and reduced the risk of breast cancer by 75%. Like estrogen, raloxifene increased the BMD of the lumbar spine and hip, but to a modest degree, equivalent to about 50% of that achieved with 0.625 mg conjugated equine estrogen. Unlike estrogen, HDL cholesterol was not increased in the raloxifene-treated subjects, but there was a decrease in total and LDL cholesterol, and triglycerides remained unaffected.

Although raloxifene has impressive inhibitory effects on the breast and endometrium, and maintains BMD, it is still not clear whether raloxifene protects the vessel wall. Also, a significant number of patients in the trial referred to previously *(6)*, experienced hot flashes, indicating the potential for CNS estrogen-antagonist-like activity *(70)*. Future clinical trials and experience will resolve these issues. Raloxifene is the forerunner of an emerging class of drugs, which, in the future, will permit specific target-tissue treatment with minimal, if any, adverse side effects.

Tibolone is a synthetic compound with estrogenic, progestogenic, and androgenic effects. This drug has been classified as a tissue-specific hormone, and has many of the attributes of raloxifene. Tibolone, however, effectively controls menopausal symptoms, but lowers HDL cholesterol *(70)*. The latter is not associated with damage to the vascular endothelium. Tibolone is still in clinical trials in the United States, but is available for clinical use in Europe and elsewhere.

CONCLUSION

It is self-evident that management of the menopause extends well beyond the treatment of hot flashes with a standard dose of estrogen. The climacteric transition influences the health and well-being of every woman in a manner unique to that individual.

Although the majority of menopausal women should be offered HT, the decision should be based on objective indications, and reassessed on an annual basis. Thus, one of two questions should be asked of the patient annually: If you are taking hormonal therapy, why? If you are not taking hormonal therapy, why not? *(40)*. Recent research has illustrated the value, and potentially increased safety, of low-dose estrogen usage, adjusted over time to the needs of the individual. For most patients, the benefits of HT outweigh the risks.

REFERENCES

1. Hammond C. Menopause and hormone replacement therapy: an overview. Obstet Gynecol 1996;87: 2S–15S.
2. Levrant SG, Barnes RB. Pharmacology of estrogens. In: Lobo RA, ed. Treatment of the Postmenopausal Woman: Basic and Clinical Aspects. Raven, New York, 1994, pp. 57–68.
3. Vermeulen A. Sex hormone status of the postmenopausal women. Maturitas 1980;2:81–89.
4. George G., Kuiper JM, Carlsson B, et al. Comparison of the ligand binding specificity and transcript tissue distribution of estrogen receptors α and β. Endocrinology 1997;138:863–870.
5. Burger HG. The endocrinology of the menopause. Maturitas 1996;23:129–136.
6. Kaunitz AM, Benrubi GI. The good news about hormonal contraception and gynecological cancer. Female Patient 1998;23:43–51.
7. Notelovitz M. Estrogen therapy and osteoporosis: principles and practice. Am J Med Sci 1997;313:2–12.
8. Arpels JC. The female brain hypoestrogenic continuum from the premenstrual syndrome to menopause. A hypothesis and review of supporting data. J Reprod Med 1996;41:633–639.
9. Speroff L, Whitcomb RW, Kempfert NJ, et al. Efficacy and local tolerance of a low-dose 7-day matrix estradiol transdermal system in the treatment of menopausal vasomotor symptoms. Obstet Gynecol 1996;88:587–592.
10. Bachman GA. A new option for managing urogenital atrophy in post-menopausal women. Cont Obstet Gynecol 1997;42:13–28.
11. Notelovitz M. Estrogen therapy in the management of problems associated with urogenital aging: a simple diagnostic test and the effect of the route of hormone administration. Maturitas 1995;22(Suppl): 31–33.
12. Bachmann, GA, Notelovitz M, Kelly SJ, et al. Long-term nonhormonal treatment of vaginal dryness. J Clin Pract Sex 1992;8:12–17.
13. Raz R, Stamm WE. A controlled trial of intravaginal estriol in postmenopausal women with recurrent urinary tract infections. N Engl J Med 1993;329:753–756.
14. Fantl JA, Cardozo L, McClish DK, et al. Estrogen therapy in the management of urinary incontinence in postmenopausal women: a meta-analysis. First Report of the Hormones and Urogenital Therapy Committee. Obstet Gynecol 1994;83:12–18.
15. Rao W, Srinvasan SR, Valdez R, et al. Longitudinal changes in cardiovascular risk from childhood to young adulthood in offspring of parents with cardiovascular disease. The Bogalusa Heart Study. JAMA 1997;278:1749–1754.
16. Wild RA. Estrogen: effects on the cardiovascular tree. Obstet Gynecol 1996;87:27S–35S.
17. Sullivan JM, Fowlkes LP. The clinical aspects of estrogen and the cardiovascular system. Obstet Gynecol 1996;87:36S–43S.

18. Campus H, Sacks FM, Walsh BW, et al. Differential effects of estrogen on low-density lipoprotein subclasses in healthy post-menopausal women. Metabolism 1993;42:1153–1156.
19. Genant HK, Lucas J, Weiss S, et al. Low-dose esterified estrogen therapy. Effects on bone, plasma estradiol concentrations, endometrium and lipid levels. Arch Int Med 1997;157:2609–2615.
20. Jewelewicz R. New developments in topical estrogen therapy. Fertil Steril 1997;67:1–12.
21. Lindoff C, Peterson F, Lecander I, Martinsson G, Åstedt B. Transdermal estrogen replacement therapy: beneficial effects on hemostatic risk factors for cardiovascular disease. Maturitas 1996;24:43–50.
22. Collins P, Shay J, Jiang C, et al. Nitric oxide accounts for dose-dependent estrogen-mediated coronary relaxation after acute estrogen withdrawal. Circulation 1994;90:1964–1968.
23. Mikkula T, Ranta V, Orpana A, et al. Hormone replacement therapy modifies the capacity of plasma and serum to regulate prostacyclin and endothelin-I production in human vascular endothelial cells. Fertil Steril 1996;66:389–393.
24. Prouder AJ, Ahmed AI, Crook D, et al. Hormone replacement therapy and serum angiotensin-converting enzyme activity in postmenopausal women. Lancet 1995;346:89–90.
25. Williams JK, Adams MR, Kloppenstein HS. Estrogen modulates responses of atherosclerotic coronary artery. Circulation 1990;81:1680–1687.
26. Field CS, Ory SJ, Wahner HW, et al. Preventive effects of transdermal 17β-estradiol on osteoporotic changes after surgical menopause: a two year placebo-controlled study. Am J Obstet Gynecol 1993;168:114–121.
27. Ettinger B, Genant HK, Steiger P, Madvig P. Low-dosage micronized 17β-estradiol prevents bone loss in post-menopausal women. Am J Obstet Gynecol 1992;166:479–488.
28. Hillard TC, Whitcroft SJ, Marsh MS, et al. Long-term effects of transdermal and oral hormone replacement on postmenopausal bone loss. Osteoporosis Int 1994;4:341–348.
29. Weiss NS, Ure CL, Ballard JH, et al. Decreased risk of fractures of the hip and lower forearm with postmenopausal use of estrogen. N Engl J Med 1980;303:1195–1198.
30. Lindsay R, Hart DM, Forrest C, Baird C. Prevention of spinal osteoporosis in oophorectomised women. Lancet 1980;2:1151–1154.
31. Bauer DC, Nevitt MC, Ettinger B, et al. Women with low serum estradiol have an increased risk of hip and vertebral fractures: a prospective study. In: Parapoulos SE, et al., eds. Osteoporosis 1996. Proceedings of the 1996 World Congress on Osteoporosis. Elsevier, Amsterdam, 1996, pp. 271–275.
32. Notelovitz M., Varner RE, Rebar RW, et al. Minimal endometrial proliferation over a two-year period in postmenopausal women taking 0.3 mg of unopposed esterified estrogens. Menopause 1997;4:80–88.
33. Birge SJ. Maintaining mental health with hormone replacement therapy. Eur Menopause J 1996;3:164–169.
34. Okhura T, Teshima Y, Isse K, et al. Estrogen increases cerebral and cerebellar blood flows in postmenopausal women. Menopause 1995;2:13–18.
35. Kampen DL, Sherwin BB. Estrogen use and verbal memory in healthy postmenopausal women. Obstet Gynecol 1994;83:979–983.
36. Ikehara R. Estrogen and Alzheimer's disease: a review and update. Prim Care Update Ob/Gyn 1997;4:228–233.
37. Potter JD. Hormones and colon cancer. J Natl Cancer Inst 1995;87:1067–1071.
38. Issa JP, Ottaviano YL, Celano P, et al. Methylation of the estrogen receptor CpG island links aging and neoplasia in human colon. Nat Genet 1994;7:536–540.
39. Newcomb PA, Storer BE. Postmenopausal hormone use and risk of large-bowel cancer. J Natl Cancer Inst 1995;87:1067–1071.
40. Notelovitz M. Hormone replacement therapy–benefits versus risks. Eur Menopause J 1996;3:186–196.
41. Gordon SF. Clinical experience with a seven-day estradiol transdermal system for estrogen replacement therapy. Am J Obstet Gynecol 1995;173:998–1104.
42. Ravnikar VA. Barriers for taking long-term hormone replacement therapy: why do women not adhere to therapy? Eur Menopause J 1996;3:90–93.
43. Stanczyk F. Structure-function relationships, potency and pharmacokinetics of progestogens. In: Lobo R, ed. Treatment of the Postmenopausal Woman: Basic and Clinical Aspects. Raven, New York, 1994, pp. 69–89.
44. Speroff L. The effect of estrogen-progestogen postmenopausal hormone replacement therapy on the cardiovascular system. Eur Menopause J 1996;3:151–163.
45. Nabulsi AA, Folsom AR, White A, et al. Association of hormone replacement therapy with various cardiovascular risk factors in post-menopausal women. N Engl J Med 1993;328:1069–1075.

46. Grodstein F. Stampfer M, Manoun J, et al. Postmenopausal estrogen and progestin use and risk of cardiovascular disease. N Engl J Med.1996;335:453–461.
47. Udoff L, Langenberg P, Adashi EY. Combined continuous hormone replacement therapy: a critical review. Obstet Gynecol 1995;86:306–316.
48. Stadberg E, Mattsson LA, Uvebrandt M. 17β-estradiol and norethisterone acetate in low doses as continuous combined hormone replacement therapy. Maturitas 1996;23:31–39.
49. Pickar JH, Thorneycroft I, Whitehead M. Effects of hormone replacement therapy on the endometrium and lipid parameters: a review of clinical trials, 1985 to 1995. Am J Obstet Gynecol 1998;178:1087–1099.
50. Archer DF, Pickar JH, Bottinglioni F. Bleeding patterns in post-menopausal women taking continuous combined or sequential regimens of conjugated estrogens with medroxyprogesterone acetate. Obstet Gynecol 1994;83:686–692.
51. Ettinger B, Selby J, Citron JT, et al. Cyclic hormone replacement therapy using quarterly progestin. Obstet Gynecol 1994;83:693–700.
52. Gambrell RD. Pathophysiology and epidemiology of endometrial cancer. In: Lobo RA, ed. Treatment of the Postmenopausal Woman. Basic and Clinical Aspects. Raven, New York, 1994, pp. 355–362.
53. Watts NB, Notelovitz M, Timmons MC, et al. Comparison of oral estrogens and estrogens plus androgens on bone mineral density, menopausal symptoms, and lipid-lipoprotein profiles in surgical menopause. Obstet Gynecol 1995;85:529–537.
54. Raisz LG, Wiita B, Artis A, et al. Comparison of the effects of estrogen alone and estrogen plus androgen on biochemical markers of bone formation and resorption in postmenopausal women. J Clin Endocrinol Metab 1996;81:37–43.
55. Honoré EK, Williams JK, Adams MR, et al. Methyltestosterone does not diminish the beneficial effects of estrogen replacement therapy on coronary artery reactivity in monkeys. Menopause 1996;3:20–26.
56. Grodstein F, Stampfer M, Goldhaber S, et al. Prospective study of exogenous hormones and risk of pulmonary embolism in women. Lancet 1996;348:983–987.
57. Wingo PA, Tong T, Bolden RA. Cancer statistics, 1995. Ca: Cancer J Clin 1995;45:16.
58. Speroff L. Postmenopausal hormone therapy and breast cancer. Obstet Gynecol 1996;87:44S–54S.
59. Stanford JL, Weiss NS, Voigt LF, et al. Combined estrogen and progestin hormone replacement therapy in relation to risk of breast cancer in middle-aged women. JAMA 1995;274:137–142.
60. Colditz GA, Hankinson SE, Hunter DJ, et al. Use of estrogens and progestins and the risk of breast cancer in postmenopausal women. N Engl J Med 1995;332:1589–1593.
61. Collaborative Group on Hormonal Factors in Breast Cancer. Breast cancer and hormone replacement therapy: collaborative reanalysis of 52,705 women with breast cancer and 101,811 women without breast cancer. Lancet 1997;350:1047–1059.
62. Henderson BE, Paganini-Hill A, Ross RK. Decreased mortality in users of estrogen replacement therapy. Arch Intern Med 1991;151:75–78.
63. Gambrell RD, Massey FM, Castaneda TA, et al. Use of the progestagen challenge test to reduce the risk of endometrial cancer. Obstet Gynecol 1980;55:732–738.
64. Morrow CP, Townsend DE eds. Synopsis of Gynecologic Oncology, 2nd ed. John Wiley, New York, 1981, pp. 133–144.
65. Paterson MEL, Wade-Evans T, Sturdee DW, et al. Endometrial disease after treatment with oestrogens and progestins in the climacteric. Br Med J 1980;1:822–824.
66. Cushing KL, Weiss NS, Voigt LF, et al. Risk of endometrial cancer in relation to use of low-bone, unopposed estrogens. Obstet Gynecol 1998;91:35–39.
67. Kearney CE, Purdie DW. Selective estrogen receptor modulators. Climacteric 1998;1:143–147.
68. Brzozowski AM, Pike AC, Dauter Z, et al. Molecular basis of agonism and antagonism in the estrogen receptor. Nature (London) 1997;389;753–758.
69. Delmas PD, Bjarnason NH, Mitlak BH, et al. Effects of raloxifene on bone mineral density, serum cholesterol concentrations and uterine endometrium in postmenopausal women. N Engl J Med 1997;337: 1641–1647.
70. Milner MH, Sinnott MM, Cooke TM, et al. A 2-year study of lipid and lipoprotein changes in postmenopausal women with tibolone and estrogen-progestin. Obstet Gynecol 1996;87:593–599.

12 Diabetes in the Elderly

Graydon S. Meneilly, MD, FRCPC,
and Daniel Tessier, MD, FRCPC

CONTENTS

EPIDEMIOLOGY

In the past few years, a number of epidemiologic studies have evaluated the incidence and prevalence of type 2 diabetes in the aged. Although these studies have used differing diagnostic criteria, they have consistently found an increased prevalence of diabetes in the elderly. The most recent data comes from the Health and Nutrition Examination Survey (HANES) III (*1*; Fig. 1). The prevalence of diabetes in patients over the age of 75 yr in the United States is approx 20%, and at least half of older people are unaware they have the disease (*2*). Although the prevalence is approx 20% in older Caucasians, it is much higher in Blacks, Hispanics, Native Indians, Micronesians, Scandinavians, Japanese, and other ethnic groups. Clearly, we are facing an epidemic of type 2 diabetes in the elderly in the next century.

From: *Contemporary Endocrinology: Endocrinology of Aging*
Edited by: J. E. Morley and L. van den Berg © Humana Press Inc., Totowa, NJ

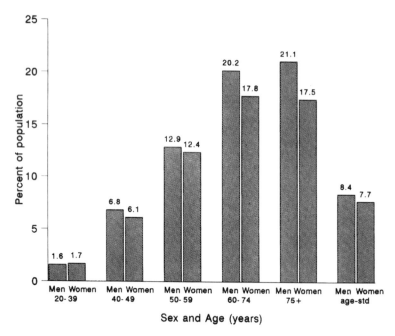

Fig. 1. Prevalence of diabetes in men and women in the U.S. population age ≥20 yr, based on HANES III (reproduced with permission from ref. *1*).

PATHOGENESIS OF DIABETES IN THE ELDERLY

It is clear that there is a strong genetic predisposition to type 2 diabetes in middle-aged patients, although the specific genes responsible have not been discovered *(3)*. This genetic predisposition appears to be equally strong in the elderly. Patients with a family history of diabetes are more likely to develop the illness as they age *(4)*. As noted above, the prevalence is high in certain ethnic groups. Elderly patients with peripheral insulin resistance and reduced glucose-induced insulin release are more likely to develop type 2 diabetes than those who have neither of these metabolic defects *(5)*. In elderly identical twins discordant for type 2 diabetes, subjects without diabetes have evidence of impaired glucose metabolism *(6)*. The data above indicate that there is a clear genetic predisposition to type 2 diabetes in the elderly.

What other factors contribute to the high prevalence of diabetes in the elderly? Normal aging is characterized by progressive alterations in glucose metabolism, including resistance to insulin-mediated glucose disposal, impaired glucose-induced insulin release, and altered regulation of hepatic glucose output *(7)*. These age-related changes interact with genetic background to explain the increasing prevalence of diabetes with aging. Lower testosterone levels in men *(8)* and higher testosterone levels in women *(9)* are risk factors for the development of diabetes. Elderly individuals who have a high intake of fat and sugar and a low intake of complex carbohydrates are more likely to develop diabetes *(10–13)*. Diabetes is more likely to develop in older people who are physically inactive, are obese, and have a central fat distribution *(6,10,14–24)*. Older people take multiple drugs, many of which may alter glucose metabolism *(25)*. Thus, genetic, physiologic, and environmental factors, working in concert, result in a high prevalence of diabetes in the elderly.

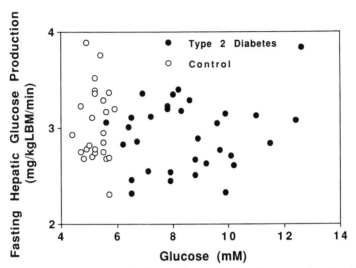

Fig. 2. Fasting hepatic glucose production in relation to fasting glucose values in elderly controls and patients with diabetes.

In middle-aged patients with type 2 diabetes, fasting hepatic glucose production is increased, glucose-induced insulin is impaired, and there is marked resistance to insulin-mediated glucose disposal *(26)*. In contrast to younger patients, fasting hepatic glucose production is normal in elderly patients with type 2 diabetes (27; Fig. 2). Glucose-induced insulin secretion is profoundly impaired in lean older people with diabetes, but is relatively preserved in obese older subjects *(27,28;* Fig. 3). Obese subjects have marked resistance to insulin-mediated glucose disposal; lean older subjects have minimal peripheral insulin resistance *(27,28;* Fig. 4). Thus, although middle-aged patients have a constellation of metabolic defects, elderly subjects with type 2 diabetes have more specific alterations in carbohydrate metabolism. The primary metabolic defect in lean elderly subjects is an impairment in glucose-induced insulin release; primary abnormality in obese elderly subjects is resistance to insulin-mediated glucose disposal. These data suggest an alteration in the therapeutic approach to older people with diabetes, with differing body composition.

Autoimmunity has an important pathogenic role in the islet-cell failure that occurs in patients with type 1 diabetes. Autoimmune phenomena may also be an important contributing factor to the marked impairment in insulin release, which occurs in lean elderly patients with type 2 diabetes, because a substantial minority of these patients have type-1-diabetes-associated human lymphocyte antigen (HLA) haplotypes and an increased frequency of islet cell and glutamic acid decarboxidase (GAD) antibodies *(29–36).* In the future, measurement of autoimmune parameters may help clinicians predict which elderly patients are likely to require insulin. In addition, if specific therapies directed against beta cell destruction may become available, measures of autoimmunity may also be useful in determining elderly subjects appropriate for such treatment.

Glucose uptake occurs by insulin-mediated and noninsulin-mediated mechanisms (glucose effectiveness). However, studies that have directly assessed glucose effectiveness in middle-aged subjects with diabetes have found conflicting results *(37).* Recently, the authors *(38)* demonstrated that glucose effectiveness is markedly impaired in elderly patients with type 2 diabetes (Fig. 5). The mechanism for this defect is unclear, but

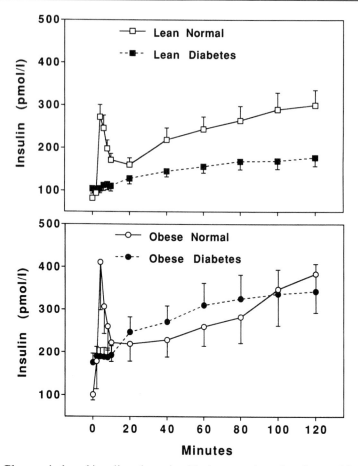

Fig. 3. Glucose-induced insulin release in elderly controls and patients with diabetes.

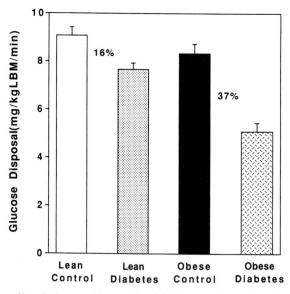

Fig. 4. Insulin-mediated glucose disposal in elderly controls and patients with diabetes.

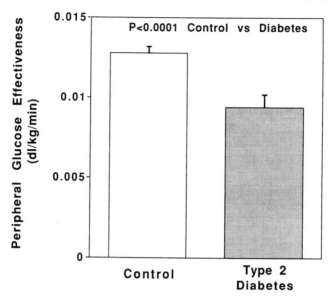

Fig. 5. Peripheral glucose effectiveness in elderly controls and patients with diabetes.

impaired glucose effectiveness clearly is a major contributing factor to elevated glucose levels in elderly patients with diabetes. Given that several interventions, including gluca-gon-like peptide-1 (GLP-1), have been shown to enhance glucose effectiveness in younger patients, these findings may have important therapeutic relevance for elderly patients with diabetes *(37)*.

Few studies have evaluated molecular biologic abnormalities in elderly patients with diabetes. The glucokinase gene is the glucose sensor for the β-cell. Defects in this gene could help to explain the impairment in glucose-induced insulin secretion that occurs in lean elderly patients with diabetes. Some studies have found that this gene acts as a marker for abnormal glucose tolerance in the elderly, but others have not *(39,40)*. Thus, it is uncertain whether defects in the glucokinase gene contribute to impaired insulin release. Insulin receptor number and affinity are normal in elderly patients, but insulin receptor tyrosine kinase activity in skeletal muscle is reduced *(41)*. However, it is unclear whether this is the result or the cause of insulin resistance and hyperglycemia in these patients. Clearly, further molecular biologic studies need to be conducted in the elderly.

PRESENTATION AND CLINICAL FEATURES

Diabetes is frequently undiagnosed in the elderly, suggesting that this illness is often asymptomatic in elderly patients. The diagnosis is usually made based on routine blood tests, or when the patient is admitted to hospital for another illness. Classic symptoms of hyperglycemia are rarely present. Glucose is not spilled into the urine until the plasma glucose is markedly elevated, because the renal threshold for glucose increases with age. Polydipsia is also less common, because thirst is impaired. When symptoms are present, they are generally atypical (failure to thrive, urinary incontinence, or delirium) *(42)*. Diabetes may present for the first time in older persons with a complication of illness, such as a myocardial infarction or stroke. Finally, nonketotic hyperosmolar coma may be the first sign of diabetes in older individuals, particularly in older nursing home patients. This probably occurs because of decreased access to water associated with osmotic diuresis, impaired thirst, and impaired cognitive function.

There are several unique syndromes that appear to occur more commonly in older patients with diabetes (43,44). Intradermal bullae of the feet that resolve spontaneously have been described (45). Painful limitation of the shoulder joints occurs frequently, and may be related to nonenzymatic glycation of proteins (46). Diabetes appears to be a risk factor for accidental hypothermia in older individuals (47). Several unusual infectious complications appear in older people with diabetes. Malignant otitis externa is a necrotizing infection caused by *Pseudomonas*, occurring almost exclusively in the elderly patient with diabetes (44). Papillary necrosis can occur in association with urinary tract infections (44). These patients may not have fever or flank pain.

Diabetic amyotrophy occurs exclusively in older men with diabetes (44). This syndrome causes asymmetric and painful weakness of the muscles of the pelvic girdle and thigh, and usually resolves spontaneously in a few months. Diabetic neuropathic cachexia is a syndrome of weight loss, depression, and painful peripheral neuropathy (48). It occurs in older patients with diabetes, and generally resolves without specific treatment in 1–2 yr.

Relatively few studies have described clinical features in elderly patients with diabetes. When compared to younger patients, elderly community-dwelling patients with diabetes are less obese, less likely to have a family history of diabetes, and more likely to be hypertensive (49). Compared to community-dwelling elderly people with diabetes, elderly nursing home patients with diabetes are less obese, more likely to be treated with diet, less likely to be treated with insulin, and have a higher incidence of renal disease, macrovascular complications, and skin infections (50). They also tend to have better glycemic control and a lower frequency of hypoglycemia, although the latter may be caused by reduced awareness of hypoglycemic warning symptoms, rather than by a truly lower number of events. Compared to nursing home residents without diabetes, elderly patients with diabetes have a higher incidence of nephropathy, retinopathy, neuropathy, macrovascular events, and urinary and soft tissue infections. These data emphasize the important effect of diabetes on morbidity in institutionalized populations.

COMPLICATIONS

Diabetes is the sixth leading cause of death among older people. This figure grossly underestimates the role of diabetes as a cause of death in elderly individuals, because, when patients die of other causes, such as cardiovascular disease (CVD), diabetes is generally not included on the death certificate. The mortality rate of older people with diabetes is 2× higher than age-matched controls without diabetes, and CVD is the principal cause of death (51). The mortality rate is related to (Hgb A_{1C}) and the long-term variability of plasma glucose (52). Diabetes also has a significant effect on function and quality of life. In longitudinal studies, diabetes is one of the strongest predictors of functional decline (53–55). Elderly patients with diabetes have a higher frequency of chronic disease, and poorer self-rated health and quality of life than age-matched controls without diabetes (56). Elderly women with diabetes, or patients on insulin, have a poorer quality of life than men or patients on oral agents (57). In addition, elderly patients with diabetes use more than twice as many hospital days and outpatient services as age-matched controls without diabetes (58–67).

Macrovascular Complications

The incidence of CVD, cerebrovascular, and peripheral vascular disease is approximately twice as high in older people with diabetes, compared to age-matched controls without diabetes *(66,68–81)*. Among patients with diabetes, the risk of these complications increases with both the age of the patient and the duration of the diabetes *(68,71, 82–86)*. The risk of macrovascular complications appears to be almost as high in patients with undiagnosed diabetes as it is in those who have known diabetes, suggesting a potential role for screening *(2)*. Among elderly patients with diabetes, the risk for CVD is increased even further by the presence of other risk factors, including hypercholesterolemia, smoking, and hypertension, suggesting that risk factor modification may be of value *(73,86–88)*.

There is a strong correlation between Hgb A_{1C} and the risk of macrovascular events in elderly patients with diabetes *(70,79,86,88-90)*. The Digami study was a randomized controlled trial that found intensive insulin therapy after myocardial infarction reduced mortality in older patients with diabetes *(91)*. These data suggest that improved glycemic control and risk factor modification may reduce the risk of macrovascular complications in the elderly, although further randomized controlled trials are required to definitively settle this issue.

Microvascular Complications

The risk of microvascular complications and peripheral and autonomic neuropathy is about twice as high in older patients with diabetes, compared to age-matched controls, and the risk of these complications increases with the age of the patient and the duration of the diabetes *(66,69–71,75,78,79,92–110)*. There are no randomized controlled trials that determine the effect of improved glycemic control on microvascular complications in the elderly. However, epidemiologic studies have found a strong association between Hgb A_{1C} and the incidence of retinopathy, neuropathy, and nephropathy *(70,79,93,108, 110,111)*, suggesting that improved glycemic control may reduce the risk of microvascular complications in older people. The incidence of retinopathy is increased in elderly patients with diabetes who have increased levels of lipoprotein(a) *(112)*. It is not known if interventions other than improved control (such as lipid-lowering agents or angiotensin-converting enzyme (ACE) inhibitors in patients with microalbuminuria) will reduce the risk of complications in this patient population.

Hypoglycemia

Hypoglycemia is the most serious complication associated with the treatment of diabetes in aged patients. The risk of severe or fatal hypoglycemia, associated with the use of oral agents or insulin, increases substantially with age *(113–121)*. In normal subjects, glucagon is the most important counterregulatory hormone. Elderly patients have a marked impairment in the glucagon response to hypoglycemia *(122*; Fig. 6). These patients lack knowledge of the warning symptoms of hypoglycemia, and have reduced awareness of autonomic warning symptoms, even when they are educated regarding these symptoms *(122,123)*. Finally, elderly patients with diabetes have impairment on tests of psychomotor performance during hypoglycemia *(122)*. Data suggest that older people with diabetes are more susceptible to hypoglycemia because of reduced secretion of counterregulatory hormones; lack of knowledge of the symptoms of hypoglycemia; impaired awareness of autonomic symptoms, even when they are educated about the

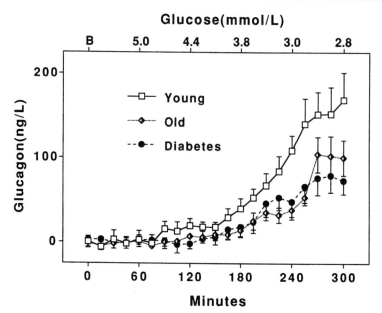

Fig. 6. Glucagon responses to hypoglycemia in healthy young, healthy old, and elderly patients with diabetes.

symptoms; and impaired psychomotor performance during hypoglycemia, which reduces the patient's ability to take appropriate steps to return blood sugar to normal.

Some younger patients with diabetes, switched from animal to human insulin, have a reduced awareness of hypoglycemic warning symptoms, and an increased frequency of hypoglycemic events. There is little data regarding animal and human insulin in the elderly. Burden *(124)* reported an elderly woman who had frequent hypoglycemic episodes when she was switched from an animal to human insulin. Berger et al. *(125)* studied 75 elderly patients who had been treated with human or animal insulin for several months, and found no difference in the frequency of hypoglycemic events between the two insulin preparations. In elderly patients with diabetes rendered hypoglycemic with animal or human insulin, the authors *(126)* found no difference in the counterregulatory hormone responses to the two insulin preparations, but awareness of autonomic and neuroglycopenic warning symptoms of hypoglycemia was greater with animal insulin.

In the future, efforts should be enhanced to reduce the frequency of severe or fatal hypoglycemia in the elderly. Potential interventions include better education about the warning symptoms of hypoglycemia, the use of alternative insulin preparations, or the use of oral agents that may be associated with a lower frequency of hypoglycemic events (*see* below under Treatment)

Cognitive Function

Compared to age-matched nondiabetic controls, elderly patients with type 2 diabetes have poorer performance on a variety of cognitive tasks, and a higher incidence of depression *(56,127,128)*. There appears to be a close correlation between levels of Hgb A_{1C}, lipid values, and blood pressure *(128,129)* and the degree of impairment in cognitive and affective function in these patients. Recent studies have found that improved glycemic control *(130,131)* results in an improvement in cognitive and affective function. The

Table 1
Diagnosis of Diabetes Mellitus

Symptoms of diabetes plus a casual[a] plasma glucose value ≥11.1 mmol/L. The classic
symptoms of diabetes include fatigue, polyuria, polydipsia, and unexplained weight loss.
OR
A fasting plasma glucose ≥7.0 mmol/L. Fasting is defined as no caloric intake for at least 8 h.
OR
The plasma glucose value in the 2-h sample of the oral glucose tolerance test is ≥11.1 mmol/L.
The test should be performed as described (National Diabetes Data Group), using a load
of 75 g anhydrous glucose.

[a]Any time of day without regard to time since last meal.

incidence of vascular dementia is increased in elderly patients with diabetes. There is an
increased risk of Alzheimer's disease (132,133), but it is not known if this increased risk
of dementia is related to glycemic control, lipid values, or blood pressure. It is possible
that improved glycemic control and risk factor modification will not only improve cognitive and affective function in the short term, but may also reduce the cumulative
incidence of vascular dementia and Alzheimer's disease in the long term.

DIAGNOSIS

Until recently, the most widely applied criteria for the diagnosis of diabetes in patients
of any age came from the National Diabetes Data Group criteria (134). These criteria
were not age-adjusted, but they were sufficiently relaxed that overdiagnosis of diabetes
in older individuals was avoided. However, the criteria lacked sufficient sensitivity, with
the consequence that a significant number of people with diabetes remained undiagnosed. The 2-h oral glucose tolerance test value above 11.1 mmol/L was based on the
potential for the development of macrovascular complications; a fasting plasma glucose
value of 7.8 mmol/L defined a greater degree of hyperglycemia than a 2-h value. Evaluation of a number of population-based studies suggested that a fasting plasma glucose of
7 mmol/L corresponded more closely to a 2-h plasma glucose of 11.1 mmol/L. The newly
revised diagnostic criteria are outlined in Table 1 (135). Diabetes can still be diagnosed
on the basis of fasting glucose, classic symptoms, and an elevated random glucose, or an
oral glucose tolerance test.

Elderly people with undiagnosed diabetes have an increased rate of complications
when compared to age-matched controls (2). This has led some to suggest widespread
screening for diabetes in elderly individuals, particularly if they have risk factors for the
development of diabetes (hypertension, obesity, history of gestational diabetes mellitus,
the presence of complications associated with diabetes mellitus, obesity, ethnicity, or
family history). There are several potential tests that could be used for screening, including fasting, random and postprandial glucose levels, an oral glucose tolerance test, Hgb
A_{1C}, glucosuria, and serum fructosamine (136,137). Although each test has its advantages and disadvantages in terms of convenience, cost, standardization of the assay, and
reliable identification of people at risk, the fasting plasma glucose is judged to be the best
compromise among these tests (135). The American Diabetes Association has recently
recommended that the fasting plasma glucose be performed every 3 yr in elderly patients
at low risk for diabetes, and annually in elderly individuals with the risk factors outlined

above *(135)*. These recommendations will be subject to change when further information becomes available.

TREATMENT GOALS

The majority of clinicians would agree that blood glucose should be reduced in elderly patients with symptoms of hyperglycemia. In general, this can be accomplished by keeping the fasting glucose below 12 mmol/L. Is there any rationale for more aggressive control of blood sugar in older patients with diabetes? The Diabetes Control and Complications Trial *(138)* found that tight control of diabetes reduced the risk of microvascular complications in young patients with insulin-dependent diabetes mellitus. Several randomized controlled trials have evaluated the effectiveness of improved glycemic control in middle-aged patients with type 2 diabetes. The University Group Diabetes Project assessed the effect of improved glycemic control on vascular complications in patients with type 2 diabetes *(139)*. The study was discontinued early, because there was a higher incidence of cardiovascular deaths in the group treated with tolbutamide. This study has been criticized on methodological grounds, and an increased cardiovascular risk for sulfonylureas has not been definitively substantiated elsewhere. A recent Japanese trial found that intensive insulin therapy in middle-aged patients with diabetes reduced the risk of microvascular complications *(140)*.

As yet, there is no data for randomized controlled trials in elderly patients to determine whether intensive control reduces the risk of long-term complications. The optimal level of glycemic control that maximizes benefit, but minimizes the risk of therapy, particularly hypoglycemia, has not been defined. The recently completed United Kingdom Prospective Diabetes Study found that improved glycemic control reduced the risk of microvascular and possibly macrovascular disease in middle-aged patients with diabetes *(140a,140b)*. Unfortunately, many of the patients enrolled in the mentioned above studies were younger than geriatricians generally manage, and had minimal comorbidity. As a consequence, the results of the studies may not be applicable to the majority of elderly patients, many of whom are frail.

In the interim, are there data from other studies that suggest that improved glycemic control improves outcome in older patients, and, if so, do the benefits outweigh the risk? As reviewed above, prospective epidemicologic studies have suggested that lower Hgb A_{1C} levels are associated with a reduced risk of macrovascular, microvascular, and other complications in older patients, as well as improved cognitive and affective function. Of more concern than complication rates for older subjects is the risk of functional disability and impaired quality of life associated with complications. The incidence of various diseases associated with disability, such as visual problems, peripheral vascular disease with amputation, myocardial infarction, and stroke, is increased in older patients with diabetes. The average 80-yr-old female in Western society has a life expectancy of approx 9 yr, but she can expect to spend 60% of this time with a major disability *(141)*. Longitudinal studies have demonstrated that diabetes is one of the strongest predictors of decline in physical function, even in very healthy older individuals *(53–55)*. If improved control reduces the risk of complications and associated functional disability, it could have a profound affect on the quality of life of older individuals.

If we accept the fact that improved glycemic control reduces the risk of complications and improves function and quality of life in older individuals, is it cost-effective? Two

Table 2
Goals of Therapy for the Elderly Patient with Diabetes

Fasting blood sugar (FBS) <7.0 mM
2-h postprandial PC <11.0 mM
Hgb A$_{1C}$ <20% above upper limit of normal

Table 3
Goals of Therapy for the Frail Elderly Patient with Diabetes

FBS <10 mM
2-h PC <15 mM
Hgb A$_{1C}$ <50% above upper limit of normal

recent cost-benefit analyses suggested that aggressive treatment of diabetes in elderly individuals is not warranted, because of the reduced life expectancy of these patients *(142–144)*. Both analyses were based on extrapolations from studies of younger subjects, only microvascular complications were considered, and the authors evaluated the benefits of control for older individuals who did not have complications. It is likely that the conclusions would have been different if data were derived from older subjects, if the effects of control on macrovascular complications were evaluated, or if the effects of improved control were assessed in patients with established complications. When cost-benefit analysis is applied in other diseases common to the elderly, the results are strikingly different. For example, treatment of hypertension in elderly patients may actually be more cost effective than in the young, because smaller numbers of subjects need to be treated to achieve benefit. It is also important to consider other potential benefits of improved glycemic control. Elderly patients with diabetes use more than twice as many outpatient services and hospital days as age-matched nondiabetic controls *(58–67)*, and there is a correlation between Hgb A$_{1C}$ values in elderly subjects and the frequency of physician visits and hospitalization for both diabetes and nondiabetes-related illnesses *(61,63)*. If improved control reduces inpatient or outpatient costs in the elderly, it would undoubtedly be cost-effective. Finally, it has been shown that, in traditional cost-benefit analysis, elderly patients appear to benefit less from life-extending treatment, because their life is felt to be worth less than that of younger patients *(145)*. Ultimately, the only way to determine if good glycemic control in the elderly is cost-effective and improves quality of life will be to conduct randomized controlled trials.

Based on the above evidence, what should the treatment guidelines be for elderly patients with diabetes? Recently, the authors developed two sets of guidelines for the control of diabetes in older people (Tables 2 and 3). These guidelines must be modified for each patient, based on his/her functional status and comorbidity.

THERAPEUTIC OPTIONS

Care of these patients is complicated by polypharmacy, multiple pathology, and alteration of the special senses, as well as a number of social factors, including social isolation and poverty. Because the patients are complex, and because the treatment of diabetes may require alterations of lifestyle, a team approach, consisting of nurse, dietician, physician, and other health professionals, is essential *(146)*. Older patients with diabetes know less about their disease than younger patients, and are also less likely to participate in an educational program *(147)*. Multidisciplinary programs aimed at improving diabetes management in older people have been shown to result in better compliance with therapy, and improved glycemic control *(147–150)*. Family members play an integral role in the care of older patients with diabetes, and involvement of family members has been shown to improve compliance with therapy *(150–151)*. When educational materials are developed for elderly patients, it is important to make sure that the print is large enough for them to read *(152)*. Knowledge of diabetes is relatively poor among staff of long-term care facilities *(153,154)*, and nursing homes frequently have few guidelines in place for the care of older patients with diabetes *(155)*. Educational programs for nursing staff can improve outcomes in elderly nursing home patients *(156)*.

Elderly patients with diabetes who have other risk factors for CVD clearly have a much higher risk of complications than those who do not (73,87,88). As a result, risk factor modification is an essential part of management. Calcium channel blockers are effective antihypertensive agents in older patients with diabetes, and do not worsen glycemic control *(157,158)*. In elderly hypertensive patients with type 2 diabetes, calcium channel blockers appear to be equivalent to the ACE inhibitors in reducing urinary protein excretion *(159)*. Recently, it has been found that middle-aged patients with type 2 diabetes and hypertension on calcium channel blockers have a greater risk of vascular events than those on ACE inhibitors *(160,161)*. Unfortunately, there are no data on patients over the age of 70 yr to determine whether a similar effect occurs. Until further data are available, prudence is warranted in the use of calcium channel blockers in elderly patients with diabetes. In the Systolic Hypertension in the Elderly Program study, low-dose chlorthalidone was an effective antihypertensive agent, and reduced the risk of major cardiovascular events in older people with diabetes *(162)*. ACE inhibitors have been found to reduce blood pressure and improve insulin sensitivity in elderly nondiabetic patients with hypertension and elderly patients with diabetes and congestive heart failure *(163,164)*.

Many elderly patients with diabetes have high lipid values. As yet, there are no data from randomized control trials in patients with diabetes over the age of 70 yr to determine whether pharmacologic treatment of lipid levels improves outcomes in these patients, although this data should be forthcoming in the near future.

DIET

A number of articles have provided guidelines for the dietary management of the older patient with diabetes *(165,166)*. However, there are few original studies regarding diet in older patients with diabetes. Horwath et al. *(167)* surveyed patients with type 2 diabetes, and found that most older patients limited simple sugars, but adherence to the latest recommendations concerning dietary fat and fiber was poor. Dietary intervention associated with weight loss was found to improve control in ambulatory obese older patients with type 2 diabetes *(168)*. However, diabetic diets did not appear to significantly improve glycemic control in frail older nursing home patients *(169)*. These diets complicated care, and increased the cost of looking after these patients.

Older patients with diabetes may be at risk for deficiency of trace elements. Short-term magnesium supplementation in elderly patients with diabetes reduces their fasting glucose levels, and increases glucose-induced release and insulin sensitivity *(170,171)*. Zinc supplements may improve wound healing, immune, and sexual function in older patients with diabetes *(172)*. A recent randomized controlled trial found that zinc supplementation in the form of bovine prostate powder lowered glucose levels and Hgb A_{1C}, and improved insulin sensitivity *(173)*.

There is a growing body of evidence that hyperglycemia is associated with increased oxidative stress. Erythrocytes from older patients with diabetes demonstrate greater basal oxidation products and greater susceptability to oxidation injury *(174)*. There is a relationship between levels of oxidative stress and insulin resistance in older people with type 2 diabetes *(175)*. In addition, supplementation with the antioxidant Vitamin C reduces insulin resistance in older patients with diabetes, and supplementation with Vitamin E improves improves glycemic control and lipid levels in these patients *(176,177)*. Further studies are needed to clearly define the role of antioxidants in the management of elderly patients with diabetes.

EXERCISE

Exercise improves glucose tolerance and increases insulin sensitivity in older people without diabetes, as well as in middle-aged patients with type 2 diabetes. Mechanisms hypothesized to increase insulin action during physical exercise in patients with diabetes include an increase in insulin regulated glucose transporters and the enzymes responsible for phosphorylation, storage, and oxidation of glucose *(178)*. Few studies have assessed the effect of exercise in elderly patients with diabetes. Skarfors et al. *(179)* conducted a randomized trial of exercise in older men with diabetes. Unfortunately, many subjects were excluded before the study, because of underlying disease, and most of the subjects dropped out before it was completed. Although exercise may be of value in older people with diabetes, further studies are needed.

α-GLUCOSIDASE INHIBITORS

α-glucosidase inhibitors are oligosaccharides that reversibly inhibit the intestinal enzymes responsible for the digestion of carbohydrates. The major side effect of these drugs is gastrointestinal intolerance. Two small, randomized controlled trials, and one large postmarketing surveillance survey have found that acarlose is well-tolerated, and results in significant reductions in Hgb A_{1C} and postprandial glucose levels in older patients with type 2 diabetes *(180–182)*. Recently, Johnston et al. *(183)* conducted a randomized controlled trial comparing Miglitol (a newer α-glucosidase inhibitor) to glyburide in elderly patients with type 2 diabetes. Hgb A_{1C} was reduced by 1% in the glyburide group, and by .5% in the Miglitol group. However, the patients on glyburide had more frequent hypoglycemic events, greater weight gain, and a greater incidence of serious cardiovascular events. Gastrointestinal side effects were common in the patients on Miglitol, but relatively few patients had to discontinue therapy. α-glucosidase inhibitors are less effective than sulphonylureas in the treatment of diabetes in older people, but may be preferred in some patients with mild diabetes, because they have a lower incidence of serious adverse effects.

METFORMIN

Metformin is the only biguanide currently available for the treatment of diabetes in North America. Age is not a risk factor for lactic acidosis with this drug, and there has never been a reported case of lactic acidosis in an older patient who had normal liver, cardiac, and renal function *(184)*. Limited data suggest that metformin is safe and effective in older patients with type 2 diabetes *(185,186)*. Metformin is a valuable drug in the management of diabetes in older obese people, because it increases insulin sensitivity, does not cause hypoglycemia, lowers lipid levels, and assists with weight loss.

THIAZOLIDINEDIONES

This is a newly developed class of oral hypoglycemic agents that lowers blood glucose by improving peripheral insulin sensitivity. The only drug in this class currently available for use is Troglitazone. Theoretically, this drug would appear to be ideal for the treatment of insulin resistance in obese elderly patients with type 2 diabetes. To date, studies have not been done to evaluate the effectiveness of this medication in older patients. Troglitazone has been associated with occasional liver dysfunction, necessitating careful monitoring of liver functions. Rosiglitazone appears to be more potent and not to produce the liver dysfunction.

INSULIN

Elderly patients make a substantial number of errors when they try to mix insulins on their own *(188,188)*. The accuracy of insulin injections has been shown to be markedly improved in older patients by using premixed preparations *(189)*. As long as a premixed insulin is used, the proportion of regular to long-acting insulin (i.e., 50:50 vs 70:30) does not seem to significantly effect glucose levels *(190)*. When older patients are started on insulin, some authors recommend one daily injection. However, hypoglycemia is more frequent in patients treated with one rather than two injections of insulin per day *(44)*. It is not clear whether there is any benefit to adding glyburide in elderly patients with diabetes who are already being treated with insulin *(191,192)*. Thus, whether a patient is placed on two daily injections of insulin or to one injection in conjunction with sulphonylureas should be based on patient and physician preference.

SULPHONYLUREAS

The kinetics of chlorpropamide and glipizide are not altered with age *(193–196)*. Peak levels of tolbutamide after a single dose are increased with age. The absorption and elimination of glyburide is reduced with age, and the pharmacodynamics of glyburide are also altered with age, because the elderly appear to have greater insulin responses to the drug *(197,198)*. The increased frequency of sulfphonylurea-induced hypoglycemia events in the elderly, and potential causes of this effect, have been detailed above. Chlorpromamide is relatively contraindicated in older patients, because, in addition to causing severe or prolonged hypoglycemia, this drug can cause the syndrome of inappropriate antidiuretic hormone secretion, an antabuse-like effect, and can interact adversely with multiple drugs *(199,200)*. The second-generation sulphonylureas appear to be free of many of the side effects of chlorpropamide, although glyburide causes a frequency of severe or fatal hypoglycemia similar to chlorpropamide. The risk of hypoglycemic events is lower in older patients treated with olbutamide, tolazamide, and gliclazide, and hypoglycemia may also be less with glipizide *(113,201–204)*. In addition to the type of sulphonylureas, other risk factors for hypoglycemia with these drugs include male sex, Black race, and multiple concomitant medications *(113,205)*.

OTHER DRUGS

A recent randomized control trial found that obese elderly patients treated with fluoxetine had significant weight loss and improved glycemic control, with no significant adverse events *(206)*. Because depression is common is older patients with type 2 diabetes, fluoxetine may be used to treat depression and improve control. No data is currently available in the elderly regarding newer therapeutic agents, such as GLP-1 rapaglinide, pramlintide, and so on.

MONITORING GLYCEMIC CONTROL

Urine glucose testing is not a reliable measure of glycemia in the elderly, because the renal threshold for glucose increases with age, and blood sugar levels must be substantially elevated before sugar spills into the urine. Elderly patients can be taught to self-monitor their blood sugar reliably, and home glucose monitoring does not significantly affect quality of life *(207,208)*. Glycosylated hemoglobin is the standard measure of long-term control (2–3 mo) in patients with diabetes, although Hgb A_{1C} values may be falsely elevated in some elderly subjects. Serum fructosamine measures glycemic control over the preceding 2–3 wk. This measure is at least as reliable as glycosylated hemoglobin in elderly patients, and may be preferred, because it costs less and is more reproducible *(209,210)*.

CONCLUSIONS

We are approaching an epidemic of diabetes in the elderly in the next millenium. Unfortunately, we still have huge gaps in our understanding of the pathogenesis and treatment of this illness in the aged, and further research is urgently needed. The recently completed United Kingdom trial in type 2 diabetes demonstrated that improved glycemic control resulted in decreased microvascular disease *(140a,140b)*. Control of hypertension was equally important for slowing the development of microvascular disease and also had a major impact on macrovascular disease. β-blockers and ACE inhibitors were equally effective. Although these studies were conducted in middle-aged subjects, the data may be directly applicable to the elderly.

REFERENCES

1. Harris MI, Flegal KM, Cowie CC, et al. Prevalence of diabetes, impaired fasting glucose, and impaired glucose tolerance in U.S. adults. Diabetes Care 1998;21:518–524.
2. Harris MI. Undiagnosed NIDDM: clinical and public health issues. Diabetes Care 1993;16:642–652.
3. Kahn CR. Banting Lecture. Insulin action, diabetogenes, and the cause of type II diabetes. Diabetes 1994;43:1066–1984.
4. Harris MI. Epidemiology of diabetes among the elderly in the United States. Clin Geriatr Med 1990;6:703–719.
5. Skarfors ET, Selinus KI, Lithell HO. Risk factors for developing non-insulin-dependent diabetes. A 10-year follow-up of men in Uppsala. Br Med J 1991;303:755–760.
6. Vaag A, Henriksen JE, Madsbad S, Holm N., Beck-Nielsen H. Insulin secretion, insulin action, and hepatic glucose production in identical twins discordant for non-insulin-dependent diabetes mellitus. J Clin Invest 1995;95:690–698.
7. Jackson RA. Mechanisms of age-related glucose intolerance. Diabetes Care 1990; 13(Suppl 2):9–19.
8. Tibblin G, Adlerberth A, Lindstedt GB, Björntorp P. The pituitary-gonadal axis and health in elderly men. Diabetes 1996;45:1605–1609.

9. Goodman-Gruen D, Barrett-Connor E. Sex hormone-binding globulin and glucose tolerance in post-menopausal women. The Rancho Bernardo Study. Diabetes Care 1997;20:645–649.
10. Feskens EJM, Bowles CH, Kromhout D. Carbohydrate intake and body mass index relation to the risk of glucose in tolerance in an elderly population. Am J Clin Nutr 1991;54:136–140.
11. Feskens EJM, Virtanen SM, Rasanen L, Tuomilehto J, Stengard J, Pekkanen J, Nissinen A, Kromhout D. Dietary factors determining diabetes and impaired glucose tolerance. Diabetes Care 1995;18:1104–1111.
12. Marshall JA, Weiss NS, Hamman RF. The role of dietary fiber in the etiology of non-insulin-dependent diabetes mellitus. The San Luis Valley diabetes study. Ann Epidemiol 1993;3:18–26.
13. Salmeron J, Asherio A, Rimm EB, Colditz GA, Spiegelman D, Jenkins DJ, et al. Dietary fiber, glycemic load, and risk of NIDDM in men. Diabetes Care 1997;20:545–550.
14. Lipton RB, Liao Y, Cao G, Cooper RS, McGee D. Determinants of incident non-insulin-dependent diabetes mellitus among blacks and whites in a national sample. The NHANES I Epidemiologic follow-up study. Am J Epidemiol 1993;138:826–964.
15. Cassano PA, Rosner B, Vokonas PS. Obesity and body fat distribution in relation to the incidence of non-insulin-dependent diabetes mellitus Am J Epidemiol 1992;136:1474–1486.
16. Travia D, Bonora E, Cacciatori V, Zenere M, Tosi F, Branzil P, et al. Study of some putative pathogenic factors of diabetes mellitus in the elderly. Arch Gerontol Geriat 1991;2(Suppl 2):219–222.
17. Morris RD, Rimm AA. Association of waist to hip ratio and family history with the prevalence of NIDDM among 25,272 adult, white females. Am J Public Health 1991;81:507–509.
18. Manson JE, Nathan DM, Krolewski AS, Stampter MJ, Willett HWC, Hennekens CH. A prospective study of exercise and incidence of diabetes among US male physicians. J Am Med Assoc 1992;268:63–67.
19. Mykkanen L, Kuusisto J, Pyorala K, Laakso M. Cardiovascular disease risk factors as predictors of type 2 (non-insulin-dependent) diabetes mellitus in elderly subjects. Diabetologia 1993;36:553–559.
20. Helmrich SP, Ragland DR, Leung RW, Paffenburger RS. Physical activity and reduced occurrence of non-insulin-dependent diabetes mellitus. N Engl J Med 1991;325:147–195.
21. Edelstein SL, Knowler WC, Bain RP, Andres R, Barrett-Connor EL, Dowse GK, et al. Predictors of progression from impaired glucose tolerance to NIDDM. Diabetes 1997;46:701–710.
22. Gurwitz J, Field TS, Glynn RJ, Manson JE, Avorn J, Taylor JO, Hennekens CH. Risk factors for NIDDM requiring treatment in the elderly. J Am Geriatr Soc 1994;42:1235–1240.
23. Mooy JM, Grootenhuis PA, de Vries H, Valkenburg HA, Bouter LM, Kostense PJ, Heine RJ. Prevalence and determinants of glucose intolerance in a Dutch Caucasian population. Diabetes Care 1995;18:1270–1273.
24. Stolk RP, Pols HA, Lamberts SWJ, de Jong PTVM, Hofman A, Grobbee DE. Diabetes mellitus, impaired glucose tolerance, and hyperinsulinemia in an elderly population. Am J Epidemiol 1997;145:24–32.
25. Pandit MK, Burke J, Gustafson AB, Minocha A, and Peiris AN. Drug induced disorders of glucose intolerance. Ann Int Med 1993;118:529–539.
26. DeFronzo RA. Lilly Lecture 1987. The triumvirate: b-cell, muscle, liver. A collusion responsible for NIDDM. Diabetes 1988;37:667–687.
27. Meneilly GS, Hards L, Tessier D, Elliott T, Tildesley H. NIDDM in the elderly. Diabetes Care 1996;19:1320–1375.
28. Arner P, Pollare T, Lithell H. Different aetiologies of type 2 (non-insulin-dependent) diabetes mellitus in obese and non-obese subjects. Diabetologia 1991;4:483–487.
29. Groop LC, Bottazzo GF, Doniach D. Islet cell antibodies identify latent type 1 diabetes in patients aged 35–75 years at diagnosis. Diabetes 1986;35:235–240.
30. Clauson P, Linnarsson R, Gottsater A, Sundkvist G, Grill V. Relationships between diabetes duration, metabolic control and β-cell function in a representative population of type 2 diabetic patients in Sweden. Diabetic Med 1994;11:794–801.
31. Tuomilehto-Wolf E, Tuamilehto J, Hitman GA, Nissinen A, Stengard J, Pekkanen S, et al. Genetic susceptibility to NIDDM and glucose tolerance are located in the HLNA region. Br Med J 1993;307:155–159.
32. Leslie RDG, Pozzilli P. Type 1 diabetes masquerading as type II diabetes. Diabetes Care 1994;17:1214–1219.
33. Gleichmann H, Zorcher B, Greulich B, Gries FA, Henrichs HR, Bertrams J, Kolb H. Correlation of islet cell antibodies and HLA-DR phenotypes with diabetes mellitus in adults. Diabetologia 1984;27:90–92.

34. Wroblewski M, Gottsater A, Lindgarde F, Fernlund P, Sundkvist G. Gender, antibodies and obesity in newly diagnosed diabetic patients aged 40–75 years. Diabetes Care 1988;21:250–255.

35. Ruige JB, Batstra MR, Aanstoot H-J, Bouter LM, Bruining GJ, de Neeling JN, Heine RJ. Low prevalence of antibodies to GAD65 in a 50- to 74-year-old general Dutch population. The Hoorn Study. Diabetes Care 1997;20:1108–1110.

36. Turner R, Stratton I, Horton V, Manley S, Zimmet P, Mackay IR, et al. UKPDS 25: autoantibodies to islet-cell cytoplasm and glutamic acid decarboxylase for prediction of insulin requirement in type 2 diabetes. Lancet 1997;350:1288–1293.

37. Best JD, Kahn SE, Ader M, Watanabe RM, Ni TC, Bergman RN. Role of glucose effectiveness in the determination of glucose tolerance. Diabetes Care 1996;19:1018–1030.

38. Forbes A, Elliott T, Tildesley H, Finegood D, Menielly GS. Alterations in non-insulin-mediated glucose uptake in the elderly patient with diabetes. Diabetes 1998;47:1915–1919.

39. McCarthy MI, Hitman GA, Hitchins M, Riikonen A, Stengard J, Nissinen A, et al. Glucokinase gene polymorphisms: a genetic marker for glucose intolerance in cohort of elderly Finnish men. Diabetic Med 1993;10:198–204.

40. Laakso M, Malkki M, Kekalainen P, Kuusisto J, Mykannen L, Deeb S. Glukokinase gene variants in subjects with late-onset NIDDM and impaired glucose tolerance. Diabetes Care 1995;18:398–400.

41. Obermajer-Kusser B, White MF, Pongratz DE, Su L, Ermel B, Muhlbacher C, et al. A defective intramolecular autoactivation cascade may cause the reduced kinase activity of the skeletal muscle insulin receptor from patients with non-insulin-dependent diabetes mellitus. J Biol Chem 1989;264: 9497–9504.

42. Gambert SR. Atypical presentation of diabetes in the elderly. Clin Geriatr Med 1990;6:721–729.

43. Morley JE, Kaiser FE. Unique aspects of diabetes mellitus in the elderly. Clin Geriatr Med 1990;6: 693–702.

44. Tattersall RB. Diabetes in the elderly—a neglected area. Diabetologia 1984;27:167–173.

45. James WD, Odom RB, Goette DKL Bullous eruption of diabetes mellitus. Arch Dermatol 1980;116: 1191–1192.

46. Friedman NA, LeBan NB. Periarthrosis of the shoulder associated with diabetes mellitus. Am J Phys Med Rehab 1989;68:12–14.

47. Neil MAW, Dawson JA, Baker JE. Risk of hypothermia in elderly patients with diabetes. Br Med J 1986;293:416–418.

48. Ellenberg M. Diabetic neuropathic cachexia. Diabetes 1974;23:418–423.

49. Pagano G, Bargero G, Bruno G. Prevalence and clinical features of known type 2 diabetes in the elderly: a population-based study. Diabetic Med 1991;11:475–478.

50. Mooradian AD, Osterveil D, Petrasek D, Morley JE. Diabetes mellitus in elderly nursing home patients. J Am Geriatr Soc 1988;36:391–396.

51. Sinclair AJ, Robert IM, Croxson SCM. Mortality in older people with diabetes mellitus. Diabet Med 1996;14:639–647.

52. Muggeo M, Verlato G, Bonora E, Ciani F, Moghetti P, Eastman R, Crepaldi G, de Marco R. Long-term instability of fasting plasma glucose predicts mortality in elderly NIDDM patients: the Verona diabetes study. Diabetologia 1995;38:672–679.

53. Seeman TE, Charpentier PT, Berkman LF, Tinetti ME, Guralnik JM, Albert M, Blazer D Rowe JW. Predicting changes in physical performance in a high-functioning elderly cohort: MacArthur studies of successful aging. J Gerontol 1994;49:M97–M108.

54. Perkowski LC, Stroup-Benham CA, Markides KS, Lichtenstein MJ, Angel, RJ, Guralnik JM, Goodwin JS. Lower-extremity functioning in older Mexican Americans and its association with medical problems. J Am Geratr Soc 1998;46:411–418.

55. Woo J, Ho SC, Yu LM, Lau J, Yuen YK. Impact of chronic diseases on functional limitations in elderly Chinese aged 70 years and over: a cross-sectional and longitudinal surgey. J Geront 1988;53: M102–M106.

56. Connell CM. Psychosocial aspects of diabetes and older adulthood: reciprocal effects. Diabetes Educ 1991;17:364–371.

57. Petterson T, Lee P, Hollis S, Young B, Newton P, Dornan T. Well-being and treatment satisfaction in older people with diabetes. Diabetes Care 1998;21:930–935.

58. Damsgard EM, Froland A, Holm N. Use of hospital services by elderly patients with diabetes. Diabetic Med 1987;4:317–321.

59. Damsgaard EM, Frøland A, Holm N. Ambulatory medical care for elderly patients with diabetes: the Frederica study of diabetic and fasting hyperglycaemic patients aged 60–74 years. Diabetic Med 1987; 4:317–321.

60. Panser LA, Naessems JM, Nobrega FT, Palumbo PJ, Ballard DJ. Utilization trends and risk factors for hospitalization in diabetes mellitus. Mayo Clin Proc 1990;65:1171–1184.

61. Rosenthal MJ, Fajardo M, Gilmore S, Morley J, Naliboff BD. Hospitalization and mortality of diabetes in older adults. Diabetes Care 1998;21:231–235.

62. Selby JV, Zhang D, Ray GT, Colby CJ. Excess costs of medical care for patients with diabetes in a managed care population. Diabetes Care 1997;20:1396–1402.

63. Gilmer TP, Manning WG, O'Connor PJ, Rush WA. The cost to health plans of poor glycemic control. Diabetes Care 1997;20:1847–1853.

64. Currie CJ, Morgan, CL, Peters JR. The epidemiology and cost of inpatient care for peripheral vascular disease, infection, neuropathy and ulceration in diabetes. Diabetes Care 1998;21:42–48.

65. Ray NF, Thamer M, Taylor T, Fehrenbach SN, Ratner R. Hospitalization and expenditures of the treatment of general medical conditions among the U.S. diabetic population in 1991. J Clin Endocrinol Metabol 1996;81:3671–3678.

66. American Diabetes Association. Economic consequences of diabetes mellitus in the U.S. in 1997. Diabetes Care 1998;21:296–309.

67. Krop JS, Powe NR, Weller WE, Shaffer TJ, Saudek CD, Anderson GF. Patterns of expenditures and use of services among older adults with diabetes. Diabetes Care 1998;21:747–752.

68. Morris AD, McAlpine R, Steinke D, Boyle DIR, Abdul-Rahim E, Boyle DI, Ebrahim AR, Vasudev N, et al. Diabetes and lower-limb amputations in the community. A retrospective cohort study. Diabetes Care 1998;21:738–743.

69. Greene DA. Acute and chronic complications of diabetes mellitus in older patients. Am J Med 1986; 80(Suppl 5A):39–53.

70. Nathan DM Singer DE, Godine JE, Perlmuter LC. Non-insulin-dependent diabetes in older patients. Am J Med 1986;81:837–842.

71. Cohen DL, Neil HAW, Thorogood M, Mann JI. A population-based study of the incidence of complications associated with Type 2 diabetes in the elderly. Diabetic Med 1991;8:928–933.

72. Welborn TA, Wearne K. Coronary heart disease incidence and cardiovascular mortality in Busselton with reference to glucose and insulin concentrations. Diabetes Care 1979;2:154–160.

73. Ford ES, DeStefano F. Risk factors for mortality from all causes and from coronary heart disease among persons with diabetes. Am J Epidemiol 1991;133:1220–1230.

74. Jarrett RJ, McCarthy P, Keen H. The Bedford survey: Ten-year mortality rates in newly diagnosed patients with diabetes, borderline patients with diabetes and normoglycaemic controls and risk indices for coronary heart disease in borderline patients with diabetes. Diabetologia 1982;22:79–84.

75. Hiller R, Sperduto RD, Podgor MJ, Ferris FL III, Wilson PWF. Diabetic retinopathy and cardiovascular disease in type II diabetes. Am J Epidemiol 1988;128:402–409.

76. Mykkänen L, Laakso M, Penttilä I, Pyörälä K. Asymptomatic hyperglycaemia and atherosclerotic vascular disease in the elderly. Diabetes Care 1992;15:1020–1030.

77. Donahue RP, Abbott RD, Reed DM, Yano K. Postchallenge glucose concentration and coronary heart disease in men of Japanese ancestry. Diabetes 1987;36:689–692.

78. Wingard DL, Barrett-Connor EL, Scheidt-Nave C, McPhillips JB. Prevalence of cardiovascular and renal complications in older adults with normal or impaired glucose tolerance in NIDDM. Diabetes Care 1993;16:1022–1025.

79. Naliboff BD, Rosenthal M. Effects of age on complications of adult onset diabetes. J Am Geriatr Soc 1989;37:838–842.

80. Abbott RD, Donahue RP, MacMahon SW, Reed DM, Yano K. Diabetes and the risk of stroke. J Am Med Assoc 1987;257:949–956.

81. Singer DE, Nathan DM, Anderson KM, Wilson PWF, Evans JC. Association of Hgb A_{1C} with prevalent cardiovascular disease in the original cohort of the Framingham heart study. Diabetes 1992;41: 202–208.

82. Davis TME, Stratton IM, Fox CJ, Holman RR, Turner R. U.K. prospective diabetes study 22. Diabetes Care 1997;20:1435–1441.

83. Sinclair AJ, Allard I, Bayer A. Observations of diabetes care in long-term institutional settings with measures of cognitive function and dependency. Diabetes Care 1997;20:778–784.

84. Klein R. Hyperglycemia and microvascular and macrovascular disease in diabetes. Diabetes Care 1995;18:258–268.
85. Vokonas PS, Kannel WB. Diabetes mellitus and coronary heart disease in the elderly. Clin Ger Med 1996;12:69–77.
86. Beks PHJ, MacKaay AJC, deVries H, de Neeling, JND, Bouter LM, Heine RJ. Carotid artery stenosis is related to blood glucose level in an elderly Caucasian population: the Hoorn study. Diabetologia 1997;40:290–198.
87. Kannel WB, McGee DL. Diabetes and glucose tolerance as risk factors for cardiovascular disease: the Framingham study. Diabetes Care 1979;2:120–126.
88. Beks PJ, MacKaay AJC, deNeeling JND, deVries H, Bouter LM, Heine RJ. Peripheral arterial disease in relation to glycaemic level in an elderly caucasian population: the Hoorn Study. Diabetologia 1995; 38:86–96.
89. Kuusisto J, Mykkänen L, Pyörälä K, Laakso M. Non-insulin-dependent diabetes and its metabolic control and important predictors of stroke in elderly subjects. Stroke 1994;25:1157–1164.
90. Kuusisto J, Mykkänen, Pyörälä, Laakso M. NIDDM and its metabolic control predict coronary heart disease in elderly subjects. Diabetes 1994;43:960–967.
91. Malmberg K. Prospective randomised study of intensive insulin treatment on long-term survival after acute myocardial infarction in patients with diabetes mellitus. Br Med J 1997;314:1512–1515.
92. Naliboff BC, Gilmore SL, Rosenthal MJ. Acute autonomic responses to postural change, Valsalva maneuver, and paced breathing in older type II diabetic men. J Am Geriatr Soc 1993;41:648–653.
93. Olivarius N de F, Andreasen AH, Keiding N, Mogensen CE. Epidemiology of renal involvement in newly-diagnosed middle-aged and elderly diabetic patients. Cross-sectional data from the population-based study "Diabetes Care in General Practice," Denmark. Diabetologia 1993;22:115–121.
94. Ohno T, Kato N, Shimizu M, Ishii C, Ito S, Tomono S, et al. Effect of age on the development or progression of albuminuria in non-insulin-dependent diabetes mellitus (NIDDM) without hypertension. Diabetes Res 1993;22:115–121.
95. Chen MS, Kao CS, Chang CJ, Wu TJ, Fu CC, Chen CJ, et al. Prevalence and risk factors of diabetic retinopathy among noninsulin-dependent diabetic subjects. Am J Ophthal 1992;114:723–730.
96. Humphrey LL, Ballard DJ. Renal complications in non-insulin-dependent diabetes mellitus. Clin Geriatr Med 1990;6:807–825.
97. Walters DP, Gatling W Mullee MA, Hill RD. The prevalence of diabetic distal sensory neuropathy in an English community. Diabetic Med 1992;9:349–353.
98. Schmidt RE, Plurad SB, Parvin CA, Roth KA. Effect of diabetes and aging on human sympathetic autonomic ganglia. Am J Path 1993;143:143–153.
99. Schmitz A. Renal function changes in middle-aged and elderly Caucasian type 2 (non-insulin-dependent) diabetic patients—a review. Diabetologia 1993;36:985–992.
100. Comi G, Lozza L, Galardi G, Ghilardi, MF, Madaglini S, Canal N. Presence of carpal tunnel syndrome in diabetes: effect of age, sex, diabetes duration and polyneuropathy. Acta Diabetol 1985;22:259–262.
101. Maser RE, Laudadio C, DeCherney GS. The effects of age and diabetes mellitus on nerve function. J Am Geriatr Soc 1993;41:143–153.
102. Wang CJ, Shen SY, Wu CC, Huang CH, Chiang CP. Penile blood flow in diabetic impotence. Urol Int 1993;50:209–212.
103. Masaoka S, Lev-Ran A, Hill LR, Vakil G, Hon EHG. Heart rate variability in diabetes; relationship to age and duration of the disease. Diabetes Care 1985;8:64–68.
104. Young MJ, Boulton AJM, Macleod AF, Williams DRR, Sonksen PH. A multicentre study of the prevalence of diabetic peripheral neuropathy in the United Kingdom hospital clinic population. Diabetologia 1993;36:150–154.
105. Stolk RP, Vingerling JR, de Jong PTVM, Dielemans I, Hofman A, Lamberts, SWJ, et al. Retinopathy, glucose, and insulin in an elderly population. Diabetes 1995;24:11–15.
106. Töyry JP, Niskanen LK, Mäntysaari MJ, Länsimies EA, Uusitupa MIJ. Occurrence, predictors, and clinical significance of autonomic neuropathy in NIDDM. Diabetes 1996;45:308–315.
107. Trautner C, Iacks A, Haastert B, Plum F, Berger M. Incidence of blindness in relation to diabetes. Diabetes Care 1997;20:1147–1153.
108. Tanaka Y, Atsumi Y, Matsuoka K, Onuma T, Tohjima T, Kawamori P. Role of glycemic control and blood pressure in the development and progression of nephropathy in elderly Japanese NIDDM patients. Diabetes Care 1995;21:116–120.

109. de Neeling JND, Beks PJ, Bertelsmann FW, Heine RJ, Bouter LM. Peripheral somatic nerve function in relation to glucose tolerance in an elderly Caucasian population: the Hoorn study. Diabetic Med 1996;13:960–966.

110. Nathan DM, Singer DE, Godine JE, Harrington CH, Perlmuter LC. Retinopathy in older type II diabetics. Diabetes 1986;35:797–801.

111. Morisaki N, Watanabe S, Kobayashi J, Kanzaki T, Takahashi K, Yokote K, et al. Diabetic control and progression of retinopathy in elderly patients: five-year follow-up study. J Am Geriatr Soc 1994;42:142–145.

112. Morisaki N, Yokote K, Tashiro J, Inadera H, Kobayashi J, Kanzaki T, et al. Lipoprotein(a) is a risk factor for diabetic retinopathy in the elderly. J Am Geriatr Soc 1994;42:965–967.

113. Shorr RI, Ray WA, Daugherty JR, Griffin MR. Individuals sulfonylureas and serious hypoglycemia in older people. J Am Geriatr Soc 1996;44:871–872.

114. Asplund K, Wilholm B-E, Lithner F. Glibenclamide-associated hypoglycemia: a report of 57 cases. Diabetologia 1983;24:412–417.

115. Sonnenblick M, Shilo S. Glibenclamide induced prolonged hypoglycemia. Age Aging 1986;15:185–189.

116. Asplund K, Wilholm B-E, Lundman B. Severe hypoglycemia during treatment with glipizide. Diabetic Med 1991;8:726–731.

117. Rump A, Stahl M, Caduff F, Berger W. 173 insulin-induzierte hypoglykamien mit spitaleinweisung. Dtsch Med Wschr 1987;112:1110–1116.

118. Weissman PN, Shenkman L, Gregerman RI. Chlorpropamide hyponatremia. N Engl J Med 1971;284:65–71.

119. Schen RJ, Benaroya Y. Hypoglycemic coma due to chlorpropamide: observations on twenty-two patients. Age Aging 1976;5:31–36.

120. Berger W, Caduff F, Pasquel M, Rump A. Die relative haufigkeit der schweren sulfopnylharnstoff-hypoglykamie in den letzten 25 jahren in der schweiz. Schweiz Med Wschr 1986;116:145–151.

121. Stepka M, Rogala H, Czyzyk A. Hypoglycemia; a major problem in the management of diabetes in the elderly. Aging 1993;5:117–121.

122. Meneilly GS, Cheung E, Tuokko H. Counterregulatory hormone responses to hypoglycemia in the elderly patient with diabetes. Diabetes 1994;3:403–410.

123. Thomson FJ, Masson EA, Leeming JT, Boulton AJ. Lack of knowledge of symptoms of hypoglycaemia by elderly diabetic patients. Age Aging 1991;20:404–406.

124. Burden AC. Awareness of hypoglycemia in diabetes. Lancet 1987;ii:1267.

125. Berger M. Human insulin: much ado about hypoglycaemia (un)awareness. Diabetologia 1987;30:829–833.

126. Meneilly GS, Milberg WP, Tuokko H. Differential effects of human and animal insulin on the responses to hypoglycemia in elderly patients with NIDDM. Diabetes 1995;44:272–277.

127. Palinkas LA, Barrett-Connor E, Wingard DL. Type 2 diabetes and depressive symptoms in older adults: a population-based study. Diabetic Med 1991;8:532–539.

128. Tun, PA, Nathan DM, Perlmuter LC. Cognitive and affective disorders in elderly patients with diabetes. Clin Geriatr Med 1990;6:731–746.

129. Elias PK, Elias MF, D'Agostino RB, Cupples LA, Wilson PW, Silbershatz H, Wolf PA. NIDDM and blood pressure as risk factors for poor cognitive performance. Diabetes Care 1997;20:1388–1395.

130. Meneilly GS, Cheung E, Tessier D, Yakura C, Tuokko H. The effect of improved glycemic control on cognifive functions in the elderly patient with diabetes. J. Gerontol 1993;48:M117–M121.

131. Gradman TJ, Laws A, Thompson LW, Reaven GM. Verbal learning and/or memory improves with glycemic control in older subjects with non-insulin-dependent diabetes mellitus. J Am Geriatr Soc 1993;41:1305–1312.

132. Leibson CL, Rocca WA, Hanson VA, Cha R, Kokmen E, O'Brien PC, Palumbo PJ. Risk of dementia among persons with diabetes mellitus: a population-based cohort study. Am J Epidemiol 1997;145:301–308.

133. Ott A, Stolk RP, Hofman A, van Harskamp F, Grobbee DE, Breterler MMB. Association of diabetes mellitus and dementia: the Rotterdam study. Diabetologia 1996;39:1392–1397.

134. National Diabetes Data Group. Classification and diagnosis of diabetes mellitus and other categories of glucose intolerance. Diabetes 1979;28:1039–1057.

135. American Diabetes Association. Report of the expert committee on the diagnosis and classification of diabetes mellitus. Diabetes Care 1988;21(Suppl I):S5–S19.

136. Cefalu WT, Ettinger WH, Bell-Farrow AD, Rushing JT. Serum fructosamine as a screening test for diabetes in the elderly: a pilot study. J Am Geriatr Soc 1993;41:1090–1094.

137. Croxson SCM, Absalom S, Burden AC. Fructosamine in diabetes screening of the elderly. Ann Clin Biochem 1991;28:279–282.
138. Diabetes Control and Complications Trial Research Group. The effect of intensive treatment on the development and progression of long-term complications in insulin-dependent diabetes mellitus. N Engl J Med 1993;329:977–986.
139. Meinert CL, Knatterud GL, Prout TE, Klimt TR. A study of the effects of hypoglycemic agents on vascular complications in patients with adult onset diabetes mellitus. Diabetes 1970;19:789–830.
140. Ohkubo Y, Kishikawa H, Araki E, Miyata T, Isami S, Motoyoshi S, et al. Intensive insulin therapy prevents the progression of diabetic microvascular complications in Japanese patients with non-insulin-dependent diabetes mellitus: a randomized prospective 6-year study. Dia Res Clin Pract 1995; 28:103–117.
140a. UK Prospective Diabetes Group. Intensive blood-glucose control with sulphonylureas or insulin compared with conventional treatment and risk of complications in patients with type 2 diabetes. Lancet 1998;352:837–853.
140b. UK Prospective Diabetes Group. Efficacy of aterolol and captopril in reducing risk of macrovascular and microvascular complications in type 2 diabetes: UKPDS 39. BMJ 1998;317:713–720.
141. Manton KG, Stallard E. Cross-sectional estimates of active life expectancy for the US elderly and oldest-old populations. J Gerontol 1991;46:S160–S182.
142. Eastman RC, Javitt JC, Herman WH, Dasbach EJ, Dong F, Manninen, D, et al. Model of complications of NIDDM. I. Diabetes Care 1997;20:725–734.
143. Eastman RC, Javitt JC, Herman WH, Dasbach EJ, Dong F, Manninen, D, et al. Model of complications of NIDDM. II. Diabetes Care 1997;20:735–744.
144. Vijan S, Hofer TP, Hayward RA. Estimated benefits of glycemic control in microvascular complications in type 2 diabetes. Ann Int Med 1997;127:788–795.
145. Avorn J. Benefit and cost analysis in geriatric care. New Engl J Med 1984;310:1294–1301.
146. Holvey SM. Psychosocial aspects in the care of elderly diabetic patients. Am J Med 1986;80(Suppl 5A): 61–63.
147. Funnell MM. Role of diabetes educator for older adults. Diabetes Care 1990;13(Suppl 2):60–65.
148. Kronsbein P, Muhlhauser I, Venhaus A, Jorgens V, Scholz V, Berger M. Evaluation of structured treatment and teaching program on non-insulin-dependent diabetes mellitus (NIDDM). Am J Public Health 1987;77:634–635.
149. Wilson W, Pratt C. The impact of diabetes education and peer support upon weight and glycemic control of elderly persons with NIDDM. Am J Public Health 1987;77:635–637.
150. Gilden JL, Hendryx M, Casia C, Singh SP. The effectiveness of diabetes education programs for older patients and their spouses. J Am Geriatr Soc 1989;37:1023–1030.
151. Silliman RA, Bhatta S, Khan A, Dukes KA, Sullivan LM. The care of older persons with diabetes mellitus: families and primary care physicians. J Am Geriatr Soc 1996;44:1314–1321.
152. Petterson T, Dornan TL, Albert T, Lee P. Are information leaflets given to elderly people with diabetes easy to read? Diabetic Med; 1994;11:111–113.
153. Leggett-Frazier N, Turner MS, Vincent PA. Measuring the diabetes knowledge of nurses in long-term care facilities. Diabetes Educator 1994;20:307–310.
154. Siegel J. Barriers to the effective use of capilllary blood glucose monitoring in extended care facilities. Diabetes Care 1990;17:381–383.
155. Funnell M, Herman W. Diabetes care policies and practices in Michigan nursing homes, 1991. Diabetes Care 1995;18:862–866.
156. Tonino RP. Diabetes education. What should health care providers in long term care facilities know about diabetes. Diabetes Care 1990;13(Suppl 2):55–59.
157. Giugliano D, Saccomanno F, Paolisso G, Ceriello A, Terella R, Varicchio M, et al. Nicardipine does not cause deterioration of glucose homeostasis in man: a placebo controlled study in elderly hypertensives with and without diabetes mellitus. Eur J Clin Pharmacol 1992;43:39–45.
158. Antonicelli R, Pagelli P, Paciaroni E. Nicardipine retard in the therapy of elderly diabetic hypertensives: final report of observational study. J Hypertension 1992;10(Suppl 2):569–572.
159. Lusardi P, Corradi L, Pasotti P, Zoppi G, Preti P, et al. Effects of amlodipine vs fosinopril on microalbuminuria in elderly hypertensive patients with type II diabetes. J Hypertension 1996;14(Suppl): S193.
160. Estacio RO, Jeffers BW, Hiatt WR, Biggerstaff SL, Gifford N, Schrier RW. The effect of nisoldipine as compared with enalapril on cardiovascular outcomes in patients with non-insulin-dependent diabetes and hypertension. N Engl J Med 1998;338:645–682.

161. Tatti P, Pahor M, Byington RP, Di Mauro P, et al. Outcome results of the fosinopril versus amlodipine cardiovascular events randomized trial (FACET) in patients with hypertension and NIDDM. Diabetes Care 1998;21:597–603.

162. Curb JD, Pressel SL, Cutler JA, Savage PJ, Applegate WB, Black H, et al. Effect of diuretic-based antihypertensive treatment on cardiovascular disease risk in older diabetic patients with isolated systolic hypertension. JAMA 1996;276:1886–1891.

163. Watson N, Sandler M. Effects of captopril on glucose tolerance in elderly patients with congestive cardiac failure. Curr Med Res Opin 1991;12:374–378.

164. Paolisso G, Gambardella A, Verza M, D'Amore A, Sgambato S, Varicchio M. ACE inhibition improves insulin-sensitivity in aged insulin-resistant hypertensive patients. J Hum Hypertens 1992;6:175–179.

165. Fonseca V, Wall J. Diet and diabetes in the elderly. Clin Geriatr Med 1995;11:613–624.

166. Reed RL, Mooradian AD. Nutritional status and dietary management of elderly diabetic patients. Clin Geriatr Med 1990;6:883–901.

167. Horwath CC, Worsley A. Dietary habits of elderly persons with diabetes. J Am Diet Assoc 1991;91:553–557.

168. Reaven GM. Beneficial effect of moderate weight loss in older patients with non-insulin-dependent diabetes mellitus poorly controlled with insulin. J Am Geriatr Soc 1985;33:93–95.

169. Coulston M, Mandelbaum D, Reaven GM. Dietary management of nursing home residents with non-insulin-dependent diabetes mellitus. Am J Clin Nutr 1990;51:67–71.

170. Paolisso G, Passariello G, Pizza G, Marrazzo R, Giunta R, Sgambato S, et al. Dietary Magnesium supplements improve B-cell response to glucose and arginine in elderly non-insulin dependent diabetic subjects. Acta Endocrinol 1989;121:16–20, 121.

171. Paolisso G, Scheen A, Cozzolino D, De Maro G, Varricchio M, D'Onofrio F, et al. Changes in glucose turnover parameters and improvement of glucose oxidation after 4-week magnesium administration in elderly non-insulin-dependent (type II) diabetic patients. J Clin Endocrinol Metab 1994;78:1510–1515.

172. Morley JE, Mooradian AD, Rosenthal MJ, Kaiser FE. Diabetes mellitus in elderly patients. Am J Med 1987;83:533–544.

173. Song MK, Rosenthal MJ, Naliboff BD, Phanumas L, Kang KW. Effects of bovine prostate powder on zinc, glucose and insulin metabolism in old patients with non-insulin-dependent diabetes mellitus. Metabolism 1998;47:39–43.

174. Aguirre F, Martin I, Grinspon D, et al. Oxidation damage, plasma antioxidant capacity, and glucemic control in elderly NIDDM patients. Free Radicals Biol Med 1998;24:580–585.

175. Paolisso G, D'Amore A, Volpe C, Balbi V, et al. Evidence for a relationship between oxidative stress and insulin action in non-insulin-dependent diabetic patients. Metabolism 1994;43:1426–1429.

176. Paolisso G, D'Amore A, Balbi V, Volpe C, et al. Plasma vitamin C affects glucose homeostasis in healthy subjects and in non-insulin-dependent diabetics. Am J Physiol 1994;266:E261–E268.

177. Paolisso G, D'Amore A, Galzerano D, Balbi V, Giugliano D, Varricchio M, D'Onofrio F. Daily vitamin E supplements improve metabolic control but not insulin secretoin in elderly type II diabetic patients. Diabetes Care 1993;16:1433–1437.

178. Ivy JL. Role of exercise training in the prevention and treatment of insulin resistance and non-insulin-dependent diabetes mellitus. Sports Med 1997;24:321–336.

179. Skarfors ET, Wegbener TA, Lithell H, Selinus I. Physical training as treatment for type 2 (non-insulin-dependent) diabetes in elderly men. A feasibility study over 2 years. Diabetologia 1987;30:930–933.

180. Orimo H, Akiguchi I, Shiraki M. Usefulness of acarbose in the management of non-insulin-dependent diabetes in the aged. In: Creutzfelt W, ed. Acarbose. Excerpta Medica, Amsterdam, 1982, pp. 348–352.

181. Johansen K. Acarbose treatment of sulfonylurea-treated non-insulin dependent diabetics. Diabete Metabol 1984;10:219–223.

182. Spengler M, Cagatay M. Evaluation of efficacy and tolerability of acarbose by postmarketing surveillance. Diab Stoffw 1992;1:218–222.

183. Johnston PS, Lebovitz HE, Coniff RF, Simonson DC, Raskin P, Munera CL. Advantages of α-glucosidase inhibition as monotherapy in elderly type 2 diabetic patients. J Clin Endocrinol Metabol 1998;83:1515–1522.

184. Knight PV, Temple G, Kessen CM. The use of metformin in the older patient. J Clin Exp Gerontol 1986;8:57–58.

185. Josephkutty S, Potter JM. Comparison of tolbutamide and metformin in elderly diabetic patients. Diabetic Med 1990;7:510–514.

186. Lalau JD, Vrmersch, Hary L, Andrejak M, Isnard F, Quichaud J. Type 2 diabetes in the elderly: an assessment of metformin (metformin in the elderly). Int J Clin Pharmacol Ther Toxicol 1990;28:329–332.
187. Puxty JAH, Hunter DH, Burr WA. Accuracy of insulin injection in elderly patients. Br Med J 1983; 287:1762.
188. Kesson CM, Bailie GR. Do diabetic patients inject accurate doses of insulin? Diabetes Care 1981;4:333.
189. Coscelli C, Calabrese G, Fedele D, Pisu E, Calderini C, Bistoni S, et al. Use of premixed insulin among the elderly. Diabetes Care 1992;15:1628–1630.
190. Brodows R, Chessor R. A comparison of premixed insulin preparations in elderly patients. Diabetes Care 1995;18:855–857.
191. Kyallastinen M, Groop L. Combination of insulin and glibenclamide in the treatment of elderly non-insulin-dependent (Type 2) diabetic patients. Ann Clin Res 1985;17:100–104.
192. Wolffenbuttel BHR, Sels, J-P JE, Rondas-Colbers GJWM, Menheere PPCA, Nieuwenhuijzen Kruseman AC. Comparison of different insulin regimens in elderly patients with NIDDM. Diabetes Care 1996;19:1326–1332.
193. Bergman U, Christensen I, Jansson B, Wilholm B-E, Ostman J. Wide variation in serum chlorpropamide concentration in outpatients. Eur J Clin Pharmacol 1980;18:165–169.
194. Kobayashi KA, Bauer LA, Horn JR, Opheim K, Wood F, Kradjan WA. Glipizide pharmacokinetics in young and elderly volunteers. Clin Pharm 1988;7:224–228.
195. Sartor G, Melander A, Schersten B, Wahlin-Boll E. Influence of food and age on the single-dose kinetics and effects of tolbutamide and chlorpropamide. Eur J Clin Pharmacol 1980;17:285–293.
196. Adir J, Miller AK, Vestal RE. Effects of total plasma concentration and age on tolbutamide plasma protein binding. Clin Pharmacol Ther 1982;31:488–493.
197. Schwinghammer TL, Antal EJ, Kubacka RT, Hackimer ME, Johnston JM. Pharmacokinetics and pharmacodynamics of glyburide in young and elderly nondiabetic adults. Clin Pharm 1991;10:532–538.
198. Jaber LA, Antal EJ, Welshman IR. Pharmacokinetics and pharmacodynamics of glyburide in young and elderly patients with non-insulin-dependent diabetes mellitus. Ann Pharmacother 1996;30: 472–475.
199. Kadowaki T, Hagura R, Kajinuma H, Kuzuya N, Yoshida S. Chlorpropamide-induced hyponatremia: incidence and risk factors. Diabetes Care 1983;6:468–471.
200. Tanay A, Firemann Z, Yust I, Abramov AL. Chlorpropamide-induced syndrome of inappropriate antidiuretic hormone secretion. J Am Geriatr Soc 1981;29:334–336.
201. Rosenstock J, Corrao PJ, Goldberg RB, Kilo C. Diabetes control in the elderly: a randomized, comparative study of glyburide versus glipizide in non-insulin-dependent diabetes mellitus. Clin Therapeutics 1993;15:1031–1040.
202. Brodows RG. Benefits and risks with glyburide and glicazide in elderly NIDDM patients. Diabetes Care 1992;15:75–80.
203. Fruhwalt T, Bohmer F. Gliclazid beim nichtinsulinpflchtigen diabetiker in der geriatrie. Schweiz Med Wochenschr 1988;138:102–106.
204. Tessier D, Dawson K, Tetrault JP, Bravo G, Meneilly GS. Glibenclamide vs glicazide in type 2 diabetes of the elderly. Diabetic Med 1994;11:974–980.
205. Chan TY, Cheung AY. Predictors of relapse in elderly diabetic patients admitted with sulphonylurea-induced severe hypoglycaemic attacks. Age Aging 1997;26:409–410.
206. Connolly VM, Gallagher A, Kesson CM. A study of fluoxetine in obese elderly patients with type 2 diabetes. Diabetic Med 1994;12:416–418.
207. Gilden JL, Casia C, Hendryx M, Singh SP. Effects of self-monitoring of blood glucose on quality of life in elderly diabetic patients. J Am Geriatr Soc 1990;28:511–515.
208. Bernbaum M, Albert SG, McGinnis J, Bursca S, Mooradian AD. The reliability of self blood glucose monitoring in elderly diabetic patients. J Am Geriatr Soc 1994;42:779–791.
209. Cefalu WT, Prather KL, Murphy WA, Parker TB. Clinical evaluation of serum fructosamine in monitoring elderly outpatient diabetics. J Am Geriatr Soc 1989;37:833–837.
210. Negoro H, Morley JE, Rosenthal MJ. Utility of serum fructosamine as a measure of glycemia in young and old diabetic and non-diabetic subjects. Am J Med 1988;85:360–364.

13

Evaluation and Management of Obesity in the Elderly

Amy Lee, MD, and Gayathri Dundoo, MD

CONTENTS

INTRODUCTION

The prevalence of obesity is growing rapidly. About one-third of the adult population in the United States is currently obese *(1)*. The percentage of older individuals is also increasing rapidly, and makes up more than 12% of the total population, encompassing approx 30 million people in the United States *(2)*. Obesity is associated with a wide range of adverse health consequences resulting in considerably increased morbidity and mortality *(3)*. The economic effect of obesity is substantial, estimated at approx 6% of the national health expenditure *(4)*. Obesity in the elderly is the result of an inability to couple energy intake with energy expenditure. The distribution of fat is a useful guideline for health risks *(5,6)*. The recommendation of a stepwise treatment plan progresses from diet through healthy nutrition to behavior and exercise for all obese elderly, and finally to the use of pharmacological treatment among obese elderly people with comorbid conditions. This chapter reviews the medical issues related to adult obesity, with particular attention directed toward the elderly.

From: *Contemporary Endocrinology: Endocrinology of Aging*
Edited by: J. E. Morley and L. van den Berg © Humana Press Inc., Totowa, NJ

Table 1
Classification of Overweight and Obesity
in Adults by BMI, Waist Circumference, and Associated Disease Risks

Classification	BMI	Classes	Men <102 cm (<40 in) Women <88 cm (<35 in)	>102 cm (>40 in) >88 cm (>35 in)
Underweight	<18.5		–	–
Normal desirable weight	8.5–24.9	0	–	–
Overweight	25.0–29.9	I	Increased	High
Obesity	30.0–34.9	II	High	Very high
	35.0–39.9	III	Very high	Very high
Extreme obesity	>40	IV	Extremely high	Extremely high

DEFINITION AND MEASUREMENT

Obesity is a condition in which the relative proportion of fat in the body is abnormally increased (body fat >25% of body wt for men and >30% of body wt for women) *(7)*. The degree of obesity can be expressed in several ways, including ratio of actual weight to desirable weight, skinfold thickness in the triceps or subscapular region, and the body mass index (BMI = weight in kilograms divided by the square of height in meters) *(7)*. Obesity and overweight measured by the BMI signify an increase of body wt above an arbitrary standard defined in relation to height. BMI has the best correlation to body fat, and has been widely used and accepted to estimate body fatness and health risks more than other techniques *(8,9)*. The waist circumference, which reflects the excess amount of fat present in the abdomen out of proportion to total body fat, is an independent predictor of obesity-related health risks.

The World Health Organization *(10)* and National Institutes of Health Expert Panel on the Identification, Evaluation, and Treatment of Obesity in Adults *(11)* proposed that individuals be classified according to their BMI (Table 1). Class I individuals have a BMI of 25–29.9 kg/m^2, and are at low risk from their obesity; class II individuals have a BMI of 30–34.9 kg/m^2, and have moderate risk associated with their obesity; class III individuals have a BMI of 35–39.9 kg/m^2 (i.e., more than 100% overweight), and are at high risk of obesity-associated complications. The sex-specific cutoffs of waist circumference can be used to identify increased relative risks for the development of obesity-related mobilities in most adults with BMI of 25–34.9 kg/m^2 (Men >102 cm, or >40 in; Women >88 cm, or >35 in). The waist circumference cutoffs lose their incremental predictive power in patients with BMI >35 kg/m^2, because these patients will exceed these cutoffs noted above *(11)*.

Because of the changes in body composition, which include decreased bone, water, and lean tissue, and increased fatness, the desirable range of BMI for each height appears to increase slightly with age, and different BMI standards may apply for individuals over the age of 65 yr *(12)*. The Committee on Diet and Health of the National Academy of Sciences proposed cutoffs for desirable BMI that rise from 21–26 at ages 45–54 yr, in increments by decade, up to 24–29 at age over 65 yr *(13,14)*. Thus, older persons are considered overweight when their BMI exceeds 30. Body fat increases with age, though the sum of the skinfolds remains constant, implying that, with aging, fat accumulates at other than the subcutaneous sites *(12)*.

PREVALENCE

In the recent population-based National Health and Nutrition Examination Surveys (NHANES), the prevalence of obesity in the United States, defined as BMI greater than 27.3 for men and 27.8 for women, is substantial; approx one-third (33.4%) of the adult population between ages 20 and 74 yr is currently overweight *(1)*. Based on height and weight (BMI) measured under standardized conditions in a series of surveys reported in NHANES, during the 10-yr period from 1982 to 1991, the mean BMI of adults age 20 to 74 yr increased from 25.3 to 26.3, and the average weight increased 3.6 kg *(1)*. In the same study, the average weight rose by 4.1 kg in Black men, 3.9 kg in White women, and 3.2 kg in Black women and White men, over the 10 yr *(1)*.

The prevalence of overweight varies by race/ethnicity, sex, and age. More women than men are overweight at any age. For all race/ethnic groups in the United States combined, 35% of adult women and 31% of adult men are overweight. The percentages of individuals classified as obese are even higher in minority populations. Excessive body wt is prominent among Black women (48.1%) and Mexican-American women (46.8%), which is estimated to be twice that of White women *(1)*. Excessive overweight is 7–12× more prevalent among women from lower socioeconomic classes than women from upper classes. Socioeconomic conditions may also explain the large differences in the prevalence of overweight among race/ethnic groups, and clearly play an important role in the development of obesity *(1,15)*.

The prevalence of obesity is also increasing in older man and women, generally because the age of the population in the United States has increased. The older American population comprises about 12% of the total population. Projections into the twenty-first century indicate that the elderly will account for 17–20% of the population by the year 2025. For both men and women, the frequency of overweight increases with age to a peak at 50–59 yr of age, and then the percentage of population who are overweight gradually declines *(1)*. It occurs less frequently in person aged >75 yr. For White and Mexican-American men, the prevalence of overweight tends to increase with each successive 10-yr increment of age, up to 60 through 69 yr *(1)*. For Mexican-American women, the highest prevalence is for women aged 40–49 yr; for White women, the highest prevalence occurs at age 50–59 yr; and for Black women, the highest prevalence is for women aged 60–69 yr *(1)*.

GENETICS

The importance of genetic factors in obesity is illustrated in the studies of twins, adoptees, and families *(16–17)*. Studies with identical twins suggest that inheritance accounts for about 70%, and environment for 30%. The correlations in body wt between adoptive mother and father and an adopted child were very low, and those between a father and his natural child or a mother and her natural child were much higher. Family studies also showed that, if both parents are obese, about 80% of the offspring will be obese. If only one parent is obese, about 40% of the offspring will be obese. If neither parent is obese, the likelihood of obesity in the offspring falls to less than 10%. Thus, genetic factors play an important role in the development of obesity, either by direct transmission, or by providing the biochemical and physiological mechanisms through which environmental factors can operate. Obesity is unlikely to be attributed to a single gene, because obesity can develop from an excess energy intake and/or reduced energy expenditure *(18,20)*.

The linkage between obesity and molecular markers for candidate genes on the basis of energy metabolism (e.g., the β_3-adrenergic receptor, the glucocorticoid receptor, and sodium/potassium-adenosine triphosphatase), obesity syndromes in humans, and obesity genes in rodents (e.g., the gene for leptin and leptin receptor) (21) are being examined among sibling pairs, extended families, and subjects within distinct ethnic or geographic populations. Isolated cases of obesity in humans have recently been identified, that result from single-gene mutations in metabolic pathways that are abnormal in genetically obese rodents, e.g., a mutation in the leptin coding sequence hypolipidemia in obese ob/ob mouse, and a mouse mutation (fat) associated with a defect in carboxypeptidase E, an enzyme that regulates energy conservation and food intake (18,20).

TECHNIQUES FOR BODY FAT ASSESSMENT

The proportion of the fat in the body can be assessed in many ways, but the most accurate are densitometry and techniques that measure isotope dilution. Measurements of body density and isotope dilution provide quantitative estimates for determining the proportion of body fat (22). Density is determined from the specific gravity of the body, that is, the weight of the body submerged under water, divided by the weight out of water. Knowing the specific gravity, one can fractionate body wt into fat and nonfat components, assuming the density of fat to be 0.915 and the density of nonfat tissues to be 1.100. A less direct technique is to estimate the volume of body water by measuring the distribution of titrated water or to measure cell mass by quantitating the naturally occurring isotope of potassium (^{40}K) in the body. Bioelectrical impedance analysis (BIA) is a relatively simple, quick, inexpensive, noninvasive, and reproducible method for estimating body composition (23). It provides an estimate of total body water (TBW). Using TBW derived from the BIA, one can estimate fat-free mass and body fat (adiposity). The estimation of body fat with BIA has a very high correlation with body fat measured by the densitometry, and is valid and accurate for measuring fat in both lean and obese subjects. Most commercial BIA machines come preprogrammed with body composition equations, which require age, weight, and stature, in addition to estimates of resistance. In research studies, more sophisticated methods, such as computer tomography (CT) scans and magnetic resonance imaging (MRI) have been used to describe body fat distribution, but these require special equipment that is expensive, time-consuming, and therefore, inappropriate for clinical use. From a practical point of view, three methods are most useful. Measurements of height and weight, expressed as the BMI provides an estimate of the degree of overweight. For fat distribution, the use of circumference at the abdomen or waist and the gluteus or hip has been helpful. Measurement of impedance (BIA) provides a quantitative estimate of total body fat.

PATHOPHYSIOLOGY

The data of caloric intake from the food consumption surveys of U.S. Department of Agriculture (USDA), Lipid Research Clinic Data (LRC), and Health and Nutrition Examination Survey I (HANES I) have shown that peak values occur in the second decade of life, followed by a gradual decline in successive decades for both women and men, indicating that the increases in body wt and body fat in older persons probably result from a greater fall in energy expenditure, rather than an increase in food intake (8).

An increase in body fat content reflects an increase in total stored energy. The amount of fat accumulated over time is the difference between food intake and energy expenditure (chiefly resting metabolism and physical activity). Homoeostatic mechanisms keep this difference in a relatively narrow range. Integrating mechanisms for the regulation of energy balance in the body include central and peripheral components. The relative constancy of energy storage is the result of the coordinate activity of these components, ranging from the hypothalamic centers to the peripheral adipocytes. The higher proportion of body fat in elderly individuals may be attributed to the mismatch between energy expenditure and intake. Their ability to adequately maintain energy homeostasis is blunted (24).

Numerous biophysiological factors regulate energy intake and expenditure. The energy balance is controlled and integrated by the central nervous system (CNS), with the key centers being in the arcuate and paraventricular nuclei and the ventromedial hypothalamus (17). Afferent neural (vagal and sympathetic) stimuli and hormonal stimuli (insulin, cholecystokinin, leptin, and glucocorticoids) related to metabolic status, are received in the hypothalamus, where they modulate the release of peptides known to affect food intake and efferent signals to the sympathetic and parasympathetic nervous system, as well as thyroid hormones, to regulate energy intake and expenditure (25,26). Weight gain and increased food intake are associated with increases in the production of triiodothyronine (T_3) from thyroxine, energy expenditure, thermic effect of eating, and sympathetic tone; weight loss or decreased food intake are associated with decreases in T_3 production, energy expenditure, postprandial thermogenesis, and sympathetic nervous system activity (27,28).

Although little is known about the age-related changes in food preferences, there is increasing evidence that obese individuals have less healthy dietary habits, and obtain more calories from foods relatively rich in fat (29,30). Obesity need not always be associated with overeating. Elevated preferences for the high-fat diet may play a role in promoting obesity. The thermic effect of food may dissipate up to 10% of the ingested calories. Fat appears to have the lowest food-induced thermic effect. In addition, fat has a higher caloric density than protein and carbohydrates, and its contribution to the palatability of foods may promote the ingestion of calories.

ENDOCRINOLOGY

Plasma insulin concentrations are proportional to the adipocyte volume (31). Insulin gains access to the CNS through a saturable transport system, and reduces food intake by inhibiting the expression of neuropeptide Y (NPY), suppressing neuronal norepinephrine reuptake, and enhancing the anorectic effects of cholecystokinin (32,33). Although it has been demonstrated that insulin may be an important humoral factor by which the periphery communicates with central body wt control mechanisms (31–34), recent evidence suggests that, in the absence of altered blood glucose concentration, physiological concentrations of insulin are unlikely to play a role in the short-term regulation of food intake (35–37). Additional studies indicate that insulin reduces food intake through an effect on leptin-mediated, and not neuropeptide-related, signaling (38).

Leptin is secreted from adipose tissue, and is a component of a regulatory loop linking fat mass to food intake and energy expenditure (39–41). Leptin acts as a blood-borne signal from adipocytes that informs the brain, through leptin receptors in the hypothalamus, about the amount of fatness, and interacts with NPY to sense and respond to alterations in energy balance *(39–41)*. NPY is synthesized in the arcuate nucleus of the hypothalamus, and is a potent central appetite stimulant. Repetitive administration of NPY into the CNS produces hyperphagia and weight gain *(42,43)*. Despite evidence of the physiologic importance of NPY in the regulation of nutritional homeostasis, NPY-knock-out mice have normal fat and food intake, with normal hyperphagia, and respond to exogenous leptin with normal or even excessive inhibition of food intake *(44)*. These findings reflect the extraordinary redundancy of systems regulating the energy balance. Leptin secretion goes up, and animals reduce their food intake and burn more calories. The investigation of a large number of obese human subjects, for both production and leptin receptor abnormalities in the gene, suggest that a genetically faulty system is rare. The available information indicates that leptin resistance is important for the development of human obesity *(45,46)*. Obese subjects are heterogeneous with respect to circulating leptin. In most of the obese subjects, circulating leptin is elevated *(45,46)*. The problem of these individuals is decreased response in the leptin receptor signaling pathway, poor penetration of the blood–brain barrier by leptin, or a less active molecular form of leptin. A small but significant group of obese persons may have relative leptin deficiency, and the administration of leptin may be useful in promoting weight loss. There is a large difference between the sexes with respect to plasma leptin *(47)*. Plasma leptin is about threefold higher in premenopausal and postmenopausal women, compared to men. Postmenopausal women have lower plasma leptin than premenopausal women, after correction for fat mass *(47)*. Leptin is probably increased by estrogen and/or progesterone, and it is likely that androgens also have a suppressive effect on plasma leptin. In females, circulating leptin is inversely related to age, and is reduced by at least one-half (53%) in subjects over age 60 yr, which can not be accounted for by increased adiposity associated with aging *(48)*. In males, leptin is positively related to aging. Testosterone supplementation lowers leptin levels in older hypogonadal males *(49)*. The leptin signaling system may be altered with age, similar to other endocrine system.

Several endocrine alterations can promote obesity. Cushing's syndrome is often associated with central obesity. A dexamethasone suppression test and a 24-h urine collection for urinary free cortisol usually determine whether a true Cushing's syndrome is present *(50)*. The recognition of iatrogenic Cushing's syndrome is important, because this syndrome is treatable by elimination of unnecessary glucocorticoid medication *(51)*. If the treatment must be continued to control the underlying disease activity, dietary therapy can be pursued to prevent further weight gain. Hypothyroidism is a rare cause of mild hypometabolism, promoting weight gain caused by edema and fat accumulation *(52)*. Iatrogenic hyperinsulinemia can result from the administration of excessive insulin to regulate glycemic control in diabetics who do not adhere to dietary therapy. An approx 2.5-kg average weight gain is observed at the time of menopause in women *(53)*. Following menopause, the gluteofemoral fat deposits decrease in size, and adiposity increases in the abdominal and breast areas *(54)*. It is unclear that the observed weight gain is the result of a metabolic effect of the loss of estrogen and progesterone, decreased physical activity, or simply increased food intake at the time of menopause. "Syndrome X" refers to a constellation of abnormalities, including obesity, hypertension, glucose intolerance, hyperlipidemia, and coagulation abnormalities, and is associated with the risks of coronary heart disease *(55,56)*. There is growing evidence indicating that the fundamental defect underlying this metabolic disorder is the combination of insulin resistance and compensatory hyperinsulinemia. It has a 50% hereditary component *(55)*. As many as 30–40% of obese type 2 noninsulin-dependent diabetics may have this syndrome *(57)*.

There is a weight-related reduction in circulating testosterone in obese males, caused by lower concentration of sex-hormone-binding globulin, which may lead to erroneous interpretation of hypogonadism *(58,59)*. The measurement of biologically active testosterone concentration is important. The dynamic responses of the male reproductive system to a challenge with gonadotropin releasing hormone remains normal.

HEALTH RISKS AND MORTALITY

Life insurance statistics suggest that excess weight is associated with increased mortality. A curvilinear relationship between BMI and medical complications, including coronary artery disease, diabetes mellitus, and all cancers for men and women, is well known. The prevalence of obesity predicts the incidence of coronary artery disease, coronary death, and congestive heart failure in men and women, independent of other risk factors. Data from the American Cancer Society show a J- or U-shaped curve, with the minimum mortality for both men and women occurring among individuals with a BMI of 22–25 kg/m^2 *(60)*. The mortality ratio increases with mild obesity, and progressively increases through moderate and severe obesity. At BMI greater than 40, the increase in mortality is exponential, and is widely referred as morbid obesity. It is also apparent that mortality increases when the BMI falls below 20 kg/m^2. At the two extremes of the U-shaped relationship between BMI and mortality, the causes of death are different. Some respiratory disease, digestive diseases, and cancer account for the extra mortality associated with low body wt (BMI <20 kg/m^2); cardiovascular diseases, diabetes mellitus, gallbladder disease, and other cancers make up the excess mortality in the overweight.

Recent studies suggest that the regional distribution of body fat is a more important correlate of the risks of cardiovascular diseases and insulin resistance-dyslipidemic syndrome, and may be a better predictor of mortality than BMI or relative weight *(61–63)*. If confirmed, this relationship may be important in the future to measure fat distribution in addition to using height–weight tables.

Recent evidence has also suggested that weight fluctuation or weight cycling, because of repeated bouts of weight loss and weight regain, may be harmful, and is associated with increased mortality *(64)*. Individuals with extreme body wt fluctuations are at higher risk of death than those with modest levels of fluctuations.

The association of obesity with increased mortality, increased risks of noninsulin-dependent diabetes mellitus (NIDDM), increased heart disease, and increased gallbladder disease has been clearly documented *(3,8*; Table 2). Although the association between obesity and various complications may differ among various age groups, with favorable health-margin-associated BMI diminishing among older people *(65)*, the degree of obesity is also very important in determining the risks from obesity *(66)*. Relative risks range between 2 and 8 when BMI exceeds 35–40 kg/m^2. Additional problems related to obesity in class IV obese individuals include cardiomegaly, Pickwickian/sleep apnea syndrome, acanthosis nigricans, and significant osteoarthritis *(65,66)*.

The major complications of obesity, including cardiovascular disease, diabetes mellitus, hypertension, and hyperlipidemias, are associated with increased abdominal fat *(3,8,61–63)*. The role for abdominal obesity as a risk for these complications is independent of BMI. Although this fat distribution pattern is more common in men, both men and

Table 2
Common Comorbidities of Obesity in the Elderly

Type 2 diabetes mellitus	Sleep apnea syndrome
Impaired glucose intolerance	Gallbladder disease
Hyperinsulinemia	Osteoarthritis of weight bearing joints
Dyslipemia	Some cancers (in women, endometrium and breast cancer)
	(In men, colon/rectum and prostate cancer)
Hypertension	Cardiomegaly/cardiomyopathy

women show increased risk of heart disease with greater abdominal fat. Localized distribution of fat can be evaluated by measuring the circumference of the abdomen (waist) and the circumference of the hip, and taking the ratio, the waist:hip ratio (WHR). The abdominal waist circumference is measured with a flexible tape placed in a horizontal plane at the level of the natural waist line, or narrowest part of the torso as seen from the anterior view. The hip circumference is measured in the horizontal plane at the level of maximal circumference, including the maximum extension of the buttocks posteriorly (7). Men tend to have more abdominal fat, giving them the android or abdominal pattern of fat distribution; women tend to have greater amounts of gluteal fat, giving them so called gynoid or gluteal pattern of fat distribution. Men may be considered at increased risk if WHR is >0.95 and women, if WHR is >0.80 (67).

The imaging methodologies of CT and MRI have allowed more accurate measurements of abdominal fat, and are helpful in distinguishing subcutaneous fat accumulation from visceral or intra-abdominal adipose tissue deposition (3,8). With these techniques, obese patients with high levels of visceral adipose tissue display a cluster of metabolic abnormalities, including marked hyperinsulinemia, glucose intolerance, hypertriglyceridemia, low high-density lipoprotein (HDL) cholesterol levels, and elevated plasma apoprotein B concentrations, as well as a greater proportion of small, dense low-density apolipoprotein particles (61–63,68–71). Accumulation of visceral fat is the best predictor of the changes in glucose tolerance and a patient's cardiovascular risk profile. Although WHR has frequently been used to estimate abdominal adiposity, recent studies have shown that waist circumference alone correlates better with visceral abdominal fat than does WHR (71). Thus, the monitoring of visceral adipose tissue accumulation appears to be critical in the evaluation of patients with obesity. The simplest predictor of atherogenic and diabetogenic visceral adipose tissue accumulation that could be used by physicians in order to identify high-risk patients is the measurement of waist circumference. With age, there is a selective accumulation of visceral fat (72). This phenomenon implies that, for any given waist circumference, older persons have a greater accumulation of visceral fat than younger persons. A waist circumference of approx 102 cm in men and 88 cm in women older than 40 yr of age is predictive of an increased visceral adipose tissue accumulation accompanied by the features of the insulin-resistance-dyslipemia syndrome (72; Table 1).

Obesity also has a number of effects on function of various organ systems. Obesity increases the work of the heart. Cardiomegaly with cardiomyopathy is associated with extremes of overweight. The increased cardiac output, stroke volume, blood volume, and cardiac size are reversible with weight loss (73). The relationship between hypertension and obesity has been widely recognized. Obesity increases the risk of developing hypertension between two- and fourfold in both men and women (3,8). Obesity is responsible for one-third of the cases of hypertension in the United States. The etiological linkage between obesity and hypertension remains under discussion and investigation. Several studies have shown that higher cardiac output with reduced venous capacitance is often observed in individuals with obesity. Insulin resistance and hyperinsulinemia may contribute to increased sodium retention and enhanced adrenergic tone. There is an average reduction of 0.5 to 1.0 mmHg for every kilogram of weight loss *(74)*. Postulated mechanisms of blood pressure reduction in response to weight loss, in hypertensive individuals with obesity, include decreased peripheral vascular resistance, decreased volume secondary to initial natriuresis and diuresis, and a decreased adrenergic tone *(75)*. Clinically significant reductions in blood pressure typically occur in obese individuals with hypertension who lose 5–10% of body wt.

It has been noted that approx 85% of all people with type 2 diabetes are obese, though this percentage appears to be lower in older persons. When obesity is uncommon, the incidence of diabetes mellitus is low; when obesity is more prevalent, diabetes increases. Impaired glucose tolerance from weight gain is accompanied by a state of insulin resistance: a decreased number of receptors that bind insulin. Insulin resistance plays a key role in increased hepatic glucose production and abnormal glucose handling in the skeletal muscle and adipose tissue *(76)*. Weight loss of 5–10% of initial body wt has been consistently shown to improve glucose tolerance. A weight loss of 10% or more is required to achieve long-term improvement in patients with type 2 diabetes *(77,78)*. Weight loss reduces both hepatic and peripheral insulin resistance in obese diabetics, and also results in improved lipid profiles. Because insulin resistance and hyperinsulinemia have been implicated in a cluster of metabolic disorders often resulting in hypertension and dyslipemia, the reduction of insulin resistance following weight loss in obese diabetics carries benefits beyond reduction of hyperglycemia.

Obesity is associated with a wide range of lipid abnormalities *(79,80)*. A reduction in HDL cholesterol may be one of the mechanisms by which obesity is associated with an increased risk of developing cardiovascular disease. Central obesity with increased abdominal visceral fat is strongly associated with dyslipidemias. It is caused by an increase in free fatty acid production in the portal circulation because of enhanced lipolysis of visceral adipocytes, resulting in abnormal lipid handling in the liver and skeletal muscle. Weight loss decreases both LDL cholesterol and triglycerides, as well as increases HDL cholesterol. It appears that a 5–10% weight loss is sufficient to result in significant improvements in lipid profile.

The increase in triglyceride storage is associated with a linear increase in the production of cholesterol, which in turn is associated with increased cholesterol secretion in bile and an increased risk of gallstone formation *(8)*.

With a moderate degree of obesity, several changes in pulmonary function may occur, including increased residual volume and increased work of breathing. Severe alveolar hypoventilation causes alveolar hypoxemia, pulmonary artery constriction, and pulmonary hypertension. The obesity hypoventilation syndrome, called the Pickwickian syndrome, with alveolar hypoventilation, hypoxemia, plethora, and somnolence, usually reflects the combination of class IV obesity and sleep apnea *(81)*.

TREATMENT

Initial treatment for the obese elderly should attempt to elevate energy expenditure through participating in regular physical activity. Energy intake should be controlled, and a balanced diet that provides daily energy deficit of about 300–500 kcal is safe and appropriate. Excessive consumption of fat should be avoided (82). Energy derived from fat should be restricted to no more than 30% of the calories, with less than 10% from saturated fat. A protein intake about of 70 g/d is desirable. One method to estimate the caloric expenditure is from desirable body wt. Energy needs are 14–19 kcal/lb (34–42 kcal/kg) in the adult male and 12–17 kcal/lb (29–38 kcal/kg) in the adult female. Desirable body wt can be calculated from the following formulas: Men (in pounds) = 106 + 6 (height in inches −60); Women = 105 + 5 (height in inches −60). A pound of body fat stores about 3500 kcal, and a caloric deficit of 300–500 kcal/d will cause the loss of 1.0 lb (0.5 kg) of fat within 1–2 wk. Other methods are the use of a normogram, which allows more precise measurement of energy requirements, based on the patient's height, weight, and age, as well as the relative extent of physical activities (8). Because of a gradual slowing in the rate of weight loss, resulting from a decrease in energy expenditure, obese patients who become frustrated during the course of weight reduction often need the physician's explanation and reassurance. Diabetic or hypertensive patients treated with drugs may need to have their dosages reduced when taking such diets. Diets that provide more than 1200 kcal/d may be reasonably used without medical supervision, and for longer periods of time. Micronutrients, such as folate, cobalamin, tocopherol (vitamin E), riboflavin (vitamin B_2), thiamine (vitamin B_1), pyridoxine (vitamin B_6) or ascorbic acid (vitamin C), may exert an inhibitory effect on osteoarthritis in the obese elderly (83). The intake of vitamins and minerals should be monitored: Prescription of supplemental vitamins and minerals is preferred for patients on dietary therapy.

Exercise is an important element of both short-term weight control and long-term maintenance of weight loss. Exercise does burn calories (8; Table 3). During sleep, approx 0.8 kcal/min is consumed. Reclining increases this level to 1.0–1.2 kcal/min, and very light activity consumes approx 1.1–2.5 kcal/min. Moderate activities expend 4.0–7.0 kcal/min, and heavy activities from 7.4 kcal/min to 12 kcal/min. The score system can be used to estimate the calories spent at various activity levels (Table 3). Exercise decreases body fat, preserves muscle mass as total weight decreases, and increases total daily energy expenditure (84,85). It may also offset the decline in resting metabolism noted with prolonged caloric restriction. Exercise interventions, such as resistance training and aerobic exercise, preserve fat-free mass, enhance aerobic capacity, increase fat oxidation, and reduce the tendency toward increasing adiposity in obese older individuals (86). Exercise itself, without significant change in body wt, can improve insulin sensitivity, and increases glucose utilization (87). Obese and diabetic patients should be encouraged to combine exercise with dieting for weight reduction.

It has been debated whether obesity in the elderly should be treated with drug intervention. There is little information regarding the effectiveness of these drugs in the treatment of the older population. When prescribing any antiobesity drug for the treatment of older individuals with obesity, it is important to consider age-related alterations in physiological functions that may affect the absorption, metabolism, and elimination, as well as the interaction, of the drugs (88).

Drugs that have been used empirically to treat obesity are of several categories, based on underlying mechanisms of the effects of the drugs on weight loss (89,90). The first category is the centrally active anorexians, which act on the serotonergic and noradrenergic systems to suppress appetite. Medications that have direct CNS effects may interact with other psychoactive drugs (e.g., antidepressants) commonly used among the elderly.

Table 3
Analysis of Physical Activity

Score	Activity	Examples	Energy expenditure (kcal/min)	
			Males	Females
0	Sleeping	<1.0	<0.9	
1	Reclining	Watching television, reading quieting.	1.0–1.2	0.9–1.1
2	Very light	Sitting or standing—typical occupational activities, e.g., painting, driving, typing, and housekeeping using labor-saving devices.	1.2–2.5	1.1–2.0
3	Light	Walking on level at 2.5–3 mph, housekeeping not using labor-saving devices, playing table tennis, golf, and volleyball, and shopping with a light load.	2.6–4.9	2.1–3.9
4	Moderate	Walking 3.4–4 mph, scrubbing floors, shopping with a heavy load, bicycling, skiing, dancing, and playing tennis.	5.0–7.4	4.0–5.9
5	Heavy	Swimming, climbing, shoveling, and playing basketball	7.5–12.0	6.0–10.0

Drugs in this class are all scheduled drugs by the Drug Enforcement Agency. The noradrenergic drugs (e.g., phentermine, mazindol, and diethypropion, and so on) increase brain catecholamine concentrations, or act directly on catecholamine receptors, to increase the activity of β-adrenergic systems (resulting in decreased appetite or increased energy expenditure), or decrease the activity of α-adrenergic systems (resulting in increased appetite or decreased energy expenditure). These drugs are unsuitable for obese patients with evidence of cardiovascular disease. The serotonergic drugs, dexfenfluramine and fenfluramine, were disapproved by the FDA for obesity treatment, because of the potential fatal side effects of pulmonary hypertension and valvular heart disease (90,91). Fluoxetine and other selective serotonin-reuptake inhibitors, used for the treatment of depression, promote some weight loss for at least 5–6 mo (92). One recent study (93) reported that fluoxetine is safe and effective in promoting weight loss and glycemic control in obese elderly with type 2 diabetes. Sibutramine, a drug with both catecholaminergic and serontoninergic agonists that decrease hunger, was approved by the FDA in early 1998, for obesity treatment (94).

The second category is drugs that affect thermogenesis and metabolism. Medications in this class are experimental in the United States, and some of these medications (caffeine and ephedrine combination) are used in European countries for weight control (95). Ephedrine may not be advisable for the treatment of elderly men with prostate hypertrophy, because of its adverse effect of vasoconstriction of the urinary sphincter. β3-adrenergic receptor agonists, and other chemicals that regulate thermogenesis in the brown adipose tissue and lipolysis in visceral fat, and to increase caloric expenditure, are currently under development. Although selective beta 3-agonist therapy, which affects energy expenditure, offers a promising strategy for the treatment in the obese elderly, future studies of potential long-term side effects are required in the older population.

The third category is drugs that inhibit the action of digestive enzymes and block the absorption of nutrients (e.g., fat) (90). Orlistat, a pancreatic lipase inhibitor that acts at the level of gut to inhibit absorption of approx one-third of the fat consumed, is currently under consideration for approval by the FDA. The side effects include reduced absorption of fat-soluble vitamins and gastrointestinal symptoms. Because inadequate nutrition and malabsorption are common in the elderly, research should address the safety of the treatment for the elderly. Metformin is an antihyperglycemic agent that has been available for the treatment of obese patients with type 2 NIDDM. One recent study confirmed the ability of metformin to reduce appetite and caloric intake in a dose-dependent manner *(96)*. Acute reduction of hyperinsulinemia is probably the mechanism by which metformin acts to suppress appetite and induce weight loss. As scientific understanding of the complex feedback loops related to obesity become more sophisticated, increasing targeted and effective pharmacological therapies are likely to become available. Given the role of leptin in the modulation of food intake, and the decline of leptin concentrations during caloric restriction, administration of leptin to promote satiety may prove useful in enhancing the long-term maintenance of weight loss.

CONCLUSION

The safest and most effective long-term nonpharmacological treatment for older persons is regular exercise combined with proper nutrition. Exercise is an important element in the weight-loss program. Exercise decreases body fat, preserves fat-free tissue and proper level of body composition, and contributes toward functional independence and a general sense of well-being for the elderly. Cautions are required in prescribing antiobesity drugs, because of the high prevalence of concurrent morbidities and polypharmacy in older individuals. Relatively modest weight loss, on the order of 5–10% of initial body wt, can result in significant health benefits and risk factor reduction. A small degree of weight loss by moderate restriction of caloric intake in the obese elderly is associated with a reduction of plasminogen activator inhibitor type-1 and an improvement in dysfibrinolysis. These changes can slow down the progression of vasculopathy in the insulin-resistance state and decrease cardiovascular disease risk in older persons with obesity *(97)*. To date, only a few long-term clinical trials have addressed the necessity of treatment of obesity in the older population *(98)*. One recent study using the bioelectrical impedance technique showed that high body fatness is an independent predictor of morbidity-related disability in older men and women *(98)*. Low fat-free mass or low muscle mass is not associated with a higher prevalence of disability. Future research studies need to be performed to determine whether interventions that are designed to induce weight loss actually decrease morbidity and mortality in the elderly.

REFERENCES

1. Kuczmarski RJ, Flegal KM, Campbell SM, Johnson CL. Increasing prevalence of overweight among US adults: the National Health and Nutrition Examination Surveys, 1960–1991, JAMA 1994;272:205–211.
2. Van Nostrand J, Furner S, Suzman R. Health data on older Americans; United States, 1992. Vital Health Statistics, vol. 3. US Department of Health and Human Services, Center for Disease Control and Prevention, National Center for Health Statistics, Hyattsville, MD, 1993.
3. Kissebah AH, Freedman DS, Peiris AN. Health risks of obesity. Med Clin North Am 1989;73:111–138.
4. Wolf AM, Colditz GA. Current estimates of the economic cost of obesity in the United States. Obes Res 1998;6:97–106.
5. Bjorntorp P. Abdominal obesity and the development of non-insulin-dependent diabetes mellitus. Diabetes Metab Rev 1988;4:615–622.

6. Bray GA. Complications of obesity. Ann Intern Med 1985;103:1052–1062.

7. Lohman TG. Skinfolds and body density and their relation to body fatness: a review. Hum Biol 1981; 53:181–225.

8. Bray GA. The Obese Patient. Major Problems in Internal Medicine, vol. 9. WB Saunders, Philadelphia, 1976.

9. Bray GA. Obesity: classification and evaluation of the obesities. Med Clin North Am 1989;73:161–184.

10. World Health Organization. Prevention and Management of the Global Epidemic of Obesity. Report of the WHO Consultation on Obesity. WHO, Geneva, 1997.

11. National Institute of Diabetes and Digestive and Kidney Diseases. Statistics Related to Overweight and Obesity. NIH Publication 96-4158. National Institutes of Health, Rockville, MD, 1996.

12. Bray GA. Overweight is risking fate: definition, classification, prevalence and risks. Ann NY Acad Sci 1987;249:14–28.

13. Committee on Diet and Health. Implication for Reducing Chronic Disease Risk. National Academy Press, Washington, DC, 1989, pp. 21–22.

14. Andres R, Elahi D, Tobin JD, et al. Impact of age on weight goals. Ann Intern Med 1985;103: 1030–1034.

15. Goldblatt PB, Moore ME,Stunkard AJ. Social factors in obesity. JAMA 1965;192:1039–1044.

16. Bray GA. The inheritance of corpulence. In: Van Itallie TB, eds. Body Weight Regulatory System: Basic Mechanisms and Clinical Implications, Raven, New York, 1981.

17. Bray GA, York DA. Hypothalamic and genetic obesity in experimental animals: an autonomic and endocrine hypothesis. Physiol Rev 1979;19:719–809.

18. Bouchard C, Bray GA, eds. Regulation of Body Weight: Biological and Behavioral Mechanisms, vol 7. John Wiley, West Sussex, UK, 1996.

19. Bouchard C, ed. Genetics of Obesity. CRC, Boca Raton, FL, 1994.

20. Bouchard C. Genetics of obesity: an update on molecular markers. Int J Obes Relat Metab Disord 1995; 19(Suppl 3):S10–S14.

21. Montague CT, Farooqi IS, Whitehead JP, et al. Congenital leptin deficiency is associated with severe early-onset obesity in humans. Nature 1997;387:903–908.

22. Buskirk ER. Underwater weighing and body density: a review of procedures. In: Brozek J, Henschel A, eds. Techniques for Measuring Body Composition. National Academy of Sciences, National Research Council, Washington, DC, 1981, pp. 148–164.

23. Pierson RN Jr, Lin DH, Phillips RA. Total body potassium in health: effects of age, sex, height, and fat. Am J Physiol 1974;226:206–208.

24. Lukaski HC, Johnson PE, Bolonchuk WW, et al. Assessment of fat-free mass using bioelectrical impedance measurements of the human body. Am J Clin Nutr 1985;41:810–817.

25. Figlewicz DP, Schwartz MW, Seeley RJ, et al. Endocrine regulation of food intake and body weight. J Lab Clin Med 1996;127:328–332.

26. Rohner-Jeanrenaud F. A neuroendocrine reappraisal of the dual-center hypothesis: its implication for obesity and insulin resistance. Int J Obes Relat Metab Disord 1995;19:17–34.

27. Danforth E Jr, Burger A. The role of thyroid hormones in the control of energy expenditure. Clin Endocrinol Metab 1984;13:581–595.

28. Landsberg L, Young JB. The role of sympathoadrenal system in modulating energy expenditure. Clin Endocrinol Metab 1984;13:475–499.

29. Romieu I, Willett WC, Stampfer MJ, et al. Energy intake and other determinants of relative weight. Am J Clin Nutr 1988;47:406–412.

30. Dreon DM, Frey-Hewitt B, Ellsworth N, et al. Dietary fat: carbohydrate ratio and obesity in middle-aged men. Am J Clin Nutr 1988;47:995–998.

31. Woods SC, Chavez M, Park CR, et al. The evaluation of insulin as a metabolic signal influencing behavior via brain. Neurosci Biobehav Rev 1996;20:39–44.

32. Bray GA. Nutrient intake is modulated by peripheral peptide administration. Obes Res 1995;3(Suppl 4): 569A–572S.

33. Schwartz MW, Finglewitz DP, Woods SC, Porte D, et al. Insulin and the central regulation of energy balance: update. Endocr Rev 1992;13:387–414.

34. Woods SC, Porte D. Insulin and the set point regulation of body weight. In: Novin D, Bray GA, eds. Hunger: Basic Mechanisms AND Clinical Implications. Raven, New York, 1976, pp. 273–280.

35. Chapman IM, Goble EA, Wittert GA, et al. Effect of intravenous glucose and euglycemic insulin infusions on short-term appetite and food intake. Am J Physiol 1998;43:R596–R603.

36. Louis-Sylvestre J, LeMagnen J. Palatability and preabsorptive insulin release. Neurosci Biobehav Rev 1980;4(Suppl 1):43–45.
37. Wood R, Kissileff HR, Pi-Sunyer FX. Elevated post-prandial insulin levels do not induce satiety in normal-weight humans. Am J Physiol 1984;247:R745–R749.
38. Kolaczynski JW, Nyce MR, Considine RV, et al. Acute and chronic effects of insulin on leptin production in humans: studies in vivo and in vitro. Diabetes 1996;45:699–701.
39. Zhang Y, Proenca R, Maffei M, et al. Positional cloning of the mouse obese gene and its human homologue. Nature 1994;372:425–432.
40. Campfield L, Smith F, Guisez Y, et al. Recombinant mouse OB protein: evidence for a peripheral signal linking adiposity and central neural networks. Science 1995;269:546–548.
41. Halaas J, Gajiwala M, Maffei M, et al. Weight reducing effects of the plasma protein encoded by the ob gene. Science 1995;269:543–546.
42. Frankish HM, Dryden S, Hopkins D, et al. Neuropeptide Y, the hypothalamus, and diabetes: insights into the central control of metabolism. Peptide 1995;16:757–771.
43. Billington CJ, Briggs JE, Harker S, et al. Neuropeptide Y in hypothalamic paraventricular nucleus: a center coordinating energy metabolism. Am J Physiol 1994;266:R1765–R1770.
44. Erickson JC, Clegg KE, Palmiter RD. Sensitivity to leptin and susceptibility to seizures of mice lacking neuropeptide Y. Nature 1996;381:415–421.
45. Francoise Rohner-Jeanrenaud, Bernard Jeanrenaud. Obesity, leptin, and the brain. N Engl J Med 1996;334:324–325.
46. Considine RV, Sinha MK, Heinman ML, et al. Serum immunoreactive-leptin concentrations in normal-weight and obese humans. N Engl J Med 1996;334:292–295.
47. Resenbaum M, Nicolson M, Hirsch J, et al. Effects of gender, body composition, and menopause on plasma concentrations of leptin. J Clin Endocrinol Metab 1996;81:3424–3427.
48. Ostlund RE, Yang JW, Klein S, et al. Relation between plasma leptin concentration and body fat, gender, diet, age, and metabolic covariates. J Clin Endocrinol Metab 1996;81:3909–3913.
49. Sih R, Morley JE, Kaiser FE, et al. Testosterone replacement in older hypogonadal men: a 12-month randomized controlled trial. J Clin Endocrinol Metab 1997;82:1661–1667.
50. Strain GW, Zumoff B, Strain JJ, et al. Cortisol production in obesity. Metabolism 1980;29:980–983.
51. Flier JS, Foster DW. Eating disorders: obesity, anorexia nervosa, and bulimia. In: Wilson JD, et al., eds. William's Textbook of Endocrinology. Philadelphia, PA, 1998, pp. 1061–1097.
52. Kyle LH, Ball M, Doolan PD. Effect of thyroid hormone on body composition in myxedema and obesity. N Eng J Med 1966;275:12–18.
53. Vermeulen A, Verdonck L. Sex hormone concentrations in postmenopausal women. Relation to obesity, fat mass, age, and years postmenopause. Clin Endocrinol 1978;9:59–64.
54. Rebuffe-Scrive M, Enk L, Crona N, et al. Fat cell metabolism in different regions in women. J Clin Invest 1985;75:1973–1976.
55. Karam JH. Type II diabetes and syndrome X: pathogenesis and glycemic management. Endocrinol Metab Clin North Am 1992;21:329–350.
56. Reaven G. Role of insulin resistance in human disease. Diabetes 1988;37:1595–1607.
57. Genest J, Cohn JS. Clustering of cardiovascular risk factors: targeting high-risk individuals. Am J Cardiol 1995;76:8A–20A.
58. Glass AR, Swerdloff RS, Bray GA, et al. Low serum testosterone and sex hormone binding globulin in massively obese men. J Clin Endocrinol Metab 1977;45:1211–1219.
59. Amtruda JM, Harman SM, Pourmotabbed G, et al. Depressed plasma testosterone and fractional binding of testosterone in obese males. J Clin Endocrinol Metab 1978;47:268–271.
60. Lew EA, Garfinkel L. Variation in mortality by weight among 750,000 men and women. J Chronic Dis 1979;32:563–567.
61. Folsom AR, Kaye SA, Sellers TA, et al. Body fat distribution and 5-year risk of death in older women. JAMA 1993;269:483–487.
62. Bjorntorp P. Regional pattern of fat distribution. Ann Int Med 1985;103:994–995.
63. Despres JP, Lemieux S, Lamarche B, et al. The insulin resistance-dyslipemic syndrome: contribution of visceral obesity and therapeutic implications. Int J Obes 1995;19:S76–S86.
64. Lissner L, Odell PM, D'Agostino RB, et al. Variability of body weight and health outcomes in the Framingham population. N Engl J Med 1991;324:1839–1844.
65. Andres R, Elahi D, Tobin JD, et al. Impact of age on weight goals. Ann Intern Med 1985:103:1030–1033.

66. Borrelli R, Isernia C, Di Biase G, et al. Mortality rate, causes and predictive factors of death in severely obese patients. Int J Vitam Nutr Res 1988;58:343–350.
67. Bouchard C, Bray GA, Hubbard VS. Basic and clinical aspects of regional fat distribution. Am J Clin Nutr 1990;52:946–950.
68. Lemieux S, Prud'homme D, Bouchard C, et al. Six differences in the relation of visceral adipose tissue accumulation to total body fatness. Am J Clin Nutr 1993;58:463–467.
69. Lemieux S, Prud'homme D, Tremblay A, et al. Anthropometric correlates to changes in visceral adipose tissue over 7 years in women. Int J Obes 1996;20:618–624.
70. Haarbo J, Marslew U, Gotfredsen A, et al. Postmenopausal hormone replacement therapy prevents central distribution of body fat after menopause. Metabolism 1991;40:1323–1326.
71. Pouliot MC, Despres JP, Lemieux S, et al. Waist circumference and abdominal sagittal diameter: rest simple anthropometric indexes of abdominal visceral adipose tissue accumulation and related cardiovascular risk in men and women. Am J Cardiol 1994;73:460–468.
72. Lemieux S, Prud'homme D, Bouchard C, et al. A single threshold value of waist girth to identify non-obese and overweight subjects with excess visceral adipose tissue. Am J Clin Nutr 1996;64:685–692.
73. Alaud-Din A, Meterissian S, Lisbona R, et al. Assessment of cardiac function in patients who were morbidly obese. Surgery 1990;108:809–920.
74. Stevens V, Corrigan S, Obarzanek E, et al. Weight loss intervention in phase I of the trials of hypertension prevention. Arch Intern Med 1993;153:849–858.
75. Kaplen NM. Clinical Hypertension, 6th ed. Williams & Wilkins, New York, 1994.
76. Unger RH, Foster DW. Diabetes mellitus. In: Wilson JD, et al., ed. William's Textbook of Endocrinology, Philadelphia, PA, 1998, pp. 973–1059.
77. Chen M, Bergman RN, Pacini G, et al. Pathogenesis of age-related glucose intolerance in man: Insulin resistance and decreased B-cell dysfunction. J Clin Endocrinol Metab 1985;60–13–20.
78. Reaven GM and Staff of the Palo Alto GRECC Aging Study Unit. Beneficial effect of moderate weight loss in older patients with non-insulin-dependent diabetes mellitus poorly controlled with insulin. Am Geriatr Soc 1985;33:93.
79. Grundy SM, Barnett JP. Metabolic and health complications of obesity. Disease-a Month 1990;36:645–658.
80. Despres JP. Lipoprotein metabolism in visceral obesity. Int J Obes 1991;15:45–52.
81. Sharp JT, Barrocas M, Chokrovertys C. The cardiorespiratory effects of obesity. Clin Chest Med 1980;1:103–108.
82. Blundell JE, Halford JCG. Pharmacological aspects of obesity treatment: towards the 21st century. Int J Obes 1995;19(Suppl 3):S51–S55.
83. Flynn MA, Irvin W, Krause G. The effect of folate and cobalamin on osteoarthritic hands. J Am Coll Nutr 1994;13:351–356.
84. Poehlamn ET, Toth MJ, Fonong T. Exercise, substrate utilization and energy requirements in the elderly. In J Obes Relat Metab Disord 1995;19(Suppl 4):S93–S96.
85. Segal KR, Pi-Sunyer FX. Exercise and obesity. Med Clin North Am 1989;3:217–236.
86. Seim HC, Holtmeier KB. Treatment of obesity in the elderly. Am Fam Physician 1993;47:1183–1189.
87. Schwartz RS. Exercise training in the treatment of diabetes mellitus in elderly patients. Diabetes Care11990;3(Suppl 2):77–85.
88. Colley CA, Lucas LM. Polypharmacy: the cure becomes the disease. J Gen Intern Med 1993;8:278–283.
89. Bray GA. Use and abuse of appetite-suppressant drugs in the treatment of obesity. Ann Intern Med 1993;119:707–713.
90. National Task Force on the Prevention and Treatment of Obesity. Pharmacotherapy in the management of obesity. JAMA 1996;276:1907–1915.
91. Khan MA, Herzog CA, St Peter JV, et al. The prevalence of cardiac valvular insufficiency assessed by transthoracic echocardiography in obese patients treated with appetite-suppressant drugs. N Engl J Med 1998;339:713–718.
92. Gray DS, Fujioka K, Bray GA, et al. A randomized double-blind clinical trial of fluoxetine in obese diabetics. Int J Obes 1992;16(Suppl 4):S67–S72.
93. Connolly VM, Gallagher A, Kesson CM. A study of fluoxetine in obese elderly patients with type 2 diabetes. Diabetic Med 1995;12:416–418.
94. Rolls BJ, Shide DJ, Thorwart ML, et al. Sibutramine reduces food intake in non-dieting women with obesity. Obes Res 1998;6:1–11.

95. Astrup A, Breum L, Toubro S, et al. The effect and safety of an ephedrine/caffeine compound compared to ephedrine, caffeine, and placebo in obese subjects on an energy restricted diet: a double-blind trial. Int J Obes 1992;16:269–277.
96. Lee A, Morley JM. Metformin decreases food consumption and induces weight loss in subjects with obesity with type II noninsulin dependent diabetes. Obes Res 1998;6:47–53.
97. Calles-Escandon J, Ballor D, Harvey-Berino J, et al. Amelioration of the inhibition of fibrinolysis in elderly, obese subjects by moderate energy intake restriction. Am J Clin Nutr 1996;64:7–11.
98. Visser M, Langlois J, Guralnik JM, et al. High body fatness, but not low fat-free mass, predicts disability in older men and women: the Cardiovascular Health Study. Am J Clin Nutr 1998;68:584–590.

Nutrition, Exercise, and Aging

David R. Thomas, MD, FACP

INTRODUCTION

Tantalizing research in nutrition in the past few years has promised the possibility of extending life span, delaying the effects of aging, preventing chronic disease, and augmenting the body's immune function. Yet, the current state of the art seems to raise more questions than solutions.

Nutritional research often seems to be proving common sense. Everyone agrees that malnutrition is bad for humans, or for any organism. The presence of malnutrition has been associated with increased mortality, more infections, and oxidative stress leading potentially to degenerative disease (1–3). Reversal of the effects of bad nutrition logically should result in demonstrable improvement in these variables.

Piecing together the complex relationship of nutrition to outcomes is difficult. Each of the components of this review—nutrition, exercise, and aging—are complex enough, individually. When combined, the degree of complexity increases logarithmically. The discussion will be limited to aged individuals, arbitrarily defined as over 65 yr old.

NUTRITION AND AGING

Aging is associated with a lower energy intake. Hallfrisch et al. (4) has shown a decline in total daily energy requirements after age 40 (Fig. 1). On average, persons over the age of 70 yr consume one-third less calories, compared to younger persons. In Fig. 2, energy intake of older men (40–74 yr old) is nearly one-third less (2100–2300 calories/d) than

From: *Contemporary Endocrinology: Endocrinology of Aging*
Edited by: J. E. Morley and L. van den Berg © Humana Press Inc., Totowa, NJ

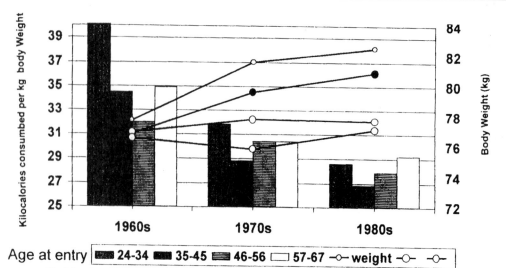

Age at entry | ▨ 24-34 ▦ 35-45 ▤ 46-56 ☐ 57-67 —○— weight —○— —○— |

Subjects decreased caloric consumption (kcal/kg body weight) for each decade, but body weight (kg) increased for each decade. *From Hallrisch et al. J Gerontology[5]*

Fig. 1. Calorie consumption and body weight.

men aged 24–34 yr old (2700 calories/d) *(5)*. Even lower caloric consumption has been reported. Sixteen to 18% of community-dwelling elderly persons consume less that 1000 kcal daily *(6)*.

Total caloric food intake is determined by energy needs *(7)*. Daily energy requirements are made up of three distinct components: the resting energy expenditure (REE), the thermic effect of food, and the thermic effect of exercise. REE decreases with age, primarily because of a decrease in muscle mass, but the other thermic effects remain relatively constant *(8)*. Active older adults have a higher REE than sedentary older adults *(9)*, and thus reach energy intakes equal to or exceeding younger persons. Lower energy expenditure in inactive older adults may be responsible for their observed lower energy intake, but the requirements for nearly all nutrients does not decline with age *(10)*.

Nutrient requirements are expressed as a Recommended Dietary Allowance (RDA). RDAs are based on the minimal requirement for 95% of the population, based on a reference male, age 25, height 5 ft 10 in, weight 150 lb, with a normal body composition *(11)*. There are no recommendations for persons older than 70 yr, because of a higher prevalence of chronic disease, insufficient data, and heterogeneity of the population. Lower energy requirements were assumed for older persons, and no adjustment for differences in sex after age 51 yr were made *(10)*.

Lower energy intakes, at times reaching levels that produce macro- and micronutrient malnutrition, are common in surveyed elderly populations. The chief reason for this decline seems to be lower energy expenditure. Neurotransmitter regulators of food intake also have been implicated in anorexia of aging. Gastrointestinal hormones, including cholecystokinin, gastrin-releasing peptide, somatostatin, and bombesin regulate satiety in humans, to varying degrees *(12)*. Changes in these regulatory hormones and their effect on malnutrition is poorly understood.

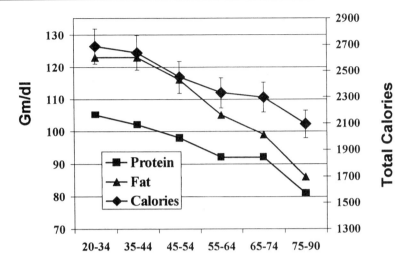

Fig. 2. Intake of protein, fat, and calories by decade.

NUTRITION AND LIFE-SPAN

Nutritional intake affects both duration and quality of life. Improvement in human life-span, and life expectancy as a society, is clearly related to improvement in nutritional status *(13)*. Life-span in individual animals is clearly related to nutrient intake. Restriction of calories, short of producing malnutrition, has been associated with increased life-span in rodents (Fig. 3; *13)*. Caloric restriction remains the only known way to consistently slow aging in higher organisms.

Whether this effect occurs in humans is controversial. Part of the difficulty stems from the fact that natural experiments or observations must substitute for controlled trials in humans. Epidemiological studies have used body mass index (BMI = weight/height^2) as a surrogate for caloric intake. The relationship between mortality and BMI has been reported as no association, inverse association, a J-shaped curve, or a U-shaped curve *(14)*. In studies adjusted for cigarette smoking and weight loss caused by illness, all-cause mortality was lower when BMI was 15–20% below the national average *(15,16)*. Weight loss of more than 5% in women 60–74 yr old was associated with a twofold increase in risk of disability over time, compared to women who did not lose weight *(17)*. This effect persisted when adjusted for age, smoking, education, study duration, and health conditions.

Short-term reductions in caloric intake (dieting) have favorable effects on blood pressure, cholesterol, and metabolic rate. These benefits require at least a 20% reduction in caloric intake *(18)*. Whether this degree of long-term caloric reduction could be sustained in elderly populations is questionable.

MALNUTRITION AND AGING

The prevalence of nutritionally related disorders in older adults depends on the population studied. The magnitude of malnutrition in community-dwelling elderly persons depends on living situation and the variables used to diagnose malnutrition. Undernutrition reportedly occurs in 5–12% of community-dwelling older persons *(19)*.

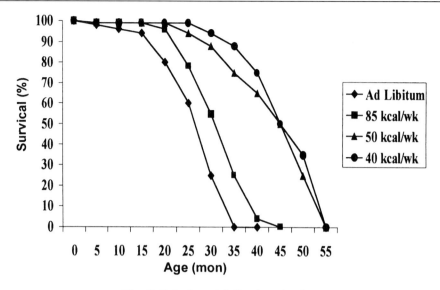

Fig. 3. Caloric restriction in animals.

Thirty to 40% of men and women over 75 yr are at least 10% underweight. Approximately 25% of males and 50% of females over 65 yr are obese (BMI >25). In dietary intake studies, 10% of men and 20% of women have intakes of protein below the RDA; one-third consume less calories than the RDA. Fifty percent of older adults have intakes of minerals and vitamins less than the RDA, and 10–30% have subnormal levels of minerals and vitamins *(20)*.

The highest prevalence of malnutrition is seen among nursing home residents. Estimates of the prevalence of protein-energy malnutrition in cross-sectional studies of nursing home patients range from 23 to 85% *(21,22)*. In a prospective study of admissions to a long-term care facility, 54% of patients were malnourished at the time of admission *(23)*. Variables widely associated with undernutrition, including body wt, midarm muscle circumference, and visceral protein levels, are low in at least 50% of nursing home patients, suggesting widespread protein-energy malnutrition. Blood levels are frequently low for both water-soluble and fat-soluble vitamins *(24)*.

Protein-calorie malnutrition is common among hospitalized older adults. In this population, ranges of malnutrition prevalence of 32–50% have been reported *(25,26)*. Nutritional status has been shown to deteriorate following hospital admission. When patients who had no current nutritional deficits and no predicted risk of developing deficits at hospital admission were followed, significant decreases in albumin, total lymphocyte count, triceps skinfold thickness, and midarm circumference occurred in all patients by 3 wk. The only nutritional parameter remaining unchanged at 3 wk was percent of ideal body wt *(27)*. Reasons for this high prevalence include poor recognition and monitoring of nutritional status *(28–30)*, and forced inadequate intake of nutrients for days at a time *(31,32)*. In this setting, severity of illness and other factors limit the patient's ability to consume an adequate diet.

Malnutrition is a risk factor for postoperative morbidity and mortality. One study *(33)* demonstrated significantly higher mortality among surgical patients with greater than 20% weight loss preoperatively. Seltzer et al. *(34)* noted a fourfold increase in complications, and a sixfold increase in mortality, among medical-surgical patients with a serum albumin less than 35 g/L.

Despite the correlations of markers for malnutrition and poor clinical outcome, it is difficult to determine whether malnutrition is casually associated with morbidity and mortality, or whether associated with age, functional status, and underlying disease. It is difficult to separate nutritional factors from confounding variables. Increased morbidity and mortality have been equally associated with many nonnutritional variables. Regression models, consisting of an activities-of-daily-living score, serum albumin, weight loss, number of medications, renal disease, income, pressure ulcers, dysphagia, and midarm muscle circumference, predict morbidity and mortality *(35)*. At 1 yr, the best predictors for mortality were the discharge serum albumin, weight loss, self-dressing ability, and discharge diagnosis of cardiac arrhythmia, in descending order. The combination of these factors was a better predictor than single individual variables *(36)*.

The most cogent proof of the effect of undernutrition in elderly populations would be a reversal of anthropomorphic and biochemical variables after replenishing nutrients. The logic of this has been tested in several studies. In a long-term care geriatric hospital, 115 of 435 (29%) newly admitted patients were malnourished by a index score *(37)*. Patients randomly received either a standard diet or standard diet plus twice daily nutritional supplementation. Thirty-nine intervention patients refused to take the supplement, and eight control patients received supplement. At 8 wk, 41% of malnourished patients who received dietary supplements improved, but only 18% of malnourished patients who did not receive nutritional supplements improved. Although improvement was demonstrated, 59% of supplemented patients did not improve during follow up. This failure rate may be higher, because patients who were offered supplementation, but refused ingestion, are not included. Both experimental and control groups showed a decrease in weight index, triceps skinfold thickness, and midarm circumference after 26 wk, although the initially nonmalnourished group who received supplemental feedings showed less decline. There were no differences in prealbumin, albumin, or antitrypsin levels between groups. The mortality rate was higher (19 vs 9%) in the initially malnourished group.

In a geriatric hospital, 87 consecutive medical patients were randomized into a placebo-controlled trial of a glucose drink plus vitamin A, B_1, B_2, B_3, and B_6 supplements. Compliance with the supplement was poor, with only one-third of subjects consuming more than 50% of the offered drink. Even when the analysis was limited to compliant subjects, there was no beneficial effect observed *(38)*. Severely malnourished patients (BMI <15 kg/m^2) were excluded in this study.

Considerable controversy surrounds the question of whether nutritional supplements in the preoperative phase can improve surgical outcome. Several small studies have demonstrated improvement in postoperative outcome with preoperative total parenteral nutrition (TPN) *(39,40)*. The largest study to date, the Veterans Administration Total Parenteral Nutrition Cooperative Study *(41)*, did not demonstrate any overall difference in morbidity and mortality between those receiving TPN and those who did not. In fact, increased infections were noted in the TPN group. Nevertheless, among the subgroup of 33 elderly patients defined as severely malnourished, using a combination of albumin and body wt, there were fewer noninfectious complications, and no increase in infectious complications among those receiving TPN. The consensus seems to be developing that delaying surgery to provide preoperative TPN is not warranted, except possibly for the severely malnourished. Even in the severely malnourished, evidence supporting pre-operative TPN is inconclusive *(42)*.

Several studies have shown a potential beneficial effect in hip surgery patients. Bastow et al. *(43)* studied 744 women with hip fractures. From this sample, 21 well-nourished patients served as a control, and 122 thin or very thin patients were randomized to receive either 1000 kcal of supplemental nasogastric feedings or no supplement. Only 43 patients completed 24–28 d of nasogastric feedings. Tube fed patients in the thin group achieved independent mobility in 10 d, compared to 12 d in the control group (*P* <0.05). The very thin nasogastric-fed group achieved independent mobility in 16 d, compared to 23 d in the control group (*P* < 0.05).

Delmi et al. provided a 254-kcal, 20-g protein oral supplement to 27 randomly selected patients with femoral neck fracture. After a mean of 32 d, the supplemented patients had a lower in-hospital complication rate (14 vs 44%, *P* <0.05), and a shorter hospital stay (24 vs 40 d, *P* <0.02) *(44)*.

These data suggest that malnutrition in elderly persons is common, associated with poor clinical outcomes, and may be reversible. The failure of controlled clinical trials to demonstrate a benefit from nutritional interventions could stem from three possibilities. First, a patient's course could be uninfluenced by nutritional interventions. Second, the nutritional state may be irreversible, or the intervention applied too late in the clinical course. Finally, methodological flaws in the study may have failed to demonstrate an effect. The effect of acute or chronic illness on the prevalence of malnutrition is difficult to distinguish. Illness and other factors limiting the voluntary intake of nutritional supplements cloud the effect of these trials. Most acute illness and many chronic diseases affect body mass and biochemical variables used to measure malnutrition. Improvement in outcomes is difficult to demonstrate in studies to date, but suggestions of an effect in patients with fractures is promising.

EXERCISE AND AGING

Most elderly persons would have to be defined as sedentary. Only 7.5% of persons 65 yr and older participate in aerobic activity. Even fewer participate in resistive exercise training *(45)*.

The most important functional change that occurs with aging is a reduction in active skeletal muscle. However, this decline in muscle mass occurs in both sedentary and active aging adults *(46–48)*. Both dynamic, static, and isokinetic muscle strength decreases with age *(49)*. A substantial 65% of older men and women report that they cannot lift 10 lb using their arms *(50)*. This decline in strength has been hypothesized to be a reason for some of the functional decline that occurs with aging *(51)*. Nonmuscle mass is relatively preserved with aging, leading to an increase in total body fat.

A research agenda has developed to ascertain whether this decline in strength and function is inevitable, or related to habitual inactivity. The muscle loss that occurs with aging has been hypothesized to result from either disease (hypogonadism, thyroid disease, growth hormone deficiency), medications (diuretics, corticosteroids), disuse, or malnutrition (Table 1; *52*).

Maximal oxygen consumption (VO_{2max}) declines with age at a rate of 3 to 8% per decade after age 30 yr *(53,54)*. The major contribution to VO_{2max} is lean muscle mass. When corrected for muscle mass, there is no important decline in VO_{2max} with aging *(55)*.

Table 1
Causes of Sarcopenia in Aging

Disease	Disuse
Hypogonadism	Malnutrition
Growth hormone	Medications
deficiency	Diuretics
Thyroid disease	Corticosteroids

Table 2
Improvement in Strength with Exercise

Ref.	Mean age	Sex	Type of exercise	Strength improvement (%)	Site
58	70	Men	Dynamic	23	Elbow
58	22	Men	Dynamic	30	Elbow
59	>65	Men	Dynamic	48	Elbow
60	65	Men	Dynamic	1107	Knee
61	69	Women	Dynamic	28–115	All
62	71	Men	Static	9–22	Knee
63	22–65	Men	Dynamic	2.9–7.5	Knee
64	90	Both	Dynamic	174	Knee

Additionally, physically active older men have a higher VO_{2max} than inactive younger men (56). Thus, although there is a decline in exercise capacity with aging, there is reason to believe that this trend is reversible.

Consistent studies in younger adults show that muscle strength and mass increases with high-intensity training (70–90% of one repetition maximum). In older men, upper arm strength has increased by 23–48% (57,58), and lower extremity strength by 107–226% (59). Similar increases, in the range of 28–115%, have been reported in older women (60). Previous studies of exercise in healthy older adults have shown only small increases in strength. Aniansson and Gustafsson (61) demonstrated a 9–22% increase in lower extremity strength at 12 wk in healthy men aged 69–74 yr. Similar results were demonstrated in men age 56–65 yr, after 15 wk of exercise (Table 2; 62).

The commonality of studies showing small vs large improvement in muscle strength has been the intensity of the exercise intervention. The data suggest that exercise programs must be high-intensity (70–90% of one repetition maximum) rather than low-intensity (against gravity) in order to produce benefit. There has been a justifiable concern about applying high-intensity exercise programs in older adults. Recent research confirms not only benefit, but also safety. The benefit of strength training has been demonstrated to exist even in frail, institutionalized, elderly men and women. After 8 wk of training in volunteers aged 90 ± 1 yr, muscle strength increased by 174 ± 31%, and midthigh muscle size by 9 ± 4.5% (63).

The benefit of exercise continues during training, and dissipates within a few weeks of ceasing exercise in both young and old adults. Thirty-two percent of the gain in muscle strength in institutionalized residents was lost within 4 wk of detraining.

A number of studies have shown a relationship between exercise and mortality. Older men who expend 500–3500 kcal/wk in exercise had lower death rates than nonexercisers

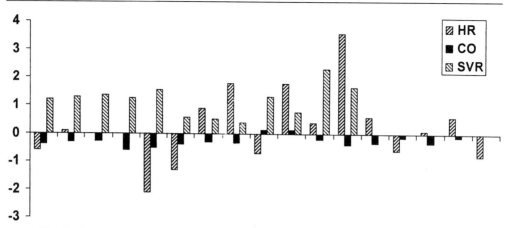

Fig. 4. Change in heart rate, cardiac output, and systemic vascular resistance at rest.

(64). The benefit of exercise seems to be independent of genetics. In a cohort study of twins (which removes genetic confounders), twins who exercised at a level of vigorous walking at least 6× monthly for 30 min were compared to twins who no or less exercise. The hazard ratio for death was 0.66 vs 0.44 (*P* = 0.005) in nonexercisers, compared to exercisers *(65)*.

Most of the data on the effect of exercise on disease is disease-specific. Cardiovascular function changes little at rest (Fig. 4), but declines at maximal exercise (Fig. 5). Exercise has been reported to benefit cardiovascular mortality. Persons over the age of 65 yr exercised by cycling at 70% of their age-adjusted maximal heart rate for 4 mo, and were then randomized to a home-exercise program with or without supervision. After 2 yr, new cardiovascular diagnoses were made in 2.5% of the supervised group, 2% of the nonsupervised group, and in 13% of the control group *(66)*. Some controversy over the relationship of exercise to cardiovascular disease continues. The Canadian Health Survey found no relationship between physical activity and coronary mortality *(67)*. The data on the cardioprotective effect of activity in women is not conclusive *(68,69)*.

Physiological control of glucose metabolism is thought to improve with exercise *(70)*. Increased activity, even of low intensity, improves insulin resistance and glycemic control *(71)*. This effect seems to reside in improved peripheral insulin action *(66,72)*. This effect is very short-lived, however: 10 d without exercise reverses the benefit *(73)*. Direct evidence for improved glucose metabolism in diabetic patients by physical training remains elusive *(74)*. Unfortunately, older patients who would benefit from help with glycemic control by exercise often are unable to exercise because of diabetic complications, such as cardiovascular or peripheral vascular disease.

Epidemiological studies show that physically active women have higher bone mineral content than less active women *(75,76)*. It is clear that exercise increases bone mineral content, and equally clear that bone mineral loss returns to baseline when exercise is stopped *(77)*. The type of exercise prescribed for osteoporosis is critical. Nonweight-bearing exercise does not affect bone loss *(78)*. No relationship between physical activity and cancer has been demonstrated *(67,79)*.

Finally, exercise as a lifetime habit may prevent premature death, because postponement of mortality results in increased life-span. Whether exercise advances life-span *per se* is not known.

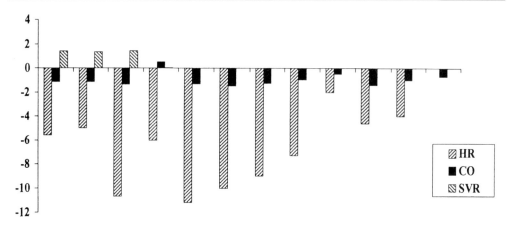

Fig. 5. Change in heart rate, cardiac output, and systemic vascular resistance at maximal resistance.

The problem associated with defining the benefit of exercise in population studies stems from difficulty in separating exercise from other variables. Because exercise may produce weight loss, improved cardiovascular fitness, and reduced blood pressure, these effects act as confounders to the outcome. Serious difficulties occur with selection bias in these studies, because persons persisting in an exercise program may be very different from the general population. The question remains whether exercise intervention can benefit large groups of sedentary persons, when the exercise must be continued indefinitely for most of their lives.

NUTRITION, EXERCISE, AND AGING

The association between nutrition and muscle function seems obvious, but the data supporting this association in older persons is sparse. Micronutrient malnutrition of magnesium, potassium, and zinc, in addition to inadequate macronutrients, may account for some muscle dysfunction, and has been shown to be reversible in younger persons *(80)*. Several studies have combined interventions aimed at improving muscle strength by nutritional supplements. Unfortunately, the results have been disappointing.

The improved muscle strength in 90 ± 1-yr-old, institutionalized persons was demonstrated, despite evidence of malnutrition in some subjects. Forty percent of these subjects were between 72 and 88% of ideal body wt, and did not meet RDA for micronutrients *(59)*.

Fiatarone et al. *(81)* randomized 100 long-term care residents, aged 87.1 ± 0.6 yr, to high-intensity exercise training. The groups were further randomized to receive 240 mL of nutritional supplementation or no supplementation. Although muscle strength increased by 113 ± 8% in the training group, the addition of a nutritional supplement did not improve outcome. In an earlier study *(82)* in 11 long-term care residents, the addition of 560 kcal of a nutritional supplement did not increase muscle strength, but computed tomography of the thigh showed more gain in muscle mass in the supplemented group. Nutritional intervention may have been too small or the observation period too short to detect a difference in outcome. When 34 healthy elderly persons who completed a daily 19-mile walk for 4 d were compared to 175 younger healthy blood donors, using two different nutritional risk instruments, undernutrition was diagnosed in 6–21% of elderly persons *(83)*.

Data such as this suggests that malnutrition either conveys no functional limitation, the intervention is not effective, or the parameters used to diagnose malnutrition are inadequate.

SUMMARY

Nutritional intake declines with aging. This seems to be primarily because of a decrease in muscle mass and resting energy expenditure. The sarcopenia that accompanies aging is probably caused by disuse, rather than abnormalities in nutrition. Malnutrition is common in elderly persons, and often fails to be recognized or corrected. Weakness and decrease in muscle mass follow severe undernutrition, and should be remedied with nutritional replenishment.

Studies clearly indicate that high-intensity resistance exercise can improve both muscle strength and muscle mass, even in very old persons. However, adding nutritional supplements to the exercise regimen do not appear to improve strength, but may increase muscle mass slightly more than nonsupplemented controls. Improvement in muscle strength may improve walking distance, stair-climbing, and balance, thus reducing falls.

REFERENCES

1. Young ME. Malnutrition and wound healing. Heart Lung 1988;17 60–67.
2. Dempsey DT, Mullen JL, Buzby GP. The link between nutritional status and clinical outcome: can nutritional intervention modify it? Amer J Clin Nutr 1988;47(Suppl 2):352–356.
3. Detsky AS, Baker JP, O'Rourke K, et al. Predicting nutrition-associated complications for patients undergoing gastrointestinal surgery. J Parenter Enteral Nutr 1987;11:440–446.
4. Hallfrisch J, Muller D, Drinkwater D, Tobin J, Andres R Continuing diet trends in men: the Baltimore Longitudinal Study of Aging (1961–1987). J Gerontol 1990;45:M186–M191.
5. McGandy RB, Barrows CH Jr, Spanias A, Meredity A, Stone JL, Norris AH. Nutrient intake and energy expenditure in men of different ages. J Gerontol 1966;21:581–587.
6. Abraham S, Carroll MD, Dresser CM, et al. Dietary intake of persons 1–74 years of age in the United States. Advance Data from Vital and Health Statistics of the National Center for Health Statistics No. G, Rockville, MD, Public Health Service, 1977.
7. Durnin JVGA. Energy intake, energy expenditure, and body composition in the elderly. In: Chandra RK, ed. Nutrition, Immunity and Illness in the Elderly. Pergamon, New York, 1985, pp. 19–33.
8. Kendrick ZY, Nelson-Steen S, Scafidi K. Exercise, aging, and nutrition. South Med J 1994;87:S50–S60.
9. Poehlman ET, McAuliffe TL, Van Houten DR, et al. Influence of age and endurance training on metabolic rate and hormones in healthy men. Am J Physiol 1990;259:E66–E72.
10. Munro HN, Suter PM, Russel RM. Nutritional requirements of the elderly. Ann Rev Nutr 1987;7:23–49.
11. Food and Nutrition Board, National Research Council. Recommended Dietary Allowances, 10th ed. National Academy Press, Washington, DC, 1990.
12. Morley JE, Silver AJ. Anorexia in the elderly. Neurobiol Aging 1988;9:9–16.
13. Fogel RW. New sources and new techniques for the study of secular trends in nutritional status, health, mortality and the process of aging. Historical Methods 1993;26:5–43.
14. Weindruch R, Sohal RS. Caloric intake and aging. N Engl J Med 1997;337:986–994.
15. Lee IM, Manson JE, Hennekens CH, Paffenbarger RS Jr. Body weight and mortality: a 27-year follow up of middle-aged adults. JAMA 1993;270:2823–2828.
16. Manson JE, Willett WC, Stampfer MJ, et al. Body weight and mortality among women. N Engl J Med 1995;33:677–685.
17. Launer LJ, Harris LT, Rumpel C, Madans J. Body mass index, weight change and risk of mobility disability in middle-aged and older women. JAMA 1994;271:1083–1098.
18. Velthuis-te Wierik EJ, van den Berg H, Schaafsma G, Hendriks HF, Brouwer A. Energy restrictions: a useful intervention to retard human ageing? Results of a feasibility study. Eur J Clin Nutr 1994;48: 138–148.
19. Sliver AJ. Malnutrition. In: Beck JC, ed. Geriatrics Review Syllabus. A Core Curriculum in Geriatric Medicine. Book 1: Syllabus and Questions. American Geriatrics Society, New York, 1991, pp. 99–104.

20. Ritchie CR, Thomas DR. Aging. In: Heimburger DC, Weinsier RL, eds. Handbook of Clinical Nutrition, 3rd ed. Mosby, St. Louis, 1997, pp. 154–164.
21. Sliver AJ, Morley JE, Strome LS, Jones D, Vickers L. Nutritional status in an academic nursing home. J Am Geriatr Soc 1988; 36:487–491.
22. Shaver HJ, Loper JA, Lutes RA. Nutritional status of nursing home patients. J Parenter Enteral Nutr 1980;4:367–370.
23. Thomas DR, Verdery RL, Gardner LD, Kant A. Prospective outcome of malnutrition in nursing home patients. J Parenter Enteral Nutr 1991;15:400–404.
24. Drinka PJ, Goodwin JS. Prevalence and consequences of vitamin deficiency in the nursing: a critical review. J Am Geriatr Soc 1991;39:1008–1017.
25. Willard MD, Gilsdorf RB, Price RA. Protein-calorie malnutrition in a community hospital. JAMA 1980, 243:1720–1722.
26. Bistrian BR, Blackburn GL, Vitale J, Cochran D, Naylor J. Prevalence of malnutrition in general medical patients. JAMA 1976;35:1567–1570.
27. Pinchcofsky GD, Kaminski MV Jr. Increasing malnutrition during hospitalization: documentation by a nutritional screening program. J Am Coll Nutr 1985;4:471–479.
28. Sullivan DH, Moriarty MS, Chernoff R, et al. Patterns of care: an analysis of the quality of nutritional care routinely provided to elderly hospitalized veterans. J Parenter Enteral Nutr 1989;13:249–254.
29. McNab H, Restivo R, Ber L, et al. Dietetic quality assurance practices in Chicago area hospitals. J Am Diet Assoc 1987;85:635–637.
30. Kamath SK, Lawler M, Smith AE, et al. Hospital malnutrition: a 33-hospital screening study. J Am Diet Assoc 1986;86:203–206.
31. Tobias AL, Van Itallie TB. Nutritional problems of hospitalized patients. J Am Diet Assoc 1977;71: 253–257.
32. Riffer J. Malnourished patients feeding rising costs. Hospitals 1986;60:86.
33. Studly HO. Percentage of weight loss: a basic indicator of surgical risk in patients with chronic peptic ulcer. JAMA 1936;106:458–460.
34. Seltzer MH, Bastidas JA, Cooper DM, Engler P, Slocum B, Fletcher HS. Instant nutritional assessment. J Parenter Enteral Nutr 1979;3:157–159.
35. Sullivan DH, Walls RC, Lipschitz DA. Protein-energy undernutrition and the risk of mortality within 1 year of hospital discharge in a select population of geriatric rehabilitation patients. Am J Clin Nutr 1991;53:599–605.
36. Sullivan DH, Walls RC, Bopp MM. Protein-energy undernutrition and the risk of mortality within one year of hospital discharge: a follow-up study. J Am Geriatr Soc 1995;43:507–512.
37. Larsson J, Unosson M, Ek A-C, Nilsson L, Thorslund S, Bjurulf P. Effect of dietary supplement on nutritional status and clinical outcome in 501 geriatric patients—a randomized study. Clin Nutr 1990; 9:179–184.
38. Hogarth MB, Marshall P, Lovat LB, Palmer AJ, Frost CG, Fletcher AE, Nicholl CG, Bulpitt CJ. Nutritional supplementation in elderly medical in-patients: a double-blind placebo-controlled trial. Age and Aging 1996;25:453–457.
39. Mullen JL, Gertney MH, Buzby GP, Goodhart GL, Rosato EF. Implications of malnutrition in the surgical patient. Arch Surg 1979;114:121–125.
40. Mullen JL, Buzby GP, Matthews DC, et al. Reduction of operative morbidity and mortality by combined preoperative and postoperative nutrition support. Ann Surg 1980;192:604–613.
41. Veterans Affairs Total Parenteral Nutrition Cooperative Study Group. Perioperative total parenteral nutrition in surgical patients. N Engl J Med 1991;325:525–532.
42. Detsky AS. Parenteral nutrition—Is it helpful? N Engl J Med 1991;325:573–575.
43. Bastow MD, Rawlings J, Allison SP. Benefits of supplementary tube feeding after fractured neck of the femur: a randomized controlled trial. Br Med J 1983;278:1589–1592.
44. Delmi M, Rapin CH, Bengoa JM, et al. Dietary supplementation in elderly patients with fractured neck of the femur. Lancet 1990;335:1013–1016.
45. Teague ML, Hunnicutt BK. An analysis of the 1990 Public Health Service physical fitness and exercise objectives for older Americans. Health Values 1989;13:15–23.
46. Aniansson A, Sperling L, Rundgren A, Lehnberg E. Muscle function in 75-year-old men and women: A longitudinal study. Scand J Rehab Med 1983; 9:92–102.
47. Davies C, Thomas D, White M. Mechanical properties of young and elderly human muscle. Acta Med Scand 1985;711(Suppl):219–226.

48. Larron L, Grimby G, Karlsson J. Muscle strength and speed of movement in relation to age and muscle morphology. J Appl Physiol 1979;46:451–456.
49. Aniansson A, Grimby G, Rundgren A. Isometric and isodinetic quadriceps muscle strength in 70-year-old men and women. Scand J Rehab Med 1980;12:161–168.
50. Jette AM, Branch LG. Impairment and disability in the aged. J Chron Dis 1985;38:59–65.
51. Jette AM, Branch LG. The Framingham Disability Study. II. Physical disability among the aging. Am J Public Health 1981;71:1211–1216.
52. Fiatarone MA, Evans WJ. The etiology and reversibility of muscle dysfunction in the aged. J Gerontol 1993;48:77–83.
53. Astrand I. Aerobic work capacity in men and women. Act Physiol Scand 1960;49S:1–5.
54. Astrand I, Astrand P-O, Hallback I, et al. Reduction in maximal oxygen uptake with age. J Appl Physiol 1973;35:649–654.
55. Fleg JL, Lakatta EG. Loss of muscle mass is a major determinant of the age-related decline in maximal aerobic capacity. Circulation 1985;72S:464.
56. Steinhaus LA, Dustman RE, Rubling RO, Emmerson RY, Johnson SC, Shearer DE, Shigeoka JW, Bonekat WH. Cardio-respiratory fitness of young and older active and sedentary men. Br J Sports Med 1988;22:163–166.
57. Moritani T, DeVries H. Potential for gross muscle hypertrophy in older men. J Gerontol 1980;35:672–682.
58. Brown AB, McCartney N, Sale DG. Postitive adaptations to weightlifting training in the elderly. J Appl Physiol 1990;69:1725–1733.
59. Frontera WR, Meredith CN, O'Reilly KP, Knuttgen HG, Evans WJ. Strength conditioning in older men: skeletal muscle hypertrophy and improved function. J Appl Physiol 1988;64:1038–1044.
60. Charette SL, McEvoy L, Pyka G, Snow-Harter C, Guido D, Weswell RA, Marcus R. Muscle hypertrophy response to resistance training in older women. J Appl Physiol 1991;70:1912–1916.
61. Anniansson A, Gustafsson E. Physical training in elderly men. Clin Physiol 1981;1:87–98.
62. Larsson L. Physical training effects on muscle morphology in sedentary males of different ages. Med Sci Sports Exerc 1982:14:203–206.
63. Fiatarone MA, Marks EC, Ryan ND, Meredith CN, Lipsitz LA, Evans WJ. High-intensity strength training in nonagenarians. Effects on skeletal muscle. JAMA 1990;263:3029–3034.
64. Paffenbarger RS Jr, Hyde RT, Wing AL, Hsieh CC. Physical activity, all-cause mortality, and longevity of college alumni. N Engl J Med 1986;314:605–613.
65. Kujala UM, Kaprio J, Sarna S, Koskenvuo M. Relationship of leisure-time physical activity and mortality: the Finnish twin cohort. JAMA 1998;279:440–444.
66. Posner JD, German KM, Gitlin LN, et al. Effects of exercise training in the elderly on the occurrence and time to onset of cardiovascular diagnoses. J Am Geriatr Soc 1990;38:205–210.
67. Arraiz GA, Wigle DT, Mao Y. Risk assessment of physical activity and physical fitness in the Canada Health Survey Mortality Follow-up Study. J Clin Epidemiol 1992;45:419–428.
68. Kannel WE, Sorlie P. Some health benefits of physical activity: the Framingham Study. Arch Intern Med 1979;139:857–861.
69. Lapidus L, Bengtsson C. Socioeconomic factors and physical activity in relation to cardiovascular disease and death: a 12-year follow-up of participants in a population study of women in Gothenburg, Sweden. Br Heart J 1986;55:295–301.
70. Tonino RP. Effect of physical training on the insulin resistance of aging. Am J Physiol 1989;256:352–356.
71. Hollenbeck CB, Haskell W, Rosenthal M, Reaven GM. Effect of habitual physical activity on regulation of insulin-stimulated glucose disposal in older males. J Am Geriatr Soc 1984;33:273–277.
72. Kahn SE, Larson VG, Beard JC, et al. Effect of exercise on insulin action, glucose tolerance, and insulin secretion in aging. Am J Physiol 1990;258:E937–E943.
73. Heath GW, Gavin JR III, Hinderliter JM, Hagberg JM, Bloomfield SM, Holloszy JO. Effects of exercise and lack of exercise on glucose tolerance and insulin sensitivity. J Appl Physiol Respir Environ Exerc Physiol 1983;55:512–517.
74. Berger M, Berchtold P. The role of physical exercise and training in the management of diabetes mellitus. Bibl Nutr Dieta 1979;27:41–54.
75. Jacobsen PC, Beaver W, Grubb SA, et al. Bone density in women: college athletes and older athletic women. J Orthop Res 1984;2:328–332.
76. Stillman RJ, Lohman TG, Slaughter MH, et al. Physical activity and bone mineral content in women aged 30 to 85 years. Med Sci Sports Exerc 1986;18:576–580.

77. Dalsky GP, Stocke KS, Ehsani AA, et al. Weight-bearing exercise training and lumbar bone mineral content in postmenopausal women. Ann Intern Med 1988;108:824–828.
78. Sinaki M, Wahner HW, Offord KP, et al. Efficacy of nonloading exercises in prevention of vertebral bone loss in postmenopausal women: a controlled trial. Mayo Clin Proc 1989;64:762–769.
79. Lindstead KD, Tonstad S, Kuzma JW. Self-report of physical activity and patterns of mortality in Seventh-Day Adventist men. J Clin Epidemiol 1991;44:355–364.
80. Russell D, Prendergast P, Darby D, Garfinkel P, Whitwell J, Jeejeebhoy K. A companson between muscles function and body composition in anorexia nervosa: the effect of refeeding. Am J Clin Nutr 1983:38:229–237.
81. Fiatarone MA, O'Neill EF, Ryan ND, Clements KM, Solares GR, Nelson ME, et al. Exercise training and nutritional supplementation for physical fraility in very elderly people. N Engl J Med 1994;330:1769–1775.
82. Meredith CN, Frontera WR, O'Reilly KP, Evans WJ. Body composition in elderly men: effect of dietary modification during strength training. J Am Geriatr Soc 1992;40:155–162.
83. Naber TH, Bree A, Schermer TRJ, Bakkeren J, Bar B, Wild G, Katan MB. Specificity of indexes of malnutrition when applied to apparently healthly people: the effect of age. Am J Clin Nutr 1997;65:1721–1725.

15   The Sympathetic Nervous System

Mark A. Supiano, MD

INTRODUCTION

Altered function of the sympathetic nervous system (SNS), whether caused by age *per se* or by age-associated disease, may contribute to impaired homeostasis in aging. The SNS occupies a central role in the maintenance of homeostasis because of its involvement in the regulation of many important physiologic functions. Age-associated alterations in SNS regulation may therefore contribute to a decline in homeostatic control. Thus, it is important to review both normal age-associated changes in the SNS and changes that result from diseases that are prevalent among the elderly.

ADRENERGIC PHYSIOLOGY

The peripheral SNS provides innervation to the entire body through its postganglionic nerves, which innervate vascular smooth muscle, endocrine glands, and cardiac tissue. This organizational structure of the SNS permits systemic, as well as organ-specific, activation. Postganglionic sympathetic nerves synthesize, store, and, when activated, release norepinephrine (NE) as their primary neurotransmitter. Activation of a SNS terminal leads to fusion of the vesicles in which NE is stored with the presynaptic nerve terminal membrane, and release of NE into the synaptic cleft. Once released, the subsequent metabolic fate of NE is quite complex: The majority of NE undergoes reuptake by the presynaptic terminal (neuronal uptake, or uptake 1), a fraction (<20%) diffuses through the extravascular space and enters the circulation (NE appearance or spillover); and a portion diffuses across the synaptic cleft, where it either functions as an agonist for

From: *Contemporary Endocrinology: Endocrinology of Aging*
Edited by: J. E. Morley and L. van den Berg © Humana Press Inc., Totowa, NJ

postsynaptic adrenergic receptors, or is transported into nonneuronal cells, where it is subsequently degraded (nonneuronal metabolism, or uptake 2). As a consequence of this complex metabolic sequence, the plasma NE concentration provides very little information about the rate of NE release and the activity of the SNS. At any given point in time, it represents the net balance between the small fraction of the released NE that enters the circulation and its active removal from the circulation.

A combination of several factors determines the physiologic response resulting from SNS activation. Presynaptic input determines the intrasynaptic NE concentration, which is a function of the frequency of sympathetic nerve impulses and depolarizing action potentials, the SNS terminal density and NE content, and the synaptic cleft width. The postsynaptic effector cell response to NE is dependent on its predominant adrenergic receptor type, their density, and their binding affinity for agonists. Adrenergic receptors are divided into two major types, α and β, based on their response to stimulation by specific pharmacologic agonists. The ultimate cellular response is dictated by the extent of receptor–effector coupling between the adrenergic receptor and its effector. For example, some adrenergic receptors are linked to the catalytic unit of adenylyl cyclase by way of a series of stimulatory and inhibitory guanine nucleotide-binding proteins (G proteins). The regulation of adrenergic receptor responsiveness is controlled in part by the level of exposure to agonists, to the extent that there is either down- or upregulation of adrenergic receptor number, or a shift in the sensitivity to agonist stimulation generally mediated by way of alterations in receptor–effector coupling.

ASSESSMENT OF SYMPATHETIC NERVOUS SYSTEM FUNCTION

Sympathetic Nervous System Activity

Given this overview of adrenergic physiology, it follows that SNS function may be defined as the integration of SNS tone or activity (the input of NE into the neuroeffector junction) with the adrenergic responsiveness of the effector cell. The necessity for direct tissue sampling to determine NE tissue-specific activity, following an infusion of radiolabeled NE until there is equilibration with intraneuronal NE stores and measuring the rate of NE turnover in SNS terminals, precludes utilizing this methodology in human investigations. Several methods have been developed to assess SNS activity in humans. For the reasons discussed in the previous subheading, measurement of plasma NE levels may not provide a reliable estimate of SNS activity in all circumstances, because they only indirectly reflect the level of NE released from SNS terminals. Regional activity of the SNS has been determined by microneurography of sympathetic nerves innervating either skeletal muscle (commonly the peroneal nerve) or an organ (e.g., renal), and recording the firing rate of sympathetic activity. Another approach has utilized the isotope dilution principle, and employs an infusion of tracer-labeled NE to achieve steady-state levels and calculate the rates of NE appearance into and removal from the circulation. This method may be used to determine either systemic or regional, organ-specific NE kinetics, depending on the site from which samples are obtained. Although this methodology permits separation of the main determinants of plasma NE concentration, and, to that end, provides a better reflection of SNS activity, the rate of NE appearance into the circulation accounts for only a small amount of the NE released from SNS terminals, and fails to account for differences in NE removal mechanisms. Moreover, this steady-state approach is a one-compartment analysis, which assumes that all NE entry is into, and removal is from, a single compartment into which NE is directly released, and from which samples are obtained. The neuroanatomy and physiology of the adrenergic system, reviewed in the previous subheading, is clearly not consistent with a single compartment system. In fact, it has been shown that the disappearance of radioisotope-labeled NE from plasma is best described by a biexponential curve, indicating that there is a minimum of two compartments into which NE is distributed *(1)*. Analysis of these data with a minimal two-compartment model, using compartmental analysis, allows information to be obtained concerning the rate of NE entry into a compartment distinct from the vascular compartment from which plasma samples are obtained, the extravascular compartment. The rate of entry into the extravascular compartment more closely approximates the rate of NE release from SNS terminals, and provides a more direct estimate of systemic SNS activity. In addition, the two-compartment model permits determination of other NE kinetic parameters, including NE spillover fraction, volume of distribution, and clearance. This approach has been used to characterize NE kinetics in a number of different conditions, for example, to study the effects of upright posture *(2)*, dietary sodium restriction *(2,3)*, and therapy with propranolol *(4)*, desipramine *(5)*, and guanadrel *(6)*.

Adrenergic Receptor Responsiveness

The assessment of adrenergic receptor responsiveness may be made at several points along the receptor–effector–target-organ signal-transduction cascade. One consideration complicating reliance on a systemic physiologic response in older individuals is the extent to which age-related alterations in the target-organ system may influence the response. For example, some studies have determined the blood pressure (BP) response to systemic infusion of α-adrenergic agonists, to attempt to assess vascular α-adrenergic receptor responsiveness. Interpretation of these results is limited by the confounding effects of baroreceptor sensitivity, cardiac function, and the interactions of other compensatory systems that regulate BP. To circumvent some of these limitations, methodologies that examine more directly the in vivo response of blood vessels to infusions of vasoactive agents have been developed. These methods include determination of the change in the diameter of a dorsal hand vein just distal to an iv infusion of drug, and measurement of blood flow by venous occlusion plethysmography, or by Doppler ultrasound, during direct intra-arterial infusions of drug. Each of these methods permits the direct assessment of vascular response to adrenergic stimulation in the absence of confounding systemic effects. The heart rate (HR) response following stimulation by β-adrenergic agonists, as a measure of cardiac β-adrenergic responsiveness, provides another example of assessment of target-organ response.

Additional details concerning signal transduction mechanisms may be obtained in in vitro systems utilizing either tissue preparations or circulating blood cells that contain adrenergic receptors (e.g., lymphocyte β_2-adrenergic receptors and platelet α_2-adrenergic receptors). Receptor-binding properties, including total receptor density, as well as the affinity state of receptors coupled to adenylyl cyclase, may be derived from radioligand binding studies *(7)*. Detailed information about the coupling state of adrenergic receptors may be derived, enabling an interpretation of a change in adrenergic responsiveness to be made at the cellular level. Additional methods are available to assess the quantity and function of stimulatory and inhibitory guanine nucleotide-binding proteins, the extent of receptor phosphorylation, and the cellular effector response (stimulation or inhibition of adenylyl cyclase activity).

Because of the age-associated alterations in SNS function discussed above, the author hypothesized that impaired downregulation of α-adrenergic responsiveness, despite a comparable level of SNS activity, could contribute to higher BP in older hypertensive humans. To test this hypothesis, the author measured systemic SNS activity (arterial plasma NE levels and the extravascular NE release rate [NE_2] derived from ^{3}H-NE kinetics studies), and α-adrenergic receptor responsiveness in platelet membranes and forearm arterial vessels in normotensive and hypertensive healthy, older subjects (age 60–75 yr). Although plasma NE levels were similar, NE_2 tended to be greater in the hypertensive group (Fig. 1). In the hypertensive group, there was greater α-agonist-mediated inhibition of platelet membrane adenylyl cyclase activity, and of the effect of intra-arterial infusions of NE to decrease in forearm blood flow (Fig. 1; *34*). These results were interpreted to be consistent with evidence for heightened systemic SNS activity, and, despite this increase, enhanced platelet membrane and arterial vasoconstrictor α-adrenergic receptor responsiveness in hypertensive, compared with normotensive, elderly humans. In addition, these results suggest that heightened level of SNS activity, in conjunction with enhanced α-adrenergic receptor response, may contribute, in part, toward the increase in peripheral vascular resistance and BP in older hypertensive humans.

Congestive Heart Failure

Impaired myocardial contractile function may lead to the clinical syndrome of CHF. There is an age-associated increase both in the incidence and prevalence of CHF *(35)*, and CHF is associated with increased morbidity and mortality *(35,36)*, and an increased frequency of hospital admissions and readmissions *(37)*. Several compensatory mechanisms, including an increase in systemic SNS activity, are invoked to increase left ventricle pump function in patients with CHF (*see* ref. *38* for review). Once invoked, there is a delicate balance between the positive effects of these compensatory mechanisms and the adverse effects that may ultimately develop as a result. The maintenance of this homeostatic balance may be even more precarious among older humans, who possess a limited functional reserve because of age-associated alterations in these systems.

The increase in SNS activity is one illustration of this situation. Activation of the SNS serves to initially increase myocardial contractile function (inotropic support), increase HR, and increase peripheral vascular resistance, to produce an increase in cardiac output and BP. As a result of coexisting age-associated alterations in SNS function, discussed above, the extent to which SNS activation compensates for myocardial contractile dysfunction in older humans may be limited. In addition, over time, enhanced SNS activity may become deleterious. Excess catecholamines may exert direct cardiotoxic effects *(39–41)*. Studies of cardiocyte cultures have demonstrated NE-mediated cytotoxicity, perhaps caused by an increase in intracellular cyclic adenosine monophosphate, and subsequent Ca^{2+} overload of the cell *(41)*. The other deleterious effect of excess SNS activity is the attenuation of β-receptor responsiveness, secondary to downregulation of myocardial β-adrenergic receptor function *(42–45)*.

The results from studies performed to characterize SNS activity in humans with CHF suggest that there is an increase in SNS activity, although none of these have focused on an older age group. An increase in plasma NE levels in CHF patients has been observed *(46,47)*, and the plasma NE level has been found to be associated with the subsequent risk of mortality *(48)*. Radiotracer kinetic studies of NE metabolism have demonstrated that

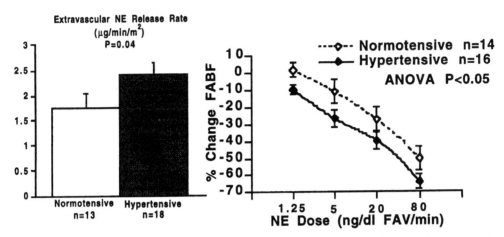

Fig. 1. A measure of systemic sympathetic nervous system activity (SNS), the rate of extravascular norepinephrine (NE) release derived from ^{3}H-NE kinetic studies was higher in the older hypertensive subject group (solid bar), compared to age-matched normotensive subjects (open bar). Despite this increase in SNS activity, the effect of intrabrachial artery NE infusions to mediate vasoconstriction (presented as the percentage change from baseline resting forearm blood flow [FABF]) was significantly greater in the older hypertensive group (closed diamonds, solid line), compared with the older normotensive group (open diamonds, dashed line), suggesting enhanced vascular α-adrenergic receptor responsiveness.

a combination of an increased appearance rate of NE into plasma, as well as a decrease in NE clearance rate from plasma, contribute to the increase in plasma NE level *(49)*. Microneurography recordings from a muscle sympathetic nerve (peroneal) have demonstrated increased muscle sympathetic nerve activity in patients with CHF *(50)*.

Experimental models of CHF have shown that cardiac β-receptor responsiveness is decreased. Several animal studies have demonstrated decreased chronotropic response to isoproterenol (ISP), downregulation of myocardial β_1-receptors, decreased ISP-stimulated myocardial adenylyl cyclase (AC) activity, decreased stimulatory G-protein (G_s), and a relative increase in inhibitory G-protein ($G_{i\alpha2}$) levels *(51–53)*. These studies have suggested that β-adrenergic receptor dysfunction in heart failure is associated with increased plasma NE levels, and subsequent uncoupling of the β_1-receptor–AC pathway. Decreased β-receptor function in humans with CHF has also been observed, although none of these studies have focused on older patients *(44,45,54)*. The overall conclusion from these studies is that there is uncoupling of the β-receptor–G protein–AC system in patients with CHF, and that this desensitization may be caused by the increase in SNS activity *(55)*.

Thus, there appear to be similar changes in SNS activity and β-adrenergic receptor responsiveness that develop both in aging and in heart failure. Given the age-associated decline in β-receptor responsiveness, an additional increase in SNS activity may not be accompanied by a further proportionate decline in β-receptor responsiveness in older CHF patients. Previous studies have not examined whether decreased chronotropic β-receptor responsiveness in older humans is related to the age-related increase in SNS activity, nor has this relationship been evaluated in older patients with CHF. To address this question, the author measured plasma NE levels as an index of SNS activity, and the amount of ISP required to produce a 25-beat/min increase above resting HR (ISP_{25}; note

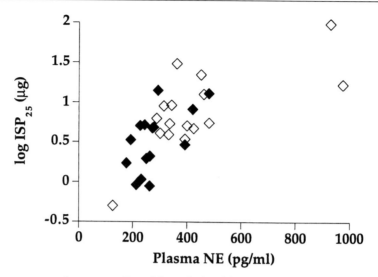

Fig. 2. There appears to be an overall positive relationship between the chronotropic response to isoproterenol (ISP$_{25}$; and the plasma norepinephrine (NE) level. Individuals from either subject group (normal systolic function, closed diamonds; and impaired systolic function, CHF, open diamonds) with higher plasma NE levels also have higher ISP$_{25}$ values (indicating a blunted chronotropic response to β-agonist stimulation).

that higher ISP$_{25}$ values reflect lower β-receptor responsiveness) calculated from the HR response to bolus ISP doses in 15 older (age >60 yr; 70 ± 2 yr) subjects with normal myocardial contractility, and 16 older (71 ± 2 yr) subjects with impaired systolic dysfunction. The older CHF group was characterized by higher levels of plasma NE (432 ± 55 vs 305 ± 24 pg/mL, $P < 0.05$) and higher ISP$_{25}$ (14.8 ± 5.8 vs 4.71 µg; $P < 0.05$). As illustrated in Fig. 2, there was an overall positive relationship identified between the plasma NE level and ISP$_{25}$, which in stepwise regression analysis was independent of age, resting HR, gender, or the presence or absence of CHF ($r = 0.705$; $P < 0.0001$) *(56)*. From these results, the author concluded that chronotropic β-receptor responsiveness is regulated appropriately by the level of SNS activity in older humans with and without CHF.

Autonomic Nervous System Dysfunction

Clinical Presentation

In contrast to the age-associated changes in SNS activity and adrenergic responsiveness discussed above, which are, in general, asymptomatic, dysfunction of the autonomic nervous system is generally symptomatic. Autonomic dysfunction may develop as a consequence of primary autonomic failure, secondary to another disease process, or because of the effects of medications that interfere with SNS function. Because the autonomic nervous system controls many key physiologic homeostatic mechanisms, the symptoms associated with its dysfunction reflect the involvement of multiple systems. Common symptoms include orthostatic hypotension, heat intolerance, constipation, urinary incontinence, erectile dysfunction, as well as neurologic features of parkinsonism or cerebellar impairment. The insidious development of these symptoms, as well as their heterogeneity, combine to complicate the diagnosis of autonomic dysfunction. Although there are no reliable estimates of the prevalence of autonomic dysfunction in the elderly, autonomic dysfunction is believed to be more common among the elderly, because of the prevalence of diseases that may be associated with autonomic dysfunction (e.g., diabetes mellitus and Parkinson's disease).

CLASSIFICATION

The classification of primary autonomic failure is determined by the constellation of symptoms grouped into categories of autonomic, parkinsonian, and cerebellar or pyramidal (57). Pure autonomic failure is defined when only autonomic symptoms are present. Orthostatic hypotension, in combination with other autonomic symptoms, is the primary manifestation. Multiple system atrophy is characterized by autonomic symptoms plus features of parkinsonism, cerebellar dysfunction, or both (mixed form). Some patients with clinical presentations consistent with Parkinson's disease may have symptoms of autonomic dysfunction. Secondary causes of autonomic dysfunction include neurologic disorders, such as spinal cord injury, and acute (e.g., Guillain-Barré syndrome) or chronic (e.g., diabetes mellitus, amyloidosis, alcohol-related) polyneuropathies. A number of medications whose mechanism of action either directly or indirectly interacts with the SNS may impair its function. Older individuals may be at increased risk of these adverse effects, because of their underlying age-associated changes in SNS function, altered drug metabolism, and interactions with other medications. Cardiovascular medications, in particular, antihypertensive drugs, which either act centrally (e.g., those that affect NE release), or which interfere with adrenergic receptor function directly, and psychiatric medications are the two drug classes most commonly associated with symptoms of autonomic dysfunction.

EVALUATION

The symptoms associated with autonomic dysfunction develop gradually, affect multiple systems, and may mimic age-associated physiologic changes. Consequently, a high index of suspicion is required when evaluating older patients for the presence of SNS dysfunction. The identification of patients who may be at greater risk for autonomic dysfunction (e.g., those with diabetes mellitus or neurodegenerative disorders) is important in this regard.

Abnormal BP regulation and orthostatic hypotension is nearly ubiquitous in patients with autonomic dysfunction. Therefore, careful measurement of supine and standing BP is an obligatory first step in the clinical evaluation when autonomic dysfunction is suspected. Because patients with autonomic insufficiency may have marked variability in BP, a stable supine BP reading is first documented. After several minutes of upright posture, a fall in systolic BP of greater than 20 mm Hg, or a fall in diastolic BP of greater than 10 mm Hg, is considered to be abnormal (58). Additional support for autonomic dysfunction is the absence of an increase in HR, especially when the BP has decreased. The balance of the physical examination is directed toward the neurological exam, to identify the presence of a pattern of neurologic features consistent with either a primary or secondary cause of autonomic dysfunction.

A number of clinical tests to assess autonomic function are available, including measures of HR variability, the pressor sensitivity to administration of adrenergic agonists, the counterregulatory response to hypoglycemia, and quantitative pupillometry. Determination of supine and upright plasma NE levels may aid in the classification of auto-

Table 1
Pathophysiological Factors in Geriatric Hypertension

Westernization, which is associated with increased salt; decreased calcium, potassium, and magnesium consumption; physical inactivity; and stress.

Increased relative adiposity with aging, which is associated with hyperinsulinemia and insulin resistance, enhanced sympathetic activity and increases peripheral vascular resistance.

Impaired ability to handle sodium, which involves a genetic decrease in the ability of the senescent kidney to excrete sodium genetic salt sensitivity, and decreased ability of the kidney to generate natriuretic substances like dopamine and prostaglandins.

Increased sympathetic nervous system activity, with increased norepinephrine levels, particularly with exercise, sleep, and upright posture.

Decreased vascular β-adrenergic vasodilatation function, leaving unopposed α-adrenergic receptor vasoconstriction in response to elevated norepinephrine levels.

Decreased endothelium vasorelaxation function.

Increased rigidity and decreased compliance of large vessels.

Hyaline degeneration within media of precapillary arterioles, resulting in decreased wall-to-lumen ratio and increased vascular resistance.

Atherosclerosis and other aging effects on the carotid and aortic baroreceptor sensitivity, resulting in enhanced sympathetic activity, increased BP lability, and increased tendency to orthostatic hypotension.

CVD morbidity and mortality, including CHD, stroke, renal disease, and mortality from all causes, increase progressively with higher levels of both SBP and DBP: These relationships are strong, continuous, independent, predictable, and clinically significant (13). Epidemiologic data demonstrate that a modest increase in BP is associated with heightened risk for CVD. In persons with SBP levels of 140–160 mmHg or DBP levels of from 85–89 mmHg, there still exists a modest risk. SBP is a greater risk factor for cardiovascular morbidity and mortality than DBP, especially in the elderly (10–13). The Multiple Risk Factor Intervention Trial demonstrated SBP elevation to be a more powerful risk factor than DBP elevation (11,19). A SBP of 160 mmHg was found to have a more significant relationship with mortality than a DBP of 95 mmHg (19).

CARDIOVASCULAR STRUCTURAL ALTERATIONS CONTRIBUTING TO HYPERTENSION

Aging in westernized cultures is often associated with functional and structural alterations of the cardiovascular system (Table 1). The elderly are more prone to orthostatic hypotension, as well as asymptomatic hypotension, both of which often accompany and complicate antihypertensive therapy (18,20). This propensity toward orthostatic hypotension is related to a number of factors. Cardiovascular structural changes associated with advancing age contribute to baroreflex dysfunction (15–20) and associated lability of BP (21), as well as a tendency toward orthostatic hypotension (22). There are also age-related physiological alterations in the vascular system that contribute to increases in peripheral vascular resistance (16), the hallmark of hypertension in the elderly (23). For example, there is a loss of β-adrenergic responsiveness in various tissues, including those of the cardiovascular system, with increasing age (24). There is, however, no such clear-cut diminution in the α-adrenergic responsivity with aging. Thus, for a given release of norepinephrine at adrenergic nerve terminals, there is a greater vasoconstrictor response from these age-related alterations in adrenergic receptor responsiveness *(18)*. The increased α-adrenergic activity may also contribute to the increased vascular smooth muscle intracellular calcium (Ca) responses and associated vascular reactivity with advancing age *(16)*. Advancing age is also associated with decreases in cardiac compliance and circulating blood volume, an increase in cardiac wall thickness, and an attenuation of the renin–angiotensin responses to various physiologic stimuli (Table 1). Enhanced rigidity and decreased elasticity and compliance of the large vessels is caused by fracturing and uncoiling of the elastic fibers in large vessels, and deposition of Ca and connective within vessel walls *(15–20)*. Because of reduced vascular compliance, the pulse generated during systole is transmitted to the aorta and its tributaries.

Aging in westernized, industrialized societies is often associated with a loss of lean body mass and an increase in adipose tissue, particularly visceral fat *(25–30)*. In females, there is an accelerated accumulation of central fat in the postmenopausal years *(31–42)*. In cross-sectional and longitudinal studies of White women, an upper-body fat distribution, as defined by high waist:to:hip ratio, is related to cardiovascular metabolic risk factors *(43–53)*. Although Black women have higher prevalences of diabetes, hypertension, and CVD than White women *(54–56)*, upper-body obesity has been reported to carry less risk for metabolic abnormalities in Black than in non-Hispanic, White, obese, nondiabetic, premenopausal women *(57,58)*. It has been suggested that this paradox may be explained by the fact that Black women accumulate abdominal fat predominantly subcutaneously rather than viscerally *(58)*, the latter being more closely associated with CHD risk factors *(59–70)*. Alternatively, risk factors for CHD in Black women, such as diabetes and hypertension, may relate differently to body fat and its distribution *(58)*. However, the effect of advancing age on differential central fat distribution vs race has not been investigated. The age-related increase in total body fat and central adiposity is greater in women than men *(31)*. Studies *(38,39)* suggest that regularly performed endurance exercise partially protects, but does not abolish, the increase in relative body fat with aging. One report indicated that, even when master athletes maintain optimal exercise volume and intensity, body fat increased by approx 2% over a 10-yr period. However, physically active men and women have less central fat than their sedentary counterparts. Exercise intervention studies *(38,41)* have demonstrated that endurance training selectively reduces central body fat. These observations are important, because central adiposity has been observed to be strongly and positively associated with CVD mortality *(42)*.

AGING, SEX HORMONES, AND BLOOD PRESSURE

CVD is the leading cause of morbidity and mortality in both men and women in the United States and other industrialized nations *(1–16)*. CVD accounts for 45% and coronary disease for one-third of all deaths in industrialized nations. Although CVD presents later in women than in men, it results in almost as many deaths in women as men, and is the leading cause of death in women by age 65 yr. Although CVD is less frequent in premenopausal women than in age-matched men counterparts, this gender difference begins to disappear after menopause, presumably because of reduced production of female sex hormones *(71)*. In the United States, the mean age of menopause is 51 yr, over 40 million women are postmenopausal, and American women live one-third of their life span after menopause *(72)*. Ovarian alterations begin at approx age 45, and are

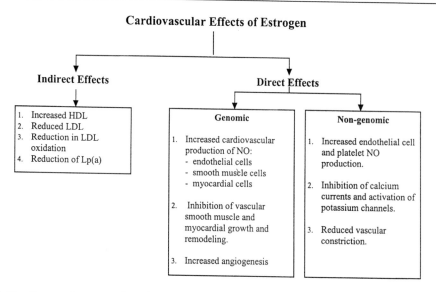

Fig. 1. Cardiovascular protective effects of estrogen. HDL indicates high-density lipoprotein; LDL, low-density lipoprotein.

accompanied by a progressive decline in the ovarian production of estradiol and progesterone *(72)*. Once menopause occurs, serum estradiol levels drop to about 10–20 pg/mL, low levels that are maintained mostly from the peripheral conversion of estrone *(72)*. The loss of estrogen, and, perhaps to a lesser extent, progesterone, accounts for most CVD observed in postmenopausal women *(72)*.

There are a number of putative mechanisms by which estradiol exerts its cardiovascular protective effects *(72)*. There are receptors for estrogen on vascular endothelial and smooth muscle cells, and estradiol exerts both genomic and nongenomic effects on these cells *(72)*. Estradiol also exerts indirect effects on the vasculature through its impact on lipoprotein metabolism (Fig 1). For example, estrogen replacement therapy in postmenopausal women increases levels of high-density lipoproteins (HDL), reduces lipoprotein(a) and low-density lipoprotein (LDL) cholesterol, and attenuates LDL oxidation *(72,73)*. However, multiple regression analysis indicates that less than 50% of the CVD protection effects of estrogen replacement therapy is afforded by its effects on lipoprotein metabolism *(53,72)*.

There is increasing evidence suggesting that estradiol exerts its cardiovascular protective effects by binding to its receptor on vascular tissue *(72)*. Estradiol receptor expression has been demonstrated in the human aorta, and heterogeneity of exists between male and female vascular tissue, and in normal and atherosclerotic vascular tissue *(72–75)*. Estradiol decreases vasoconstriction, in part, by stimulating the release of vasodilators, such as nitric oxide and prostacyclin, from the vessel wall (Fig. 1; *72,76*). Because these vasodilators, particularly nitric oxide, attenuate platelet aggregation and vascular growth, this appears to be one mechanism by which estradiol exerts its antiatherogenic effects *(72)*. Atherosclerotic arteries of women demonstrate significantly diminished estradiol receptors *(77)*, further suggesting that the antiatherosclerotic effects of estradiol are mediated through cardiovascular estrogen receptors.

A gender-specific association between elevations in BP and metabolic abnormalities exists in women *(51,72)*. Androgen excess in women may promote insulin resistance/

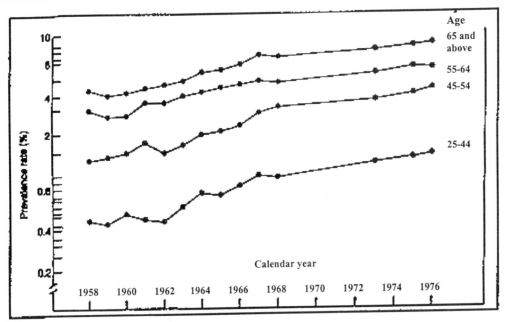

Fig. 2. Prevalence of diabetes mellitus by age and calendar year. Data from the National Center for Health Statistics.

hyperinsulinemia and central obesity, glucose intolerance, hyperuricemia, dyslipidemia, and hypertension *(43,46,48,51,60–70).* In particular, it appears that elevated serum levels of dehydroepiandrosterone sulfate is a significant risk factor for elevated BP and associated metabolic cardiovascular risk factors in women *(51).*

Age-related increases in hypertension parallel increases in CVD in the United States and other industrialized countries. Following adolescence, men have a significantly higher prevalence of hypertension than women until 50–60 yr of age, at which time the prevalence is similar in men and women *(78).* Indeed, the absolute number of women with hypertension is greater than that for men, because of the greater longevity of women *(72).* Despite the fact that women with hypertension outnumber men, relatively few large, controlled, interventional and hypertensive trials have been conducted in women. Exceptions include prospective clinical trials, such as the SHEP *(99),* the Treatment of Mild Hypertension Study Trial *(80),* and the Antihypertensive and Lipid-Lowering Treatment to Prevent Heart Attack Trial (ALLHAT) *(81).* The studies have included postmenopausal, as well as premenopausal, women, but precise hormonal status has not been delineated. Gender-specific analysis of the SHEP and the Treatment of Mild Hypertension Study trials has shown equal benefits between women and men treated for hypertension. The ongoing ALLHAT contains a substantial number of women, as well.

DIABETES AND ASSOCIATED HYPERTENSION

The prevalence of type 2 diabetes increases with age, and this disease is present in nearly one in five North Americans aged ≥65 yr *(16,82–85;* Fig. 2). According to the National Diabetes Data Group criteria *(84),* an increased incidence of noninsulin-dependent diabetes mellitus has been seen in the United States in each decade past 40 yr. Fasting plasma glucose levels have been reported to rise 1–2 mg/dL for each decade past 40 yr *(85).*

CHD is the leading cause of mortality in type 2 diabetes, including elderly subpopulations, in whom CHD is already an in dependent, prevalent condition *(86,87)*. Data from the Rancho Bernardo Study of elderly community-dwelling persons indicate that asymptomatic ischemic heart disease, documented by resting electrocardiograms, was 1.80× more common in women with type 2 diabetes, and 1.75× more common in men with type 2 diabetes, than in an age-matched control population *(89)*. Diabetes also increases the likelihood of stroke in the elderly, and mortality is substantially higher in diabetic persons who suffer from myocardial infarction or stroke, compared to nondiabetic persons.

Diabetes and hypertension are associated diseases that increase with age in industrialized societies *(88–90)*. Data obtained from death certificates show that hypertensive disease has been implicated in 4.4% of deaths coded to diabetes, and diabetes was involved in 10% of deaths coded to hypertensive disease. Indeed, an estimated 35–75% of diabetic cardiovascular and renal complications can be attributed to hypertension *(88–90)*. Hypertension also contributes to diabetic retinopathy, which is the leading cause of newly diagnosed blindness in the United States *(88–90)*. For these reasons, hypertension and diabetes should be recognized and treated early and aggressively.

Both diabetes and hypertension increase CHD risk via a number of mechanisms. As recently reviewed *(53,89)*, these disorders are individually associated with increased platelet aggregation, a procoagulent state, and atherogenic lipoprotein profiles. Further, all of these co-existing conditions contribute to endothelial dysfunction and increased vascular reactivity, which are the hallmarks of hypertension in diabetics, particularly elderly diabetic persons *(88–90)*. Further, it appears that hyperglycemia, *per se*, may exacerbate the cardiovascular and renal disease associated with these disorders *(88–90)*.

DYSLIPIDEMIA

Secondary and primary prevention trials need to encompass more persons over the age of 65 yr. Lipoprotein patterns (HDL, LDL, and triglyceride levels) have been demonstrated to be predictors of cardiovascular death in elderly women *(91)*. The pooled data in 25 populations from 22 cohort studies has indicated that total cholesterol and LDL cholesterol levels were significantly related to fatal CHD in both men and women across a broad age range, and into older populations (>65 yr); however, relative risk decreased with increasing age *(92)*. Because CHD is more prevalent among older persons, as well as in those with diabetes and hypertension, the cholesterol treatment panel has indicated that age is not a contraindication to cholesterol-lowering therapy. Further, one small study in Italy *(93)* indicates that 1 yr of cholesterol lowering therapy was associated with either arrest or regression of atherosclerotic plaques in elderly patients with hypercholesterolemia. Nevertheless, primary prevention trials in middle-aged men suggest that at least 2 yr are required before a reduction in CHD becomes manifest *(92–94)*. In elderly diabetic hypertensive patients with a prior CHD event, the benefits may be manifested earlier *(94)*; however, adequately sized, controlled trials in this population are yet to be performed.

TREATMENT

Lifestyle Modification

Weight reduction, more physical activity, and moderation of dietary salt and alcohol intake may be effective in lowering BP in many elderly patients. Indeed, lifestyle modifications should be initiated as an alternative to drug therapy for most elderly patients with hypertenson. A weight-reduction program that includes supervised regular aerobic physical activity, and a reduction in caloric intake, is appropriate for many elderly patients who weigh more than 10% above their ideal body wt *(1,95–97)*. A regular physical activity program may improve tissue insulin sensitivity, lower triglyceride levels, raise HDL cholesterol, and lower BPs in elderly hypertensive patients *(98–101)*. Moderate restriction of salt intake is prudent in elderly hypertensive persons, because these individuals have a high prevalence of salt sensitivity. Thus, the Joint National Committee (JNC)-VI guideline of restricting salt intake to less than 6 g sodium chloride (2.3 g sodium) daily is an appropriate goal in these patients, as noted in the working group report *(102)*. Furthermore, daily alcohol consumption should be limited to no more than two glasses of wine (8 oz), two beers (24 oz), or two shots of whiskey (2 oz). Even though cigarette smoking and dietary saturated fat and cholesterol are not directly implicated in raising BP, elderly patients with hypertension also should be advised to avoid cigarette smoking, and to reduce dietary intake of saturated fat and cholesterol, especially if they have dyslipidemia. Adequate dietary intake of potassium, Ca, and magnesium should be maintained for general health, even though reduced intake of these minerals may not lower BP *per se*. Lifestyle modifications may offer multiple benefits at little cost and with minimal risk: Even when not adequate in themselves to control hypertension, these behavioral changes may reduce the number and doses of antihypertensive medications needed to manage the condition. Lifestyle modifications are particularly helpful in patients who have other risk factors, such as diabetes mellitus and dyslipidemia. If lifestyle modifications are unsuccessful in achieving goal BP, then antihypertensive drug therapy should be instituted.

Pharmacologic Therapy

Antihypertensive therapy should be begun more cautiously in elderly patients, because these persons are more sensitive to volume depletion, and to sympathetic inhibition, than are younger individuals. Elderly patients may have impaired baroreflexes that make them more susceptible to postural hypotension; for this reason, BP should always be measured in the standing, as well as the supine and sitting, positions, and antihypertensive treatment should be initiated with smaller doses than those used in younger patients. Increases in dosage should also be smaller, and spaced at longer intervals, than might be appropriate for younger patients. Large controlled studies have shown that elderly patients tolerate antihypertensive medications when administered cautiously *(103–105)*.

Polypharmacy is common in the elderly. Adverse drug reactions are 2–3× more common in older patients than in younger. Further, decreased renal function, contracted blood volume, and altered drug metabolism may all predispose the elderly to adverse drug reactions. Nonsteroidal anti-inflammatory drugs (NSAIDs) are potentially very toxic in elderly patients *(106)*. The escalating use of these drugs support the notion that NSAIDs are effective drugs in the treatment of the many clinical conditions for which they are prescribed. At the same time, however, the number of patients at risk for adverse events related to the use of these agents is rapidly expanding. This concern is further heightened by the availability of ibuprofen and, most recently, of NSAIDS over-the-counter *(106)*.

One study *(106)* examined the effects of ibuprofen and a thiazide diuretic on renal water handling in otherwise normal young and old volunteers given a water load. Three d of hydrochlorothiazide (100 mg/d) was found to impair both free water clearance and the ability to elaborate a maximally dilute urine. A delay in the recovery of serum osmolality was noted in both the young and old, but to a significantly greater extent in the older subjects. When the young subjects were given a water load after treatment with ibuprofen together with the thiazide, free water clearance and serum osmolality were reduced even further, to a degree similar to that seen in the elderly subjects on the thiazide regimen alone . It was postulated that thiazide-induced hyponatremia, known to occur in some elderly patients, may be related, in part, to lower renal prostaglandin production. It can be expected that a greater number of elderly patients will be taking a combination of NSAIDs and hydrochlorothiazide, given the efficacy of thiazide diuretics in the treatment of hypertension in the geriatric population.

All classes of antihypertensive drugs have been shown to be effective in lowering BP in older patients. Diuretics and β-blockers have been shown to reduce cardiovascular morbidity and mortality in large clinical trials. A small dose, 12.5–25 mg/d, of a thiazide diuretic, such as chlorthalidone or hydrochlorothiazide, should be considered as first-line therapy in geriatric patients (107). They have been used in many large trials that have documented reduction in cardiovascular morbidity and mortality. Diuretics are also the only class of antihypertensive drug currently recommended for initial therapy that tends to cause a disproportionately great reduction in SBP. They are the least expensive of the various classes of antihypertensive drugs that are effective as monotherapy. Type 2 diabetes mellitus is increasingly common with aging; therefore, more elderly people are at risk of developing hyperglycemia and other metabolic abnormalities associated with the syndrome of insulin resistance (including hypertriglyceridemia and a low HDL cholesterol concentration) than would be expected in younger people. However, there is no proof, as yet, from clinical trials that the use of diuretics has resulted in any increase in drug-induced diabetes mellitus (108–112).

In SHEP, the metabolic changes were also minimal, although significantly different between the active and placebo groups (112). The gout was more likely to occur with active therapy. Diabetes also occurred more often with active treatment than with placebo, but the difference was not significant (29 vs 20 cases, respectively); 28 actively treated patients needed oral hypoglycemic agents, compared with 18 on placebo (112). In the Swedish Trial in Old Patients with Hypertension, the adverse clinical and biochemical events were minor, and not substantively different from those patients treated with diuretics or β-blockers (113). In the Medical Research Council (MRC) trial, diuretics were better tolerated than β-blockers (110).

β-blockers, like thiazide diuretics, have been evaluated in large, controlled clinical trials that have documented that active antihypertensive therapy can reduce cardiovascular events. However, in the MRC trial, the group given a β-blocker as initial therapy showed no significant reduction in events, compared with the group receiving placebo (110). These agents should be employed in elderly patients that have had myocardial infarctions (secondary prevention), because they reduce the risk of a subsequent event and sudden death (111). β-blockers should be used with some caution in elderly patients with peripheral vascular disease, bradycardia and conduction problems, glucose and lipid abnormalities, congestive heart failure, obstructive lung disease, depression, and allergic rhinitis.

Angiotensin-converting enzyme (ACE) inhibitors are generally well tolerated in elderly patients, but they appear to be slightly less effective monotherapeutic agents than diuretics and Ca channel blockers, perhaps because geriatric hypertension is a low-renin, salt-sensitive type of hypertension. Although ACE inhibitors are particularly useful in hypertensive patients who also have congestive heart failure *(114,115)*, they should be used cautiously in patients with renal dysfunction, type IV renal tubular acidosis, and those taking NSAIDs, because of the risk of hyperkalemia and worsening of kidney function.

Ca antagonists may be useful antihypertensives in some older patients with relative contraindications to some of the other classes of antihypertensive drugs (e.g., chronic airways disease, cough, significant renal disease, or gout). Concerns regarding Ca antagonists in the elderly include cardiovascular effects of these agents, edema, and constipation. Other potential antihypertensive agents in the elderly include peripheral and central α-blockers and combination α/β-blockers. The recent Systolic Hypertension-Eur study *(116)* demonstrated a reduction in CVD mortality in elderly patients with isolated systolic hypertension, utilizing a Ca antagonist. Thus, the JNC-VI includes long-acting Ca antagonists as an appropriate class of drugs to treat the elderly *(102)*.

REFERENCES

1. Sowers JR. Hypertension in the elderly. Am J Med 1987;82:1–8.
2. Bush TL. The epidemiology of cardiovascular disease in postmenopausal women. Ann NY Acad Sci 1990;592:262–271.
3. Stuck SE, Siu AL, Wieland GD, Adams J, Rubenstein LZ. Comprehensive geriatric assessment: a meta-analysis of controlled trials. Lancet 1993;342:1032–1036.
4. Robinson JG, Leon AS. The prevention of cardiovascular disease: emphasis on secondary prevention. Med Clin North Am 1994;18:69–98.
5. Scott M, Owen P, Porter P. Prevalence of adults with no known risk factors for coronary heart disease. Behavioral risk factor surveillance system, 1992. MMWR 1994;43:61–66.
6. Stamler J, Wentworth D, Neaton JD. Is the relationship between serum cholesterol and risk of premature death from coronary heart disease continuous and graded? Findings in 356,222 primary screenees of the Multiple Risk Factor Intervention Trial MRFIT. JAMA 1986;256:2823–2828.
7. Lau J, Antman EM, Jimenez-Silva J, Kuplnick B, Mosteller F, Chalmers TC. Cumulative meta-analysis of therapeutic trials for myocardial infarction. N Engl J Med 1992;327:248–254.
8. Adult Treatment Panel II. Second report of the Expert Panel on Detection, Evaluation, and Treatment of High Blood Cholesterol in Adults. Circulation 1994;89:1336–1340.
9. Malenka DJ, Baron JA. Cholesterol and coronary heart disease: the importance of patient-specific attributable risk. Arch Intern Med 1988;148:2247–2252.
10. Vokonas PS, Kannel WB, Cupples L.A. Epidemiology and risk of hypertension in the elderly: the Framingham study. J Hypertens 1988;6(Suppl I):S3–S9.
11. Applegate WB. The relative importance of focusing on elevations of systolic versus diastolic blood pressure: a definitive answer at last. Arch Int Med 1992;152:1162–1166.
12. Sowers JR, Khoury S, Imam K. Therapeutic approach to hypertension in the elderly. Primary Care 1991;18:593–604.
13. Applegate WB, Sowers JR. Elevated systolic blood pressure: increased cardiovascular risk and rationale for treatment. Am J Med 1996;100(Suppl 3A):S3–S9.
14. Perry HM, Smith WM, McDonald RH. Morbidity and mortality in the Systolic Hypertension in the Elderly Program (SHEP) pilot study. Stroke 1989;20:4–13.
15. Kuramato K, Matsushito S, Kuwajimi I. The pathogenetic role of elderly hypertension. Jpn Circ J 1981;45:833–843.
16. Sowers JR, Farrow SL. Treatment of elderly hypertensive patients with diabetes, renal disease, and coronary heart disease. Am J Geriatr Cardiol 1996;5:57–70.
17. Sowers JR, Mohanty PK. Effects of advancing age on cardiopulmonary baroreceptor function in hypertensive men. Hypertension 1987;10:274–279.
18. Sowers JR, Mohanty PK. Norepinephrine and forearm vascular resistance responses to tilt and cold pressor test in essential hypertension: effects of aging. Angiology 1989;40:872–879.
19. Fleich JH, Hooker CS. The relationship between age and relaxation of vascular smooth muscle in the rabbit and rat. Circ Res 1976;38:243–249.

20. Shimada K, Kitazumi T, Sadakane N, Ogura H, Ozawa T. Age-related changes of baroreflex function, plasma norepinephrine, and blood pressure. Hypertension 1985;7:113–117.
21. Khoury S, Yarows S, O'Brian T, Sowers JR. Ambulatory blood pressure monitoring in a nonacademic setting: effects of age and sex. Am J Hypertens 1992;5:616–623.
22. Sowers JR, Rubenstein LZ, Stern N. Plasma norepinephrine responses to posture and isometric exercise with age in the absence of obesity. J Gerontol 1983;38:315–317.
23. Gambert SR, Duthie EH. Effect of age on red cell membrane sodium-potassium dependent adenosine triphosphatase activity in healthy men. J Gerontol 1983;38:23–28.
24. Van Brummelen P, Buhler FR, Kiowski W. Age-related increase in cardiac and peripheral vascular responses to isoproterenol: studies in normal subjects. Clin Sci 1981;60:571–577.
25. Borkan GA, Norris AH. Fat redistribution and the changing body dimensions of the adult male. Hum Biol 1977;49:495–514.
26. Flynn MA, Nolph GB, Baker AS, Martin WM, Krause G. Total body potassium in aging humans: a longitudinal study. Am J Clin Nutr 1989;50:713–717.
27. Durning J, Womerskly J. Body fat assessed from total body density and its estimation from skin fold thickness: measurements in 481 men and women aged from 16 to 72 years. Br J Nutr 1974;32:77–97.
28. Sowers JR, Standley PR, Ram JL. Insulin resistance, carbohydrate metabolism, and hypertension. Am J Hypertens 1991;4:466S–472S.
29. Fukagawa NK, Bandini LG, Young JB. Effect of age on body composition and resting metabolic rate. Am J Physiol 1990;259:E233–E238.
30. Sowers JR, Sowers PS, Peuler JD. Role of insulin resistance and hyperinsulinemia in development of hypertension and atherosclerosis. J Lab Clin Med 1994;123:647–652.
31. Poelman ET, Toth MJ, Bunyard LB, Gardner AW, Donalson KE, Colman E, Fonong T, Ades PA. Physiological predictions of increasing total and central adiposity in aging men and women. Arch Int Med 1995;155:2443–2448.
32. Zamboni M, Armellini F, Milani MP. Body fat distribution in pre- and postmenopausal women: metabolic and anthropometric variables and their inter-relationships. Int J Obes 1992;16:495–504.
33. Mantzoros CS, Georgiadis EI, Young R, Khoury S, Evagelopoulou K, Katsilambros K, Sowers JR. Relative androgenicity and blood pressure levels of young, healthy females. Am J Hypertens 1995;8: 606–614.
34. Carey DG, Jenkins AB, Campbell LV, Freund J, Chisholm DJ. Abdominal fat and insulin resistance in normal and overweight women. Diabetes 1996;45:633–638.
35. Dowling HJ, Pi-Sunyer FX. Race dependent health risks of upper-body obesity. Diabetes 1993;42: 537–543.
36. Albu JB, Murphy L, Frager DH, Johnson JA, Pi-Sunyer FX. Visceral fat and race-dependent health risk in obese nondiabetic premenopausal women. Diabetes 1997;46:456–462.
37. Banerji MA, Lebowitz J, Charken RL, Gordon D, Kral JG, Lebowitz HE. Relationship of visceral adipose tissue and glucose disposal is independent of sex in black NIDDM subjects. Am J Physiol 1997;273:E425–E432.
38. Kohrt WM, Obert KA, Holloszy JO. Exercise training improves fat distribution patterns in 60- to 70-year-old men and women. J Gerontol 1992;47:M99–M105.
39. Troisi RJ, Heinold JW, Vokonas PS, Weiss ST. Cigarette smoking, dietary intake, and physical activity: effects on body fat distribution: the Normative Aging Study. Am J Clin Nutr 1991;53:1104–1111.
40. Wing RR, Matthews KA, Kuller LH, Meilahn EN, Plantinga P. Waist to hip ratio in middle-aged women: associations with behavioral and psychological factors and with changes in cardiovascular risk factors. Arterioscler Thromb 1991;11:1250–1257.
41. Schwartz RS, Shuman WP, Larson V. The effect of intensive endurance exercise training on body fat distribution in young and older men. Metabolism 1991;40:545–551.
42. Folsom AR, Kaye SA, Sellers TA. Body fat distribution and 5-year risk of death in older women. JAMA 1993;269:483–487.
43. Evans DJ, Hoffman RG, Kalkoff RK, Kissebah AH. Relationship of body fat tipography to insulin sensitivity and metabolic profiles in premenopausal women. Metabolism 1984;33:68–75.
44. Lapidus L, Bengtson C, Larsson B, Peunert B. Distribution of adipose tissue and risk of cardiovascular disease and death: a 12-year follow up of participants in the population study of women in Gothenburg, Sweden. Br Med J 1984;289:1257–1263.
45. Lundgren H, Bengtsson C, Blohme G, Lapidus L, Sjostrom L. Adiposity and adipose tissue distribution in relation to incidence of diabetes in women: results from a prospective population study in Gothenburg, Sweden. Int J Obes 1989;13:413–423.

46. Després JP, Moorjan, S, Farland M, Tremblay A, Lapien P, Nadeun A, Pinault S, Thereault G, Borrchard C. Adipose tissue distribution and plasma lipoprotein levels in obese women important of intra-abdominal fat. Arteriosclerosis 1989;9:203–210.
47. Zamboni M, Armellini F, Milani MP. Body fat distribution in pre- and postmenopausal women: metabolic and anthropometric variables and their inter-relationships. Int J Obes 1992;16:495–504.
48. Busby MJ, Bellantoni MJ, Tobin JD, Muller DC, Kafonik SD, Blackman MR. Glucose tolerance in women: the effects of age, body composition, and sex hormones. J Am Geriatr Soc 1992;40:497–502.
49. Landin K, Lönnroth M, Krotkiewski M, Holm G, Smith U. Increased insulin resistance and fat cell lipolysis in obese but not lean women with a high waist/hip ratio. Eur J Clin Invest 1990;20:530–536.
50. Bonaro E, DelPrato S, Bonadonna G. Total body fat content and fat topography are associated differently with in vivo glucose metabolism in non-obese and obese nondiabetic women. Diabetes 1992;41:1151–1159.
51. Flack JM, Sowers JR. Epidemiologic and clinical aspects of insulin resistance and hyperinsulinemia. Am J Med 1991;91(Suppl 1A):11S–21S.
52. Carey DG, Jenkins AB, Campbell LV, Freund J, Chisholm DJ. Abdominal fat and insulin resistance in normal and overweight women. Diabetes 1996;45:633–638.
53. Sowers JR. Diabetes mellitus and cardiovascular disease in women. Arch Intern Med 1998;158:617–621.
54. Kumanyika S. Obesity in black women. Epidemiol Rev 1987;9:31–50.
55. Bonham GS, Brock DB. The relationship of diabetes with race, sex, and obesity. Am J Clin Nutr 1985;41:776–783.
56. Manolio TA, Pearson TA, Wenger NK. Cholesterol and heart disease in older persons and women. Review of an NHLBI workshop. Ann Epidemiol 1992;2:161–176.
57. Dowling HJ, Pi-Sunyer FX. Race dependent health risks of upper-body obesity. Diabetes 1993;42:537–543.
58. Albu JB, Murphy L, Frager DH, Johnson JA, Pi-Sunyer FX. Visceral fat and race-dependent health risk in obese nondiabetic premenopausal women. Diabetes 1997;46:456–462.
59. Banerji MA, Lebowitz J, Charken RL, Gordon D, Kral JG, Lebowitz HE. Relationship of visceral adipose tissue and glucose disposal is independent of sex in black NIDDM subjects. Am J Physiol 1997;273:E425–E432.
60. Jensen M, Haymond M, Rizza R. Influence of body fat distribution on free fatty acid metabolism in obesity. J Clin Invest 1989;83:1168–1173.
61. Pouliot MC, Després JP, Nadeau A, Moorjani S, Prud'homme D, Lupien PJ. Visceral obesity in men. Associations with glucose tolerance, plasma insulin, and lipoprotein levels. Diabetes 1992;41:826–834.
62. Spiegelman D, Israel RG, Bouchard C, Willett WC. Absolute fat mass, percent body fat, and body-fat distribution: which is the real determinant of blood pressure and serum glucose? Am J Clin Nutr 1992;55:1033–1044.
63. Björntorys P. Abdominal fat distribution and disease: an overview of epidemiology data. Ann Med 1992;24:15–18.
64. Tchernof A, Lamarchi B, Prud'homme A. The dense LDL phenotype: association with plasma lipoprotein levels, visceral obesity, and hyperinsulinemia in men. Diabetes Care 1996;19:629–637.
65. Goodpaster BH, Thaete FL, Simoneau JA, Kelley DE. Subcutaneous abdominal fat and thigh muscle composition predict insulin sensitivity independently of visceral fat. Diabetes 1997;46:1579–1585.
66. Abate N, Garg A, Peshock RM, Stray-Dunderson J, Grundy SM. Relations of generalized and regional adiposity to insulin sensitivity in men. J Clin Invest 1995;96:88–98.
67. Abate N, Garg Q, Peshock RM, Stray-Gunderson J, Adams-Huet B, Grundy SM. Relationship of generalized and regional adiposity to insulin sensitivity in men with NIDDM. Diabetes 1996;45:1684–1693.
68. Sowers JR, Sokol RJ, Standley PR, Kruger M, Mason BA, Sowers PS, Cotton DB. Insulin resistance and increased body mass index in women developing hypertension in pregnancy. Nutr Metab Cardiovasc Dis 1996;6:141–146.
69. Conway NJ, Janovski SZ, Avila NA, Hubbard VS. Visceral adipose tissue differences in black and white women. Am J Clin Nutr 1995;61:765–771.
70. Lovejoy JC, Bretonne JA, Klemperer M, Tulley R. Abdominal fat distribution and metabolic risk factors: effects of race. Metabolism 1996;45:1119–1124.
71. Stampfer MJ, Colditz GA, Willett WC. Postmenopausal estrogen therapy and cardiovascular disease. Ten-year follow-up from the nurses' health study. New Engl J Med 1991;325:756–762.
72. Skafar DF, Xu R, Morales J, Ram J, Sowers JR. Female sex hormones and cardiovascular disease in women. J Clin Endocrin Metab 1998;82:3913–3928.

73. Walsh BW, Schiff E, Rosner B. Effects of postmenopausal estrogen replacement on the concentrations and metabolism of plasma lipoproteins. N Engl J Med 1991;325:1196–1204.
74. Knauthe R, Diel P, Hagele-Haratung C. Sexual dimorphism of steroid hormone receptor messenger ribonucleic acid expression and hormonal regulation in rat vascular tissue. Endocrinology 1996;137: 3220–3227.
75. Losordo DW, Kearney M, Kim EA. Variable expression of the estrogen receptor in normal and atherosclerotic coronary arteries of premenopausal women. Circulation 1994;89:1501–1510.
76. Hayashi T, Yamada K, Esaki T. Estrogen increases endothelial nitric oxide by a receptor mediated system. Biochem Biophys Res Commun 1995;214:847–855.
77. Orimo A, Inoue S, Ikegami A. Vascular smooth muscle cells as targets for estrogen. Biochem Biophys Res Commun 1993;195:730–736.
78. Hanes DS, Weir MR, Sowers JR. Gender considerations in hypertension pathophysiology and treatment. Am J Med 1996;101(Suppl 3A):10S–21S.
79. Skafar DF, Xu R, Morales J, Ram J, Sowers JR. Female sex hormones and cardiovascular disease in women. J Clin Endocrinol Metab 1997;82:3913–3918.
80. Lewis CE, Grandits GA, Flack J, McDonald R, Elmer PJ. Efficacy and tolerance of antihypertensive treatment in men and women with stage 1 diastolic hypertension. Arch Intern Med 1996;156:377–385.
81. Davis BR, Cutler JA, Gordon DJ, Furberg CD, Cushman WC, et al., for the ALLHAT Research Group. Rationale and design for the Antihypertensive and Lipid-Lowering Treatment to Prevent Heart Attack Trial (ALLHAT). Am J Hypertens 1996;9:342–360.
82. Harris MI, Hadden WC, Knowler WC, Bennett PH. Prevalence of diabetes and impaired glucose tolerance and plasma glucose levels in U.S. population aged 20–74 years. Diabetes 1987;36:523–534.
83. Wingard DL, Sinsheimer P, Barrett-Connor EL, McPhillips JB. Community-based study of prevalence of NIDDM in older adults. Diabetes Care 1990;13:3–8.
84. Wilson PWF, Anderson KM, Kannel WB. Epidemiology of diabetes mellitus in the elderly. Am J Med 1986;80(Suppl 5A):3–9.
85. Goldberg AP, Coon PJ. Non-insulin-dependent diabetes mellitus in the elderly. Influence of obesity and physical inactivity. Endocrinol Metab Clin North Am 1987;16:843–865.
86. Aronow WS, Herzig AH, Etienne F, D'Alba P, Ronquillo J. 41 Month follow-up risk factors correlated with new coronary events in 708 elderly patients. J Am Geriatr Soc 1989;37:501–506.
87. Barrett-Connor EL, Cohn BA, Wingard DL, Edelstein SL. Why is diabetes mellitus a stronger risk factor for fatal ischemic heart disease in women than in men? The Rancho Bernardo Study. JAMA 1991;265:627–631.
88. The National High Blood Pressure Education Program Working Group. Report on hypertension in diabetes. Hypertension 1994;23:145–158.
89. Sowers JR, Epstein M. Diabetes mellitus and hypertension: an update. Hypertension 1995;26(Part 1): 869–879.
90. Sowers JR, Epstein M. Diabetes mellitus and hypertension, emerging therapeutic perspectives. Cardiovasc Drug Rev 1995;13:149–210.
91. Bass KM, Newschaffer CJ, Klag MJ, Bush TL. Plasma lipoprotein levels as predictors of cardiovascular death in women. Arch Intern Med 1993;153:2209–2215.
92. Manolio TA, Pearson TA, Wenger NK, Barrett-Connor E, Payne GH, Harlan WR. Cholesterol and heart disease in older persons and women. Review of an NHLBI workshop. Ann Epidemiol 1992;2: 161–176.
93. Terranova R, Luca S. Effects of treatment with Simvastatin in elderly patients with primary hypercholesterolemia. Riv Eur Sci Med Farmacol 1993;15:163–170.
94. Davenport J, Whittaker K. Secondary prevention in elderly survivors of heart attacks. AFP 1988; 38:216–224.
95. Applegate WB, Miller ST, Elam JT, Cushman WC, Derwi DE, Brenner A, Graney MJ. Nonpharmacologic intervention to reduce blood pressure in older patients with mild hypertension. Arch Intern Med 1992;152:1162–1166.
96. Schaefer EJ, Lichtenstein AH, Lamon-Fava S, Contois JH, Li Z, Rasmussen H, McNamara JR, Ordovas JM. Efficacy of a National Cholesterol Education Program Step 2 diet in normolipidemic and hypercholesterolemic middle-aged and elderly men and women. Arterioscl Throm Vasc Biol 1995;15:1079–1085.
97. Hagberg JM, Montain SJ, Martin WH, Ehsani AA. Effect of exercise training on 60–89-year-old essential hypertensives. Am J Cardiol 1989;64:348–353.
98. Tran ZV, Weltman A. Differential effects of exercise on serum lipids and lipoproteins levels seen with changes in body weight. JAMA 1985;254:919–924.

99. Lavie CJ, Milani RV. Effects of cardiac rehabilitation programs on exercise capacity, coronary risk factors, behavioral characteristics, and quality of life in a large elderly cohort. Am J Cardiol 1995;76: 177–179.

100. Wood PD, Stefanick ML, Dreon D. Changes in plasma lipids and lipoproteins in overweight men during weight loss through dieting as compared with exercise. N Engl J Med 1988;319:1173–1179.

101. Kasim S, Maxwell MM, Dornfeld L, Sowers JR. The effects of marked caloric restriction on lipoprotein lipase-activators in obese subjects. Nutr Res 1986;6:773–783.

102. The Joint National Committee on Prevention, Detection, Evaluation, and Treatment of High Blood Pressure and the National High Blood Pressure Education Program Coordinating Committee. The Sixth Report. Arch Intern Med 1997;157:2413–2446.

103. Goldstein G, Matterson BJ, Cushman WC, Reda DJ, Freis ED, Ramirez EA, et al., for the Department of Veterans Affairs Cooperative Study. Treatment of hypertension in the elderly. II. Cognitive and behavioral function. Hypertension 1990;15:361–369.

104. Ekbom I, Dahlof B, Hasson L, Lindholm LH, Schersten B, Wester P-O. Antihypertensive efficacy and side effects of three beta-blockers and a diuretic in elderly hypertensives: a report form the STOP-Hypertension study. J Hypertens 1992;10:1525–1530.

105. Fletcher A, Amery A, Birkenhager W, Bulpitt C, Clement D, de Leeuw P, et al. Risk and benefits in the trial of the European Working Party on High Blood Pressure in the Elderly. J Hypertens 1991;9: 226–230.

106. Palmer BF. Renal complications associated with use of nonsteroidal anti-inflammatory agents. J Invest Med 1995;43:516–533.

107. Clark BA, Shannon RP, Rosa RM, Epstein FH. Increased susceptibility to thiazide-induced hyponatremia in the elderly. J Am Soc Nephrol 1994;5:1106–1111.

108. Moser M, Gifford RW. Hypertension: steps forward and steps backward. Arch Intern Med 1993;153: 1843–1846.

109. Veterans Administration Cooperative Study Group on Antihypertensive Agents. Comparison of propranolol and hydrochlorothiazide for the initial treatment of hypertension. I: Results of short-term titration with emphasis on racial differences in response. JAMA 1982;248:1996–2003.

110. Medical Research Council Working Party. Medical Research Research Council trial of treatment of hypertension in older adults. Br Med J 1992;304:405–412.

111. Yusef S, Wittes J, Probstfield J. Evaluating effects of treatment in subgroups of patients within a clinical trial: the case of non-Q-wave myocardial infarction and beta-blockers. Am J Cardiol 1990;66: 220–222.

112. The Systolic Hypertension in the Elderly Program (SHEP) Cooperative Research Group: Prevention of stroke by antihypertensive drug treatment in older persons with isolated systolic hypertension: final results of SHEP. JAMA 1991;265:3255–3264.

113. Dahlof B, Lindholm LH, Hannson L, et al. Morbidity and mortality in the Swedish Trial in Old Patients with Hypertension (STOP-Hypertension). Lancet 1991;338:1281–1285.

114. SOLVD Investigators. Effect of enalapril on mortality and the development of heart failure in asymptomatic patients with reduced left ventricular ejection fractions. N Engl J Med 1992;327:685–691.

115. Pfeffer MA, Braunwald E, Moy JLA, et al. Effect of captropril on mortality and morbidity in patients with left ventricular dysfunction after myocardial infarction. N Engl J Med 1992;327:669–677.

116. Staessen JA, Fagard R, Thijs L, et al., for the Systolic Hypertension-Europe (Syst-Eur) Trial Investigators. Morbidity and mortality in the placebo-controlled European Trial on isolated systolic hypertension in the Elderly. Lancet 1997;360:757–764.

Index

A

Adrenergic receptor responsiveness,
  aging effects, 238, 239
  assessment, 237
  congestive heart failure role, 241
Aging theories,
  programmed theories,
    finite cell division theory, 3, 4
    immune theory, 3
    neuroendocrine theory, 2, 3
    overview, 1, 2
  wear and tear theories,
    DNA damage theory, 6
    error catastrophe theory, 5, 6
    free radical theory, 4, 5
    glycosylation theory, 6, 7
    rate of living theory, 5
Aldosterone, aging changes, 81, 82
Alzheimer's disease,
  diabetes association, 189
  estrogen therapy, 168–169
  fluid balance, 87
Angiotensin, aging changes, 81, 82
Angiotensin-converting enzyme inhibitors,
  diabetes treatment, 192
  fluid balance side effects, 85
  hypertension treatment, 256–257
ANH, *see* Atrial natriuretic hormone
Antidepressants,
  diabetes treatment in elderly, 195, 215
  fluid balance side effects, 85
Antidiuretic hormone, *see* Arginine vasopressin
Antioxidant supplements, diabetes treatment
  in elderly, 193
Arginine supplementation, growth hormone
  release in elderly, 33
Arginine vasopressin (AVP),
  aging effects,
    gender differences, 79
    levels, 77–79
    response in aging, 76, 77, 79, 80
  syndrome of inappropriate antidiuretic
    hormone secretion, 84–86

urinary incontinence treatment, 87
Atherothrombosis, estrogen therapy, 166, 167
Atrial natriuretic hormone (ANH),
  aging effects,
    levels, 80, 81
    response, 81
  regulation of secretion, 80
Atrophic vaginitis, estrogen therapy, 165, 166
Autonomic nervous system dysfunction,
  classification, 243
  clinical presentation, 242, 243
  evaluation, 243, 244
  management, 244

AVP, *see* Arginine vasopressin

B

Balding, testosterone effects, 139
BIA, *see* Bioelectrical impedance analysis
Bioelectrical impedance analysis (BIA),
  body fat assessment, 208
Bisphosphonates,
  osteoporosis treatment, 105
  Paget's disease of bone treatment, 109,
    110, 120–122
Blood pressure, *see* Hypertension
BMD, *see* Bone mineral density
BMI, *see* Body mass index
Body composition,
  aging changes, 28, 73.74, 226
  fat assessment, 208
  growth hormone effects, 28, 30, 34
  water composition, 73, 74
Body mass index (BMI),
  classifications, 206
  nutrition in elderly, 14, 15
Bone mineral density (BMD),
  see also Osteoporosis,
  clinical guidelines based on findings, 99, 100
  exercise effects, 228
  interpretation, 96–98
  loss in aging, 93, 94